Signs and Symptoms Analysis from a Functional Perspective

A Question by Question Guide

Second Edition

Signs and Symptoms Analysis from a Functional Perspective-
A Question by Question Guide
Second Edition

Dicken Weatherby, N.D.

Bear Mountain Publishing • Jacksonville, OR

Signs and Symptoms Analysis from a Functional Perspective- A Question by Question Guide
2nd Edition

Bear Mountain Publishing
1-541-631-8316

ISBN 0-9761367-2-4

Warning - Disclaimer
This book is designed to provide information in regard to the subject matter covered. It is sold with the understanding that the publisher and the author is not liable for the misconception or misuse of information provided. The purpose of this book is to educate. Information contained in this book should not be construed as a claim or representation that any treatment, process or interpretation mentioned constitutes a cure, palliative, or ameliorative. The interpretation is intended to supplement the practitioner's knowledge of their client. It should be considered as adjunctive support to other diagnostic medical procedures.

Printed in the United States of America

Table of Contents

QUESTION BY QUESTION GUIDE TO THE NAQ

Appendix: Diet and Lifestyle Handouts (continued)

Acknowledgments

Signs and Symptoms Analysis from a Functional Perspective- A Question by Question Guide has incorporated tests from a variety of practitioners without prejudice to degree. The author has used signs, indicators, and concepts from Medicine, Osteopathy, Naturopathy, Chiropractic, Oriental Medicine, Biochemistry, and Nutrition.

The author would specifically like to thank the following practitioners for their contributions either from specific tests that are referenced or major concepts that are used in this guide.

Terence Bennett, D.C.
Erin P. Boeger, Nutritionist
Frank Chapman, D.O.
Arthur Coca, M.D.
Major B. Dejarnette, D.O., D.C.
Scott Ferguson, ND
George Goodheart, D.C.
Gray L. Graham, C.N.T.
Jeremy Kaslow, M.D.
Dietrich Klinghart, M.D., Ph.D.
Royal Lee, D.D.S
Nicolai Lennox, D.C.
Dale Migliaccio, D.C.
Owen W. Miller, N.D.
David Overton, PA-C
Michael Owen, D.C.
Melvin Page, D.D.S.
Frances Pottenger, M.D.
Weston Price, D.D.S.
Robert E. Ridler, D.C.
Alexander Schauss, Ph.D.
Dickson Thom, D.D.S., N.D.
Paul Varnas, D.C.
Linda Warren, N.D.
Steven Sandberg-Lewis, ND
Deborah L. Wilcox, B.S., C.H.t.

Disclaimer

Information contained in this book should not be construed as a claim or representation that any process or product mentioned constitutes a cure, palliative, or ameliorative. Procedures and products are intended to supplement the client's metabolic status and should be considered as adjunctive support to other medical procedures.

Introduction

Signs and Symptoms Analysis from a Functional Perspective- A Question by Question Guide is an excellent tool for not only gathering information on the client's initial visit but also for re-assessing your client's progress on a regular basis. Please refer to the beginning chapter, which will tell you how you can use the book to make your interpretation of the questionnaire.

Signs and Symptoms Analysis from a Functional Perspective- A Question by Question Guide is not meant to be used to make a diagnosis and the information filled out by the client is not meant to take the place of a medical history, physical examination and appropriate lab work. This book and the Nutritional Assessment Questionnaire software are to be used by licensed health care professionals.

This book goes over each question and its significance, along with tools for further assessment, sample protocols and diet and lifestyle suggestions. It is an additional tool for refining your information gathering and for individualizing the best course of treatment for your client.

RESOURCES

Many of the tools for further assessment mentioned in the manual are covered in Dr. Weatherby's "*Foundations of Functional Diagnosis Training Program*", an in-depth 11 Module training covering Dr. Weatherby's "Four Quadrants of Functional Diagnosis". For more information please visit www.FunctionalDiagnosis.com.

If you wish to analyze blood chemistries from a functional perspective, consider Dr. Weatherby's pioneering Blood Chemistry Analysis Software program. Full details at www.BloodChemSoftware.com. Or consider using "*Blood Chemistry and CBC Analysis- Clinical Laboratory Testing from a Functional Perspective*" by Dicken Weatherby, ND and Scott Ferguson, ND. This book is available from Amazon.com and www.BloodChemistryAnalysis.com.

If you wish to get more information on some of the in-office tests recommended in this book e.g. the urine indican and sediment test, the Oxidata test, and the zinc taste test you should consider using "In-Office Lab Testing- Functional Terrain Analysis" by Dicken Weatherby, N.D. and Scott Ferguson, ND. This book is full of many easy to use in-office lab tests and is also available from Amazon.com and www.BloodChemistryAnalysis.com.

**If you wish to increase your knowledge of Functional Diagnosis please consider signing up for our "Functional Diagnosis" Electronic Newsletter.
Visit http://www.BloodChemistryAnalysis.com for more details.**

Weatherby & Associates

Signs and Symptoms Analysis from a Functional Perspective- A Question by Question Guide is brought to you by Weatherby & Associates, LLC, and distributed by Emperors Group, LLC, an educational corporation providing Health Care Professionals with resources (seminars, software, books, and online training) to effectively integrate Functional Diagnosis into their practice.

Mission Statement

Weatherby & Associates, LLC and Emperors Group, LLC are committed to helping Health Care Professionals make the most of the tests they are already using and take their diagnostic skills to the next level.

We are guided by:

- A profound respect for the teachings of the alternative medical pioneers
- A commitment to the concepts of biochemical individuality
- The belief that within each of us lies an innate intelligence that will guide us

SIGNS AND SYMPTOMS ANALYSIS FROM A FUNCTIONAL PERSPECTIVE- A QUESTION BY QUESTION GUIDE

2ND EDITION

DICKEN WEATHERBY, N.D.

Dr. Dicken Weatherby is a native of England and has studied, practiced, and taught medicine in Europe and the United States. He received his Naturopathic Medical Degree from National College of Naturopathic Medicine in 1998. He is actively involved in research, writing and education, and makes his home in Southern Oregon. Dr. Weatherby is the co-author of *Blood Chemistry and CBC Analysis– Clinical Laboratory Testing from a Functional Perspective, In-Office Lab testing- Functional Terrain Analysis, The Complete Practitioner's Guide to Take-Home Testing,* and *The Complete Physical Exam Reporting System.* He is also the creator of *the Blood Chemistry Software Program at* http://www.BloodChemSoftware.com

For more information on other books by Dr. Weatherby and Dr. Ferguson please visit www.BloodChemistryAnalysis.com or e-mail Info@BloodChemistryAnalysis.com

For more information on Dr. Weatherby's Blood Chemistry Software program please visit http://www.BloodChemSoftware.com

Nutritional Assessment Questionnaire 1.5

Name: ______________________________ **Date:** ____/____/____

Birth Date: ____________________ **Gender:** __________

Please list your five major health concerns in order of importance:

1. ______________________
2. ______________________
3. ______________________
4. ______________________
5. ______________________

Notes:

PART I

Read the following questions and circle the number that applies:

KEY: **0 = Do not consume or use**
1 = Consume or use 2 to 3 times monthly
2 = Consume or use weekly
3 = Consume or use daily

DIET

58

1. 0 1 2 3 Alcohol
2. 0 1 2 3 Artificial sweeteners
3. 0 1 2 3 Candy, desserts, refined sugar
4. 0 1 2 3 Carbonated beverages
5. 0 1 2 3 Chewing tobacco
6. 0 1 2 3 Cigarettes
7. 0 1 2 3 Cigars/pipes
8. 0 1 2 3 Caffeinated beverages
9. 0 1 2 3 Fast foods
10. 0 1 2 3 Fried foods
11. 0 1 2 3 Luncheon meats
12. 0 1 2 3 Margarine
13. 0 1 2 3 Milk products
14. 0 1 Radiation exposure (0=no, 1=yes)
15. 0 1 2 3 Refined flour/baked goods
16. 0 1 2 3 Vitamins and minerals
17. 0 1 2 3 Water, distilled
18. 0 1 2 3 Water, tap
19. 0 1 2 3 Water, well
20. 0 1 2 3 Diet often for weight control

LIFESTYLE

12

21. 0 1 2 3 Exercise per week (0 = 2 or more times a week, 1 = 1 time a week, 2 = 1 or 2 times a month, 3 = never, less than once a month)
22. 0 1 2 3 Changed jobs (0 = over 12 months ago, 1 = within last 12 months, 2 = within last 6 months, 3 = within last 2 months)
23. 0 1 2 3 Divorced (0 = never, over 2 years ago, 1 = within last 2 years, 2 = within last year, 3 = within last 6 months)
24. 0 1 2 3 Work over 60 hours/week (0 = never, 1 = occasionally, 2 = usually, 3 = always)

MEDICATIONS **Indicate any medications you're currently taking or have taken in the last month (0=no, 1=yes):**

54

25. 0 1 Antacids
26. 0 1 Antianxiety medications
27. 0 1 Antibiotics
28. 0 1 Anticonvulsants
29. 0 1 Antidepressants
30. 0 1 Antifungals
31. 0 1 Aspirin/Ibuprofen
32. 0 1 Asthma inhalers
33. 0 1 Beta blockers
34. 0 1 Birth control pills/implant contraceptives
35. 0 1 Chemotherapy
36. 0 1 Cholesterol lowering medications
37. 0 1 Cortisone/steroids
38. 0 1 Diabetic medications/insulin
39. 0 1 Diuretics
40. 0 1 Estrogen or progesterone (pharmaceutical, prescription)
41. 0 1 Estrogen or progesterone (natural)
42. 0 1 Heart medications
43. 0 1 High blood pressure medications
44. 0 1 Laxatives
45. 0 1 Recreational drugs
46. 0 1 Relaxants/Sleeping pills
47. 0 1 Testosterone (natural or prescription)
48. 0 1 Thyroid medication
49. 0 1 Acetaminophen (Tylenol)
50. 0 1 Ulcer medications
51. 0 1 Sildenafal citrate (Viagra)

PART II **(See key at bottom of page)**

Section 1

55

52. 0 1 2 3 Belching or gas within one hour after eating
53. 0 1 2 3 Heartburn or acid reflux
54. 0 1 2 3 Bloating within one hour after eating
55. 0 1 Vegan diet (no dairy, meat, fish or eggs) (0=no, 1=yes)
56. 0 1 2 3 Bad breath (halitosis)
57. 0 1 2 3 Loss of taste for meat
58. 0 1 2 3 Sweat has a strong odor
59. 0 1 2 3 Stomach upset by taking vitamins
60. 0 1 2 3 Sense of excess fullness after meals
61. 0 1 2 3 Feel like skipping breakfast
62. 0 1 2 3 Feel better if you don't eat
63. 0 1 2 3 Sleepy after meals
64. 0 1 2 3 Fingernails chip, peel or break easily
65. 0 1 2 3 Anemia unresponsive to iron
66. 0 1 2 3 Stomach pains or cramps
67. 0 1 2 3 Diarrhea, chronic
68. 0 1 2 3 Diarrhea shortly after meals
69. 0 1 2 3 Black or tarry colored stools
70. 0 1 2 3 Undigested food in stool

KEY: 0=No, symptom does not occur
1=Yes, minor or mild symptom, rarely occurs (monthly)
2=Moderate symptom, occurs occasionally (weekly)
3=Severe symptom, occurs frequently (daily)

Section 2

68

71. 0 1 2 3 Pain between shoulder blades
72. 0 1 2 3 Stomach upset by greasy foods
73. 0 1 2 3 Greasy or shiny stools
74. 0 1 2 3 Nausea
75. 0 1 2 3 Sea, car, airplane or motion sickness
76. 0 1 History of morning sickness (0 = no, 1 = yes)
77. 0 1 2 3 Light or clay colored stools
78. 0 1 2 3 Dry skin, itchy feet or skin peels on feet
79. 0 1 2 3 Headache over eyes
80. 0 1 2 3 Gallbladder attacks (0=never, 1=years ago, 2=within last year, 3=within past 3 months)
81. 0 1 Gallbladder removed (0=no, 1=yes)
82. 0 1 2 3 Bitter taste in mouth, especially after meals
83. 0 1 Become sick if you were to drink wine (0=no, 1=yes)
84. 0 1 Easily intoxicated if you were to drink wine (0=no, 1=yes)
85. 0 1 Easily hung over if you were to drink wine (0=no, 1=yes)
86. 0 1 2 3 Alcohol per week (0=<3, 1=<7, 2 =<14, 3=>14)
87. 0 1 Recovering alcoholic (0=no, 1=yes)
88. 0 1 History of drug or alcohol abuse (0=no, 1=yes)
89. 0 1 History of hepatitis (0=no, 1=yes)
90. 0 1 Long term use of prescription/recreational drugs (0=no, 1=yes)
91. 0 1 2 3 Sensitive to chemicals (perfume, cleaning agents, etc.)
92. 0 1 2 3 Sensitive to tobacco smoke
93. 0 1 2 3 Exposure to diesel fumes
94. 0 1 2 3 Pain under right side of rib cage
95. 0 1 2 3 Hemorrhoids or varicose veins
96. 0 1 2 3 Nutrasweet (aspartame) consumption
97. 0 1 2 3 Sensitive to Nutrasweet (aspartame)
98. 0 1 2 3 Chronic fatigue or Fibromyalgia

Section 3

47

99. 0 1 2 3 Food allergies
100. 0 1 2 3 Abdominal bloating 1 to 2 hours after eating
101. 0 1 Specific foods make you tired or bloated (0=no, 1=yes)
102. 0 1 2 3 Pulse speeds after eating
103. 0 1 2 3 Airborne allergies
104. 0 1 2 3 Experience hives
105. 0 1 2 3 Sinus congestion, "stuffy head"
106. 0 1 2 3 Crave bread or noodles
107. 0 1 2 3 Alternating constipation and diarrhea
108. 0 1 2 3 Crohn's disease (0 =no, 1=yes in the past, 2=currently mild condition, 3=severe)
109. 0 1 2 3 Wheat or grain sensitivity
110. 0 1 2 3 Dairy sensitivity
111. 0 1 Are there foods you could not give up (0=no, 1=yes)
112. 0 1 2 3 Asthma, sinus infections, stuffy nose
113. 0 1 2 3 Bizarre vivid dreams, nightmares
114. 0 1 2 3 Use over-the-counter pain medications
115. 0 1 2 3 Feel spacey or unreal

Section 4

58

116. 0 1 2 3 Anus itches
117. 0 1 2 3 Coated tongue
118. 0 1 2 3 Feel worse in moldy or musty place
119. 0 1 2 3 Taken antibiotic for a total accumulated time of (0=never, 1= <1 month, 2= <3 months, 3= >3 months)
120. 0 1 2 3 Fungus or yeast infections
121. 0 1 2 3 Ring worm, "jock itch", "athletes foot", nail fungus
122. 0 1 2 3 Yeast symptoms increase with sugar, starch or alcohol
123. 0 1 2 3 Stools hard or difficult to pass
124. 0 1 History of parasites (0=no, 1=yes)
125. 0 1 2 3 Less than one bowel movement per day
126. 0 1 2 3 Stools have corners or edges, are flat or ribbon shaped
127. 0 1 2 3 Stools are not well formed (loose)
128. 0 1 2 3 Irritable bowel or mucus colitis
129. 0 1 2 3 Blood in stool
130. 0 1 2 3 Mucus in stool
131. 0 1 2 3 Excessive foul smelling lower bowel gas
132. 0 1 2 3 Bad breath or strong body odors
133. 0 1 2 3 Painful to press along outer sides of thighs (Iliotibial Band)
134. 0 1 2 3 Cramping in lower abdominal region
135. 0 1 2 3 Dark circles under eyes

Section 5

75

136. 0 1 History of carpal tunnel syndrome (0=no, 1=yes)
137. 0 1 History of lower right abdominal pains or ileocecal valve problems (0=no, 1=yes)
138. 0 1 History of stress fracture (0=no, 1=yes)
139. 0 1 2 3 Bone loss (reduced density on bone scan)
140. 0 1 Are you shorter than you used to be? (0=no, 1=yes)
141. 0 1 2 3 Calf, foot or toe cramps at rest
142. 0 1 2 3 Cold sores, fever blisters or herpes lesions
143. 0 1 2 3 Frequent fevers
144. 0 1 2 3 Frequent skin rashes and/or hives
145. 0 1 Herniated disc (0=no, 1=yes)
146. 0 1 2 3 Excessively flexible joints, "double jointed"
147. 0 1 2 3 Joints pop or click
148. 0 1 2 3 Pain or swelling in joints
149. 0 1 2 3 Bursitis or tendonitis
150. 0 1 History of bone spurs (0=no, 1=yes)
151. 0 1 2 3 Morning stiffness
152. 0 1 2 3 Nausea with vomiting
153. 0 1 2 3 Crave chocolate
154. 0 1 2 3 Feet have a strong odor
155. 0 1 2 3 History of anemia
156. 0 1 2 3 Whites of eyes (sclera) blue tinted
157. 0 1 2 3 Hoarseness
158. 0 1 2 3 Difficulty swallowing
159. 0 1 2 3 Lump in throat
160. 0 1 2 3 Dry mouth, eyes and/or nose
161. 0 1 2 3 Gag easily
162. 0 1 2 3 White spots on fingernails
163. 0 1 2 3 Cuts heal slowly and/or scar easily
164. 0 1 2 3 Decreased sense of taste or smell

KEY: 0=No, symptom does not occur	2=Moderate symptom, occurs occasionally (weekly)
1=Yes, minor or mild symptom, rarely occurs (monthly)	3=Severe symptom, occurs frequently (daily)

Section 6

22

165. 0 1 Experience pain relief with aspirin (0=no, 1=yes)
166. 0 1 2 3 Crave fatty or greasy foods
167. 0 1 2 3 Low- or reduced-fat diet (0=never, 1=years ago, 2=within past year, 3=currently)
168. 0 1 2 3 Tension headaches at base of skull
169. 0 1 2 3 Headaches when out in the hot sun
170. 0 1 2 3 Sunburn easily or suffer sun poisoning
171. 0 1 2 3 Muscles easily fatigued
172. 0 1 2 3 Dry flaky skin or dandruff

Section 7

39

173. 0 1 2 3 Awaken a few hours after falling asleep, hard to get back to sleep
174. 0 1 2 3 Crave sweets
175. 0 1 2 3 Binge or uncontrolled eating
176. 0 1 2 3 Excessive appetite
177. 0 1 2 3 Crave coffee or sugar in the afternoon
178. 0 1 2 3 Sleepy in afternoon
179. 0 1 2 3 Fatigue that is relieved by eating
180. 0 1 2 3 Headache if meals are skipped or delayed
181. 0 1 2 3 Irritable before meals
182. 0 1 2 3 Shaky if meals delayed
183. 0 1 2 3 Family members with diabetes (0=none, 1=1 or 2, 2=3 or 4, 3=more than 4)
184. 0 1 2 3 Frequent thirst
185. 0 1 2 3 Frequent urination

Section 8

81

186. 0 1 2 3 Muscles become easily fatigued
187. 0 1 2 3 Feel exhausted or sore after moderate exercise
188. 0 1 2 3 Vulnerable to insect bites
189. 0 1 2 3 Loss of muscle tone, heaviness in arms/legs
190. 0 1 2 3 Enlarged heart or congestive heart failure
191. 0 1 2 3 Pulse below 65 per minute (0=no, 1=yes)
192. 0 1 2 3 Ringing in the ears (Tinnitus)
193. 0 1 2 3 Numbness, tingling or itching in hands and feet
194. 0 1 2 3 Depressed
195. 0 1 2 3 Fear of impending doom
196. 0 1 2 3 Worrier, apprehensive, anxious
197. 0 1 2 3 Nervous or agitated
198. 0 1 2 3 Feelings of insecurity
199. 0 1 2 3 Heart races
200. 0 1 2 3 Can hear heart beat on pillow at night
201. 0 1 2 3 Whole body or limb jerk as falling asleep
202. 0 1 2 3 Night sweats
203. 0 1 2 3 Restless leg syndrome
204. 0 1 2 3 Cracks at corner of mouth (Cheilosis)
205. 0 1 2 3 Fragile skin, easily chaffed, as in shaving
206. 0 1 2 3 Polyps or warts
207. 0 1 2 3 MSG sensitivity
208. 0 1 2 3 Wake up without remembering dreams
209. 0 1 2 3 Small bumps on back of arms
210. 0 1 2 3 Strong light at night irritates eyes
211. 0 1 2 3 Nose bleeds and/or tend to bruise easily
212. 0 1 2 3 Bleeding gums especially when brushing teeth

Section 9

78

213. 0 1 2 3 Tend to be a "night person"
214. 0 1 2 3 Difficulty falling asleep
215. 0 1 2 3 Slow starter in the morning
216. 0 1 2 3 Tend to be keyed up, trouble calming down
217. 0 1 2 3 Blood pressure above 120/80
218. 0 1 2 3 Headache after exercising
219. 0 1 2 3 Feeling wired or jittery after drinking coffee
220. 0 1 2 3 Clench or grind teeth
221. 0 1 2 3 Calm on the outside, troubled on the inside
222. 0 1 2 3 Chronic low back pain, worse with fatigue
223. 0 1 2 3 Become dizzy when standing up suddenly
224. 0 1 2 3 Difficulty maintaining manipulative correction
225. 0 1 2 3 Pain after manipulative correction
226. 0 1 2 3 Arthritic tendencies
227. 0 1 2 3 Crave salty foods
228. 0 1 2 3 Salt foods before tasting
229. 0 1 2 3 Perspire easily
230. 0 1 2 3 Chronic fatigue, or get drowsy often
231. 0 1 2 3 Afternoon yawning
232. 0 1 2 3 Afternoon headache
233. 0 1 2 3 Asthma, wheezing or difficulty breathing
234. 0 1 2 3 Pain on the medial or inner side of the knee
235. 0 1 2 3 Tendency to sprain ankles or "shin splints"
236. 0 1 2 3 Tendency to need sunglasses
237. 0 1 2 3 Allergies and/or hives
238. 0 1 2 3 Weakness, dizziness

Section 10

29

239. 0 1 Height over 6' 6" (0=no, 1=yes)
240. 0 1 Early sexual development (before age 10) (0=no, 1=yes)
241. 0 1 2 3 Increased libido
242. 0 1 2 3 Splitting type headache
243. 0 1 2 3 Memory failing
244. 0 1 Tolerate sugar, feel fine when eating sugar (0=no, 1=yes)
245. 0 1 Height under 4' 10" (0=no, 1=yes)
246. 0 1 2 3 Decreased libido
247. 0 1 2 3 Excessive thirst
248. 0 1 2 3 Weight gain around hips or waist
249. 0 1 2 3 Menstrual disorders
250. 0 1 Delayed sexual development (after age 13) (0=no, 1=yes)
251. 0 1 2 3 Tendency to ulcers or colitis

KEY:	
0=No, symptom does not occur	2=Moderate symptom, occurs occasionally (weekly)
1=Yes, minor or mild symptom, rarely occurs (monthly)	3=Severe symptom, occurs frequently (daily)

Section 11 48

252. 0 1 2 3 Sensitive/allergic to iodine
253. 0 1 2 3 Difficulty gaining weight, even with large appetite
254. 0 1 2 3 Nervous, emotional, can't work under pressure
255. 0 1 2 3 Inward trembling
256. 0 1 2 3 Flush easily
257. 0 1 2 3 Fast pulse at rest
258. 0 1 2 3 Intolerance to high temperatures
259. 0 1 2 3 Difficulty losing weight
260. 0 1 2 3 Mentally sluggish, reduced initiative
261. 0 1 2 3 Easily fatigued, sleepy during the day
262. 0 1 2 3 Sensitive to cold, poor circulation (cold hands and feet)
263. 0 1 2 3 Constipation, chronic
264. 0 1 2 3 Excessive hair loss and/or coarse hair
265. 0 1 2 3 Morning headaches, wear off during the day
266. 0 1 2 3 Loss of lateral 1/3 of eyebrow
267. 0 1 2 3 Seasonal sadness

Section 12 – Men Only 27

268. 0 1 2 3 Prostate problems
269. 0 1 2 3 Difficulty with urination, dribbling
270. 0 1 2 3 Difficult to start and stop urine stream
271. 0 1 2 3 Pain or burning with urination
272. 0 1 2 3 Waking to urinate at night
273. 0 1 2 3 Interruption of stream during urination
274. 0 1 2 3 Pain on inside of legs or heels
275. 0 1 2 3 Feeling of incomplete bowel evacuation
276. 0 1 2 3 Decreased sexual function

Section 13 – Women Only 60

277. 0 1 2 3 Depression during periods
278. 0 1 2 3 Mood swings associated with periods (PMS)
279. 0 1 2 3 Crave chocolate around periods
280. 0 1 2 3 Breast tenderness associated with cycle
281. 0 1 2 3 Excessive menstrual flow
282. 0 1 2 3 Scanty blood flow during periods
283. 0 1 2 3 Occasional skipped periods
284. 0 1 2 3 Variations in menstrual cycles
285. 0 1 2 3 Endometriosis
286. 0 1 2 3 Uterine fibroids
287. 0 1 2 3 Breast fibroids, benign masses
288. 0 1 2 3 Painful intercourse (dysparenia)
289. 0 1 2 3 Vaginal discharge
290. 0 1 2 3 Vaginal dryness
291. 0 1 2 3 Vaginal itchiness
292. 0 1 2 3 Gain weight around hips, thighs and buttocks
293. 0 1 2 3 Excess facial or body hair
294. 0 1 2 3 Hot flashes
295. 0 1 2 3 Night sweats (in menopausal females)
296. 0 1 2 3 Thinning skin

Section 14 30

297. 0 1 2 3 Aware of heavy and/or irregular breathing
298. 0 1 2 3 Discomfort at high altitudes
299. 0 1 2 3 "Air hunger" or sigh frequently
300. 0 1 2 3 Compelled to open windows in a closed room
301. 0 1 2 3 Shortness of breath with moderate exertion
302. 0 1 2 3 Ankles swell, especially at end of day
303. 0 1 2 3 Cough at night
304. 0 1 2 3 Blush or face turns red for no reason
305. 0 1 2 3 Dull pain or tightness in chest and/or radiate into right arm, worse with exertion
306. 0 1 2 3 Muscle cramps with exertion

Section 15 13

307. 0 1 2 3 Pain in mid-back region
308. 0 1 2 3 Puffy around the eyes, dark circles under eyes
309. 0 1 History of kidney stones (0=no, 1=yes)
310. 0 1 2 3 Cloudy, bloody or darkened urine
311. 0 1 2 3 Urine has a strong odor

Section 16 30

312. 0 1 2 3 Runny or drippy nose
313. 0 1 2 3 Catch colds at the beginning of winter
314. 0 1 2 3 Mucus producing cough
315. 0 1 2 3 Frequent colds or flu (0=1 or less per year, 1=2 to 3 times per year, 2=4 to 5 times per year, 3=6 or more times per year)
316. 0 1 2 3 Other infections (sinus, ear, lung, skin, bladder, kidney, etc.) (0=1 or less per year, 1=2 to 3 times per year, 2=4 to 5 times per year, 3=6 or more times per year)
317. 0 1 2 3 Never get sick (0 = sick only 1 or 2 times in last 2 years, 1 = not sick in last 2 years, 2 = not sick in last 4 years, 3 = not sick in last 7 years)
318. 0 1 2 3 Acne (adult)
319. 0 1 2 3 Itchy skin (Dermatitis)
320. 0 1 2 3 Cysts, boils, rashes
321. 0 1 2 3 History of Epstein Bar, Mono, Herpes, Shingles, Chronic Fatigue Syndrome, Hepatitis or other chronic viral condition (0 = no, 1 = yes in the past, 2 = currently mild condition, 3 = severe)

KEY: 0=No, symptom does not occur; 1=Yes, minor or mild symptom, rarely occurs (monthly); 2=Moderate symptom, occurs occasionally (weekly); 3=Severe symptom, occurs frequently (daily)

Manual Analysis of the NAQ

The Nutritional Assessment Questionnaire was first designed to be assessed using a sophisticated computer analysis program. This provided the practitioner with a number of comprehensive reports that could assist them to make further assessments and nutritional recommendations to their clients. However, there are many practitioners who would rather not rely on a computer program and have requested that I write a section in this second edition to help them do a manual assessment. This section of the ***Question by Question Guide to the Nutritional Assessment Questionnaire*** is written for them.

How to use the NAQ

The NAQ is one of the best data gathering tools available. It has saved me and my clients many hours of history taking and provides an incredible tool to track data over a longer period of time. I call this "history taking in motion". Many practitioners spend a lot of time gathering that initial history. However, that valuable data is often relegated to the back of the file and never referred to again. The NAQ allows you to ask relevant history questions in an easy to use questionnaire and enables you to ask the same questions at a later date to see how much change there has been. In medicine we are always looking for change and this tool is one of the best ways I know of to monitor changes in the symptom burden of the client.

The NAQ is also an excellent tool to encourage compliance in clients. How many of us have had the experience of putting together an excellent protocol for a client's migraine headaches only to have the client return in 3 weeks saying that the headaches have not changed. By using the NAQ the client themselves answers the questions and the questionnaire gathers the information for analysis. You can sit down with the client and point out that yes, their headaches have not completely resolved but they reported on their initial NAQ that their headaches were a 3 (a severe symptom that occurs frequently) and on their next NAQ they had reported that the same symptom had dropped down to a 1 (a minor or mild symptom, rarely occurs). This client is more likely to comply with your recommendations.

How to do a manual analysis of the NAQ

As you are probably aware the NAQ has been broken down into two main parts and each part is broken down into sub sections. There are a specific number of questions in each section and a maximum total score for each section. The questionnaire has a place at the top of each section that indicates the maximum score that can be recorded for each section.

For instance the Upper Gastrointestinal System has 19 questions that are asked on the questionnaire. If a client answered a 3 to each and every question on that section they would have a maximum symptom count of 55. This number reflects the maximum symptom count in that section or body system. The symptom burden in this case is extraordinarily high.

The table below breaks the questionnaire down into each of its individual sections and lists the maximum symptom count for each section. It also indicates how many questions are in each section. These two numbers are going to be used to evaluate the severity of symptom burden for each system and also give you a sense of the total symptom burden.

Section	Maximum symptom count for each section	Number of questions in each section
Diet	58	20
Lifestyle	12	4
Upper GI System	55	19
Liver and Gallbladder	68	28
Small Intestine	47	17
Large Intestine	58	20
Mineral Needs	75	29
Essential Fatty Acids	22	8
Sugar Handling	39	13
Vitamin Need	81	27
Adrenal	78	26
Pituitary	29	13
Thyroid	48	16
Men Only	27	9
Women Only	60	20
Cardiovascular	30	10
Kidney and Bladder	13	5
Immune System	30	10
Total	**830**	**294**

Evaluating the Symptom Burden

The best way to get a general assessment of the symptom burden for any particular system is to look at the total symptom count for each system and then divide that by the number of questions in that section. The closer the fraction gets to 1 the greater the severity. It is time to treat and further assess that system the closer the fraction gets to 1.

The following is an example of how to evaluate the symptom burden in a particular system:

A client has filled in their NAQ and you note that the symptom count for the sugar handling section appears to be high. The following example will illustrate how to evaluate the symptom burden for a typical sugar handling section on a NAQ:

Section 7 – Sugar Handling 39

173. 0 1 2 **3** Awaken a few hours after falling asleep, hard to get back to sleep
174. 0 1 **2** 3 Crave sweets
175. 0 1 **2** 3 Binge or uncontrolled eating
176. 0 1 **2** 3 Excessive appetite
177. 0 1 2 **3** Crave coffee or sugar in the afternoon
178. 0 1 2 **3** Sleepy in afternoon
179. 0 1 **2** 3 Fatigue that is relieved by eating
180. 0 1 2 **3** Headache if meals are skipped or delayed
181. 0 **1** 2 3 Irritable before meals
182. 0 1 **2** 3 Shaky if meals delayed
183. 0 **1** 2 3 Family members with diabetes (0=none, 1=1 or 2, 2=3 or 4, 3=more than 4)
184. 0 **1** 2 3 Frequent thirst
185. 0 **1** 2 3 Frequent urination

Total symptom count in this section: 26
Total number of questions in this section: 14
The symptom burden for the sugar handling section for this client = 1.87 (26/14)

The symptom burden for this particular case is severe because the symptom burden is way above 1. This is a significant finding and the underlying cause of the blood sugar dysregulation must be further assessed and treated. Suggestions of further assessment can be found in the individual sections further in the book.

Evaluating the total body symptom burden

You can use the same principle when evaluating the total body symptom burden. The best way to evaluate the total body symptom burden is to add up the symptom count for each section and divide that number by the total number of questions on the NAQ. I recommend that you do not include the medication count in this calculation as it just reflects a straight yes or no and will not add anything to your evaluation.

If the number is above 1 you know that the client is under fairly significant burden from their symptoms. The significance increases as the number increases above 1. Assessing total body symptom burden can very helpful when you are doing serial NAQs. You want to see the number decrease over time.

Breakdown of the Sections of the NAQ
Part I of the NAQ

Part I deals with Diet, Lifestyle, and Medications that your clients may be taking. It is often easy to gloss over this section and head into Part II, which covers the organ systems. I think that this is a mistake. I find Part I a very helpful tool for uncovering hidden diet and lifestyle related factors that are obstructing my clients' journey to health and wellness. It is also a great way to track prescription and over-the-counter drug use. It can also be used to track dietary and lifestyle changes that you ask your clients to make over the course of treatment. I use part I of the NAQ to steer my initial history intake. I ask the client to go into more detail on the dietary related questions they answer. This is a wonderful way to begin the consult.

Diet

The diet section has 20 questions that ask about general dietary history. Take the time to look in the diet section later in this book. I go into detail about each of the questions on the Diet section. As I mentioned above, this is an excellent place to start the re-education process for your clients. I will often tie in symptoms from part II with the questions they answer in the diet section. For instance, a client has a heavy symptom burden in the sugar handling section. They get sleepy in the afternoon, crave sweets, have headaches if meals are skipped, get irritable if meals are skipped, and crave coffee in the afternoon. I would then turn to the diet section and see what elements in their diet may contribute to these symptoms. They may eat refined sugar daily, drink caffeinated beverages, use artificial sweeteners, and consume refined flour on a daily basis. Connecting lifestyle and diet choices in with symptomology is a very effective way of creating change.

Lifestyle

The lifestyle section of the NAQ asks four very important questions:

1. Are you exercising?
2. Have you changed jobs recently?
3. Have you had a change in marital state recently?
4. How much do you work in a given week?

These questions are related to the stress levels a client is under. Hans Selye, the "father" of modern stress physiology put tremendous stock in the lifestyle factors that caused daily stress on the body.

Are you exercising?
The question "Are you exercising?" has a dual purpose. It identifies if the client is exercising at all. Moderate exercise is an important way to de-stress. You can begin the conversation about the importance of exercise with the clients who answer a 3 on the questionnaire (never exercise, or less than once a month). Please see the chapter on this question in the Lifestyle section of the book for a brief description on the benefits of exercise for your clients.

The other question it asks is whether or not the client may be over exercising. Research has shown that many people exercise too much. This puts considerable stress on the body, which has a difficult time recovering. Dr. Schwarzbein, in her seminal work ***"Schwarzbein Principle 2: The transition"*** documents the dangers of over exercise in terms of blood sugar control and adrenal burnout. I ask a client who answer 0 to this question (I exercise 2 or more times a week) very specific questions related to their exercise:

1. What type of exercise they do?
2. How much recovery time do they give between sessions?
3. What ratio of cardio to resistance training?
4. Do they incorporate stretching, yoga or core muscle work into their exercise?
5. Do they get sore between exercise sessions?
6. Do they get muscle cramps?
7. How much water do they drink?

The answers to these questions can help the client create a more balanced exercise regime. Also tie in the answers to the Part II questions to see how much of their symptom burden is being aggravated by their exercise routine.

The other 3 questions are directly related to the severity of stress that a client may be under. Clients who answer 3 on these three questions (changed jobs within last 2 months, divorced within last 6 months, and always work over 60 hours/week) are under a tremendous amount of stress. Expect to see a significant symptom burden in the sugar handling, adrenal, and thyroid section in part II.

Exposure to long, daily bouts of sustained stress put tremendous burden on the adrenals causing first an elevated cortisol level followed by a decreased level as the body passes through a stage of maladaptation to stress that leads eventually to outright adrenal dysregulation. This in turn contributes to blood sugar dysregulation as the body has a hard time regulating insulin levels, which leads to abnormal blood sugar swings. Sustained adrenal stress is one of the major causes of a dysfunctional thyroid. High levels of stress lead to the creation of a substance called reverse T3, which inhibts the creation and activity of active thyroid hormone.

Medications

It is very difficult to remember to ask your clients about every drug they may be taking. The NAQ is a great tool to assess the medications your clients are taking. I always glance at the medication section of the NAQ and am prompted to ask for specifics about any medications they are taking. I ask questions such as:

1. How long have you been taking this medication?
2. Who is the prescribing physician?
3. When was the last time you saw this doctor about this medication?
4. What condition is this medication meant to be addressing?
5. Do you notice any unusual symptoms associated with this medication?
6. Do you get routine lab work to make sure that your liver, kidneys and red blood cells are coping with this medication?
7. Are you interested in trying to reduce your dependence on your medication?

Note well: Only the prescribing physician has the right to change or alter a client's medication.

Part II of the NAQ

Part II of the NAQ focuses on the organ systems of the body and is organized according to a very specific system called the "Foundations of Health".

Foundations of Health

Part II of the Nutritional Assessment Questionnaire is organized according to a functional hierarchy called the Foundations of Health. You will notice that the digestive system is placed at the top of the list ahead of say the kidney and bladder section. This is not to say that the kidney and bladder are any less important to optimum health. It has been noted over many years that the body heals in very clear patterns. It is possible to clear up kidney and bladder dysfunction by first assessing and treating any dysfunction in the digestive system. You can have a tremendous impact on kidney function by increasing the level of available macro and micro nutrients in the body through optimizing digestion, by increasing the levels of Essential fatty Acids (EFAs) in the body by optimizing the gallbladder function, and by cleaning up the liver.

The foundations of health include:

1. Proper diet,
2. Adequate sleep,
3. Proper stress management,
4. Optimal digestion, absorption, and utilization of nutrients,
5. Adequate elimination,
6. Optimal tissue minerals,
7. Balanced essential fatty acids,
8. Proper blood sugar regulation,
9. Optimal hydration,
10. Adequate vitamin levels,
11. Balanced adrenals, thyroid and sex hormones,
12. Good cardiovascular health,
13. Balanced kidney, bladder, and immune systems.

It is important to focus the most attention on the symptom burden that is highest up the functional hierarchy. Even though a client may have a high priority in the cardiovascular system, it would be best to focus the most attention on the high priority in the liver gallbladder system for instance. Assessing and correcting the symptom burden in the liver gallbladder system will have a strong impact on the cardiovascular system.

The following sections will explain the relevance of a high symptom burden in the systems that are covered in part II of the NAQ.

1. Upper Gastrointestinal Section

The upper gastrointestinal (GI) system refers to the stomach and pancreas. This is one of the primary areas of dysfunction in the body. It is placed first on the NAQ because it has the highest priority in the foundations of health. Many dysfunctions in the body will resolve themselves once the upper GI has been appropriately assessed and treated. In my experience you cannot expect to resolve problems further down the digestive system without addressing stomach acidity.

The stomach adds hydrochloric acid and pepsin to help digest the food. The food then moves to the first part of the small intestine, or duodenum. There the pancreas adds enzymes to digest protein, fat and carbohydrate, and the gall bladder secretes bile to help emulsify fats.

Problems with digestion in the stomach and duodenum include inadequate production of hydrochloric acid (also called "hypochlorhydria"), pancreatic enzymes and bile salts. If this initial phase of digestion is inadequate, nutrients will not be absorbed, the GI tract can become irritated and yeast and other improper flora can grow in the lower bowel.

Assessing the symptom burden of the upper GI:

Symptom count	Significance
6 – 9	Low priority
10 – 14	Moderate priority
Above 15	High Priority

When the symptom burden of the upper GI approaches 15 or higher, then there is a need for further assessment and treatment. This signifies that there is significant distress in the upper GI. This may be caused by functional hypochlorhydria, with a concomitant zinc or thiamine insufficiency, a problem with gastric inflammation and a concomitant Helicobacter pylori infection, or ulceration. Poor digestion can be the beginning of digestive problems, fatigue, nutrient deficiency, obesity, food cravings, and allergies. It can also be the cause of irritable bowel, colitis, and Crohn's disease.

Refer to the explanation on each individual question in this book and follow the general guidelines below to further assess the upper GI.

Assessing the Upper GI (stomach function)

Further assessment	1. Check Ridler HCL reflex for tenderness 1 inch below xyphoid and over to the left edge of the rib cage 2. Check for tenderness in the Chapman reflex for the stomach and upper digestion located in 6th intercostal space on the left 3. Check for a positive zinc tally: A client holds a solution of aqueous zinc sulfate in their mouth and tells you if and when they can taste it. An almost immediate very bitter taste indicates the client does not need zinc. Clients who are zinc deficient will report no taste from the solution. 4. Gastric acid assessment using Gastrotest 5. Increased urinary indican levels

Assessing the Upper GI (exocrine pancreatic function)

Further assessment	1. Check Ridler enzyme point for tenderness 1 inch below xyphoid and over to the right edge of the rib cage 2. Check for tenderness in the Chapman reflex for the pancreas located in the 7th intercostal space 3. Increased urinary sediment levels

Supplemental Support for Upper GI

1. Betaine HCL, Pepsin, and Pancreatin 2. Pancreatic Enzymes 3. Bromelain, cellulase, lipase, and amylase 4. Beet juice, taurine, vitamin C and pancreolipase 5. Water soluble fiber and other nutrients to support colon health 6. Lactobacillus acidophilus and Bifidobacterium bifidus

NOTES:

2. Liver and Gallbladder Section

The liver has over 500 known functions. It is involved with digestion, the endocrine system, controlling blood sugar, and protein and fat metabolism. The liver also produces a substance called bile that is stored in the gallbladder. Bile is essential for proper fat emulsification and is also a major route of elimination for the body. Gallbladder dysfunction is very common in the developed world, hence the reason why this section is so high up the foundational hierarchy.

The amounts of chemicals we are exposed to are unprecedented in history. The average American consumes 10 pounds of chemical food additives each year. Add to that the chemical burden caused by food sprayed with pesticides and from air and water pollution, you can see that our chemical burden is considerable.

The body has systems designed to eliminate waste and to detoxify poisons. The liver chemically converts toxins to be easily eliminated by the kidneys. Detoxification is an ongoing process. The sheer volume of chemicals in the environment and in the diet has caused many people to reach their threshold of tolerance, which has adversely affected their health.

When the body is burdened with more chemicals than it can efficiently detoxify, chronic health problems can occur. Problems like allergies, skin problems, digestive problems, headaches, fatigue, joint pain and a variety of ailments can be caused by chemical exposure. Theron Randolph, MD, and early researcher of chronic allergies, was convinced that the increased incidence of allergies and other chronic health problems in the latter half of the 20th century is due to the amount of chemicals we are exposed to on a day-to-day basis.

The gallbladder will become more and more compromised as the liver becomes more dysfunctional. The gallbladder stores the bile and when stimulated by the appropriate response (fat and protein in the GI and from the influence of cholecystokinin) will contract and pump bile into the lumen of the GI tract. However, a couple of conditions exist that greatly impact the function of the gallbladder. Mild liver damage due to fatty deposits within the functional units of the liver itself can greatly impact the production of bile. This leads to a situation called biliary insufficiency. Some of the common causes of biliary insufficiency include changes in metabolism within the liver itself. This is most often caused by the consumption of excess hydrogenated or trans fatty acids, excess refined foods, oxidative stress, and low fat diets. Other causes include overt liver damage due to hepatitis, chemical damage to the liver and liver cirrhosis.

Another condition that affects the biliary system is a condition called biliary stasis. This is a condition of progressive solidification and thickening of the bile itself within the gallbladder. This is often due to a low fat diet that does not provide adequate stimulation for bile release from the gallbladder. The hormone cholecystokinin (CCK) will not be released if there is no fat in the lumen and the gallbladder will receive no stimulation to contract and release bile. This causes a Supersaturation of the bile within the gallbladder; if left unchecked this can lead to overt stone formation. Other causes of biliary stasis include a decrease in bile acid formation and decreased phosphatidylcholine secretion.

Assessing the symptom burden of the Liver and Gallbladder:

Symptom count	Significance
7 – 11	Low priority
12 – 17	Moderate priority
Above 18	High Priority

When the symptom burden of the Liver Gallbladder section approaches 18 or higher, then there is a need for further assessment and treatment. This signifies that there is significant distress in the Liver and/or Gallbladder. This may be caused by detoxification problems that can significantly affect the functioning of the liver, biliary insufficiency, biliary stasis, a low fat diet, or the consumption of hydrogenated oil.

Refer to the explanation on each individual question in this book and follow the general guidelines below to further assess the liver gallbladder system.

Assessing Liver dysfunction

Further assessment	1. Check for tenderness in the Chapman reflex for the liver-gallbladder located over the 6th intercostal space on the right side 2. Check for tenderness in the Liver point located on the 3rd rib, 3 " to the right of the sternum, at the costochondral junction. 3. Check for tenderness underneath the right rib cage 4. Assess for Hepato-biliary congestion with the Acoustic Cardiogram (ACG), which will show post-systolic rounding due to increased backpressure on the pulmonic and aortic valve. It may also show through to the tricuspid valve if chronic. 5. Decreased uric acid on a blood chemistry panel is an indication for molybdenum deficiency, a sign of Phase II liver detoxification dysfunction. 6. Increased SGOT, SGPT on a blood chemistry panel 7. Various labs do liver detoxification panels

Assessing Gallbladder dysfunction

Further assessment	1. Check for tenderness underneath the right rib cage 2. Check for tenderness and nodulation on the web between thumb and fore-finger of right hand 3. Check for tenderness in the Chapman reflex for the liver-gallbladder located over the 6th intercostal space on the right side 4. Blood chemistry and CBC testing for SGOT, SGPT, GGT 5. Increased urinary sediment levels, especially calcium oxalate levels, which are typically elevated in these cases

Supplemental Support

1. Beet juice, taurine, vitamin C and pancreolipase with or without bile salts
2. Nutrients to support Phase II liver detoxification
3. Herbs that cleanse the liver
4. Glutathione, cysteine, and Glycine
5. Powdered detoxification support formula

3. Small Intestine Section

The small intestine is the site for further digestion and also absorption and assimilation of the majority of nutrients. It is split up into 3 distinct areas: the Duodenum, Jejunum, and Ileum. About 90% of all absorption takes place in the small intestines. However, success in the small intestine is dependent on proper setup from the stomach, gallbladder, and pancreas. Dysfunction in any one of these systems will lead to the production of metabolic toxins. The bacterial flora in the small intestine feasts on maldigested nutrients and produce metabolic toxins that cause considerable damage to the lining of the small intestine leading to problems such as leaky gut syndrome and malabsorption. The small intestine becomes a great place for potentially pathogenic to take up residence as the terrain in the small intestine begins to deteriorate.

The small intestine is about 10 feet in length, but its surface area is far larger. Some estimates suggest that the surface area of the small intestine is about the size of a tennis court due to the presence of the villi and microvilli, microscopic projections out into the lumen of the small intestine. The small intestine continues the digestive process using mechanical digestion of localized segments that contract and mix up the chime with digestive juices and brings the chime in direct contact with the mucosa for nutrient absorption. Chemical digestion in the small intestine is from the joint efforts of bile, pancreatic and intestinal juices.

Some of the functional disorders that affect the small intestine include:

1. Bowel toxemia, which is the production of metabolic toxins that can damage the mucosa,
2. Dysbiosis: bacterial, fungal or parasitic infections,
3. Malabsorption, a condition whereby the absorptive surface of the lumen of the small intestine is reduced from the size of a tennis court to the size of a small parking space,
4. Leaky gut syndrome, a condition marked by the emergence of gaps between the cells of the small intestine. Large molecules that would normally be blocked from entering into direct systemic absorption can flow freely into the blood stream setting up immune and allergy like reactions.
5. Allergies/intolerances and sensitivities. These are directly associated with small intestine health. Please see the small intestine section later in the book for an in-depth explanation of the small intestine's role in allergies and sensitivities.

Assessing the symptom burden of the Small Intestine:

Symptom count	Significance
5 – 7	Low priority
8 – 15	Moderate priority
Above 16	High Priority

When the symptom burden of the Small Intestine section approaches 16 or higher, then there is a need for further assessment and treatment. This signifies that there is significant distress in the Small Intestine. This may be caused by dysbiosis, bowel toxemia, malabsorption, leaky gut syndrome, or allergies.

Refer to the explanation on each individual question in this book and follow the general guidelines below to further assess the Small Intestine.

Assessing Small intestine dysfunction

Further assessment	1. Check for tenderness in the Chapman reflex for the colon located bilaterally along the iliotibial band on the thighs. Palpate the colon for tenderness and tension. Tenderness in the colon can relate to a dysfunction upstream in the small intestine. 2. Check for tenderness in the Chapman reflex for the small intestine located on the 8th, 9th and 10th intercostal spaces near the tip of the rib. 3. Check the Bennet reflex for the small intestine. Palpate four quadrants in a 2" to 3" radius around the umbilicus for tenderness and tension. 4. Increased urinary indican levels 5. Stool analysis- either comprehensive digestive analysis or a parasite profile 6. Decreased secretory IgA on stool analysis

Supplemental Support

1. Micro Emulsified Oregano
2. Nutrients that heal the intestines
3. L-glutamine
4. Betaine HCL, Pepsin, and pancreatin
5. Water soluble fiber and nutrients to support colon health Gut healing nutrients and demulscents
6. Multiple nutrients that support the immune system
7. Lactobacillus acidophilus and Bifidobacterium bifidus
8. Gut healing nutrients and demulscents

NOTES:

4. Large Intestine Section

The large intestine is the area in the GI where water is reabsorbed back into the body. The liquid chyme is transformed into feces, which consists of water, inorganic salts, sloughed off epithelial cells, and bacteria. The expulsion of feces through the colon requires optimal peristaltic function. The bacterial environment in the colon can synthesize certain nutrients including vitamin B1, B2, B12, and vitamin K. It is important to have adequate amounts of fiber in the diet because the bacteria act on the fiber to produce butyric acid, which is one of the main sources of fuel for the cells that make up the colonic mucosa.

Success in the large intestine is dependent on optimal function in the rest of the digestive tract. Resolving issues of hypochlorhydria, pancreatic insufficiency, bowel toxemia, dysbiosis, leaky gut syndrome, and malabsorption will have tremendous effects on the colonic health.

Some of the main areas of dysfunction in the large intestine include:

1. Sluggish colon (constipation)
2. Rapid bowel transit (Diarrhea)
3. Dysbiosis- bacterial and parasitic
4. Bowel toxemia
5. Yeast overgrowth

Assessing the symptom burden of the Large Intestine:

Symptom count	Significance
6 – 9	Low priority
10 – 15	Moderate priority
Above 16	High Priority

When the symptom burden of the Large intestine section approaches 16 or higher, then there is a need for further assessment and treatment. This signifies that there is significant distress in the large intestine. This may be caused by a sluggish colon, a fast bowel transit time, dysbiosis, bowel toxemia, or a yeast overgrowth in the colon.

Refer to the explanation on each individual question in this book and follow the general guidelines below to further assess the large intestine.

Assessing Large Intestine dysfunction

Further assessment	1. Have a client check their bowel transit time. Give 6 "00" caps of activated charcoal and ask them to record how long it takes for the black to appear and to go completely away. Various dyes, including beets, sweetcorn and un-popped popcorn can also be used. 2. Assess the client's hydration status. Have client stand with hands by their side and check and palpate the veins in the right hand. Have them slowly raise their hand to heart level and see if the veins still stick out. Veins that are only just visible or not visible at all are a sign of dehydration.

	3. Increased urinary indican and sediment levels 4. Stool analysis- either comprehensive digestive analysis or a parasite profile 5. Check for tenderness in the Chapman reflex for the colon located bilaterally along the iliotibial band on the thighs. 6. Palpate the colon for tenderness and tension. 7. Check for tenderness in the Chapman reflex for the small intestine located on the 8th, 9th and 10th intercostal spaces near the tip of the rib. Also palpate four quadrants in a 2" to 3" radius around the umbilicus for tenderness and tension 8. Decreased secretory IgA on stool analysis

Supplemental Support

1. Water soluble fiber and nutrients to support colon health
2. Nutrients that heal the intestines
3. Betaine HCL, Pepsin, and pancreatin
4. Larch arabinogalactans
5. Micro Emulsified Oregano
6. Beet juice, taurine, vitamin C and pancreolipase
7. Bromelain, cellulase, lipase, and amylase

NOTES:

5. Mineral Needs Section

No discussion of minerals can be done without first addressing calcium needs and calcium supplementation. A major part of the NAQ Mineral Needs section deals with the signs and symptoms of calcium insufficiency. Calcium is the most abundant mineral in the human body. Of the two to three pounds of calcium contained in the average body, 99% is located in the bones and teeth. Calcium is needed to form bones and teeth and is also required for blood clotting, transmission of signals in nerve cells, and muscle contraction. The importance of calcium for preventing osteoporosis is probably its most well-known role.

Many in the healing arts feel that calcium deficiency is widespread and almost everyone would benefit from a daily calcium supplement. Our experience indicates that **the inability to use calcium available in the diet is far more wide-spread than simple calcium deficiency**. When a calcium need is identified through subjective indications or through laboratory analysis, the lack of synergists or metabolizing agents may be locus to the problem. Always rule out the need for magnesium, phosphorus, vitamin A, B, and C, unsaturated fatty acids, iodine, and the inability to absorb calcium from the diet (hypochlorhydria) as the possible reason(s) for the calcium need.

Many doctors feel that an increased serum calcium indicates poor fat emulsification and decreased serum calcium indicates poor fatty acid utilization.

Common subjective indications of calcium needs are:

1. Frequent skin rashes or hives,
2. Muscle cramps at rest (especially leg or toe cramps while sleeping),
3. Soft fingernails,
4. Frequent nose bleeds,
5. Increased fever with a mild cold or virus,
6. Frequent hoarseness,
7. Irritability,
8. High or low blood pressure.

Some of the main causes for calcium insufficiency include:

1. Arthritis
2. Blood loss
3. Decreased absorption
4. Decreased intake especially if eating SAD (Standard American Diet)
5. High intake of sodium
6. High intake of sugar
7. High phosphorus
8. Hypochlorhydria
9. Lead toxicity

The mineral section of the NAQ covers more than just calcium insufficiency. It covers the major symptoms associated with mineral insufficiency in general. Minerals may be depleted under several conditions. Individuals who eat a lot of sugar and refined foods tend to excrete minerals in their urine; this is compounded by the fact that a refined diet is very low in minerals in the first place. Stress and stimulation of the adrenal glands tend to increase the secretion of hormones that cause a loss of minerals. It has been argued that the use of chemical fertilizers and soil erosion is responsible for the produce of today being lower in mineral content than vegetables grown in decades past.

The following section outlines the importance of the major macro and micro minerals to human physiology.

Boron: Boron is a trace mineral that may influence hormones, especially estrogen. It is used in many products to enhance bone strength in those experiencing osteoporosis.

Calcium: Necessary for bone health. It is also necessary for muscles to relax after contraction. Calcium may be needed by people who suffer from leg cramps or by women who suffer from menstrual cramps. Low calcium can be a reason for poor growth in children. It may be helpful for clients with high blood pressure. High calcium intake may reduce the risk for colon cancer.

Copper: Copper is a common cofactor in enzymes that break down and build up body tissue, help with blood clotting and enable the adrenal glands to work properly.

Copper is necessary (along with vitamin C) for the integrity of skin and connective tissue. It is necessary for the production of myelin (necessary for nerve function). Copper deficiency can lead to arthritis, arterial disease, loss of pigmentation, myocardial disease and neurologic effects. Copper deficiency can lead to an anemia that will not respond to iron supplementation (interestingly, too much copper can also lead to altered iron metabolism and also cause an anemia).

Copper, in high levels, can be toxic. High levels of copper can deplete zinc and iron. Excess zinc, iron or molybdenum intake can deplete copper. There is some evidence that an imbalance between zinc and copper (favoring copper) may lead to attention-deficit/hyperactivity disorder (ADHD) and aggressive behavior in general.

Chromium: Chromium is part of glucose tolerance factor (GTF). GTF increases the effectiveness of insulin. It is a useful nutrient for both hypoglycemic (low blood sugar) individuals and for diabetics. Chromium deficiency is fairly common in the United States because the mineral is difficult to absorb. Deficiency can lead to severe glucose intolerance (problems handling sugar, sugar cravings). Chromium may also play a role in protein and fat metabolism. There is some evidence that taking adequate chromium may help to prevent atherosclerotic plaques.

Iodine: Iodine aids the development and functioning of the thyroid gland. It is found in seawater and in soil on the coasts of the world. The world's "goiter belts," like the American Midwest, are areas that are far from the ocean with soil that is deficient in iodine. Adding iodine to salt eliminates the symptoms of goiter. According to Broda Barnes, MD, iodizing salt is not adequate to eliminate hypothyroidism in these areas and that people in land-locked areas may still need more iodine (*Hypothyroidism, the Unsuspected Illness,* by Broda Barnes and Lawrence Galton, Harper Collins Publishers, Inc., 1976).

The condition of hair, nails, skin and teeth are dependent on adequate thyroid function. Poor thyroid function can lead to problems like high cholesterol and immune system problems. People with poor thyroid function often feel cold when others do not, have trouble losing weight, may cry for no reason, feel fatigue, be depressed, lack motivation, have swelling of their ankles, catch colds easily or lack sex drive. Iodine also has the effect of thinning mucus and can be used to relieve sinus pressure.

Iron: The primary use of iron is in making red blood cells. Low iron can create microcytic anemia (an anemia with small red cells) however, not all anemias are the result of low iron. Symptoms of iron deficiency anemia (and other types of anemia) include weakness, fatigue, pallor (being pale), becoming out of breath on exertion, palpitation, coldness and loss of sensation in the extremities, and a sense of being overly tired. Iron deficiency can cause people to eat things like clay, starch, salt, cardboard, and ice.

Magnesium: Magnesium is a cofactor for many enzymes that are involved with metabolizing and converting the components of food. Magnesium facilitates at least 300 such enzymes.

Magnesium is nature's muscle relaxer. It is useful for relieving all kinds of muscle tension, including menstrual cramps, muscle cramps, and general muscle tension. It is necessary for the production of bone. Magnesium deficiency is also a source of heart arrhythmias. Low magnesium is also responsible for many of the symptoms of premenstrual syndrome (PMS). Low magnesium may also be responsible for mood swings associated with the menstrual cycle. For menstrual issues, magnesium is much more effective when given with vitamin B_6. In fact, B_6 and magnesium generally work together in many enzyme systems.

Magnesium helps with glucose tolerance and fat metabolism. Magnesium deficiency has been linked to increased triglycerides and cholesterol. Magnesium, along with vitamin B_6, is useful for the prevention of kidney stones.

Manganese: Manganese deficiency can lead to skeletal abnormalities, impaired growth, depressed reproductive function and defects of lipid and carbohydrate metabolism. Low manganese levels may be responsible for some seizures in epileptics. Manganese deficiency can also weaken ligaments and discs. It is necessary for proper function of the pituitary gland.

Molybdenum: Molybdenum is an important mineral cofactor for three important enzymes which the body uses to detoxify various chemicals. This mineral is commonly deficient in individuals who are sensitive to chemicals and smoke.

Selenium: Selenium functions as an antioxidant. In other words, it helps protect your cells. It also necessary for adequate thyroid function. Some studies show that selenium supplementation increases resistance to viral infections. Selenium deficiency in animal studies has lead to hair loss, growth retardation, reproductive failure, and pancreatic problems.

Zinc: Zinc is important for use in hundreds of enzyme systems production. Low zinc levels in children can be a cause of poor growth.

Zinc deficiency can cause delayed sexual maturation, impotence, low sperm counts, loss of hair, glossitis, nail dystrophy, night blindness, impaired sense of taste and smell, depression, compulsive behavior, and decreased appetite (even to the point of anorexia).

Imbalance between copper and zinc (too much copper in relation to zinc) may be linked to ADHD and aggressive or antisocial behavior. There may be a link between diarrhea and zinc deficiency.

Zinc is also important for immune function; letting a zinc tablet slowly dissolve in your mouth is a very effective treatment for a sore throat. Zinc deficiency can lead to depressed thymic activity.

The cornea is the tissue with the highest zinc concentration and is affected by zinc deficiency. Dry, irritated eyes can result from low zinc levels.

Assessing the symptom burden of the Mineral Needs Section:

Symptom count	Significance
8 – 12	Low priority
13 – 19	Moderate priority
Above 20	High Priority

When the symptom burden of the Mineral Needs section approaches 20 or higher, then there is a need for further assessment and treatment. This signifies that there is significant distress in the systems that help regulate the mineral balance in the body. This may be caused by an inability to absorb minerals from the diet, essential fatty acid insufficiency, adrenal hormone imbalance, systemic pH issues, vitamin D insufficiency, and general hormone imbalance.

Refer to the explanation on each individual question in this book and follow the general guidelines below to further assess for the mineral needs in your clients.

Assessing Mineral Insufficiency

Further assessment	1. Assess for mineral deficiency using Tissue Mineral Assessment Test. Place a standard blood pressure cuff around the largest portion of the client's calf muscle (sitting). Instruct the client to let you know when they feel the onset of cramping pain and gradually inflate the cuff. Stop and deflate immediately when they have cramping pain. Less than 200 mmHg is considered deficient in minerals. Use neurolingual testing to challenge the body with several types of magnesium to see if this raises threshold above 200mmHg. 2. Check for a positive zinc tally: A client holds a solution of aqueous zinc sulfate in their mouth and tells you if and when they can taste it. An almost immediate very bitter taste indicates the client does not need zinc. Clients who are zinc deficient will report no taste from the solution. 3. Check client's urine for the loss of type 1 collagen (several labs offer this test often called Bone Resorption Assessment) 4. Check client's urine for calcium loss (Sulkowitch test). 5. Check serum calcium, phosphorous, sodium, potassium and uric acid levels.

	6. Assess for mineral insufficiency by using Dr. Kane's mineral assessment tests. 7. Assess the impact of mineral deficiencies on the body's acid buffering capacities by using Dr. Bieler's salivary pH acid test.

Supplemental Support

1. Alkaline Ash minerals (Calcium, Magnesium,Potassium)
2. Calcium and Magnesium formula with or without parathyroid tissue
3. Emulsified Vitamin E drops
4. Multiple nutrients to support bone health
5. Multiple mineral without iron or copper
6. Betaine HCL, Pepsin, and pancreatin
7. Mixed fatty acids (walnut, hazelnut, sesame, and apricot)

NOTES:

6. Essential Fatty Acids Section

A lot has been written and broadcast about the dangers of eating fat. Doctors, athletic trainers, and dieticians are recommending low-fat diets. What has been lost in the midst of all of this advice is that fat is actually a necessary component of your diet. You need fats and oils for a properly functioning immune system, integrity of the skin and mucus membranes and absorption of fat-soluble vitamins (vitamins A, E, D, and K). Not all fats are created equal. Some need to be avoided; some are a vital component of a healthy diet. Most Americans need to add a source of essential fatty acids to their diets; so avoiding fats completely is not always a good idea.

Essential fatty Acids (EFAs) are just that, essential. You need to have them in order to live. Unfortunately most people in the so-called developed Western world are commonly deficient in essential fatty acids for a variety of reasons. One of the main causes of essential fatty acid deficiency is the consumption of hydrogenated and partially-hydrogenated oils. Hydrogenation is a process in which hydrogen is bubbled through an oil, turning it into a solid. Unfortunately, it changes the chemistry of the oil so that it is unusable by the body. Hydrogenating oil turns a liquid oil into a solid fat with a very long shelf-life—good for food processors, bad for your health. The fats created are called "trans fats" and they can create health problems.

Trans fats not only cause health problems of their own, they prevent the essential fatty acids from being properly utilized by tying up the enzymes necessary for their metabolism. In fact, one common sign of trans fats creating problems is a craving for fried food, or snacks fried in oil, like potato chips. The body is actually craving the essential oil it needs, but when deep-fried food is substituted it "gums-up" the works, creating a more severe deficiency than if the fried food was never consumed.

Encourage your clients to absolutely avoid all forms of hydrogenated and partially hydrogenated oils. As time passes, we keep finding out more and more bad things about hydrogenated oil and fried foods.

Some of the many problems associated with Trans fats include:

1. Women with higher levels of trans fats in their cells are much more likely to develop breast cancer than those with low levels.
2. High levels of trans fats create platelet aggregation, which is the beginning of the plaque associated with coronary heart disease.
3. Pain and inflammation become much worse for clients who consume hydrogenated oils. They chemically prevent the formation of natural anti-inflammatory substances that are normally produced by the body. If you suffer from chronic pain or have recently been injured, strictly avoid hydrogenated oil.
4. Trans fats are incorporated into the cells and affect the integrity of the cellular membrane. This makes the cell less resistant to bacteria and viruses. They are a source of immune system problems.
5. There may be a link between trans fats and ADD, depression and fatigue. Brain and nerve tissue have a high content of fat. Some researches believe that when trans fats

are incorporated into the nerve cells they affect certain functions, creating problems like ADD and depression.

6. Muscle fatigue and skin problems are also linked to hydrogenated oils. Trans fats cause the muscles to fatigue easily. Since the myelin sheath is largely composed of fat, trans fats may affect function of the nervous system and there may be a connection to attention-deficit disorder (ADD).
7. Most chips and fried snacks contain hydrogenated oils. Hydrogenated oils are found in a lot of packaged foods like crackers, cereals, and even bread. They are in margarine, mayonnaise and a lot of bottled salad dressings. Read labels.
8. Not all fats are bad for you. Permissible fats include raw nuts (not roasted), virgin or extra virgin olive oil and avocados.

Encourage your clients to eat foods that contain essential fatty acids. Raw nuts and seeds and cold water fish (like salmon) are good sources of essential fatty acids. Your doctor may have some specific suggestions for you. Clients suffering from chronic pain and inflammation should ***strictly avoid hydrogenated oil and trans fats***. For that matter, they should go easy on meat products since they too may contribute to inflammation.

Another reason for essential fatty acid deficiency is the prevalence of low-fat diets. Americans are so afraid of fat that they will consume sugar and all manner of chemicals if the food promises to be low in fat. The problem isn't the amount of fat we eat as much as it is the quality of the fat we eat.

Assessing the symptom burden of Essential Fatty Acids Section:

Symptom count	Significance
3 – 4	Low priority
5 – 6	Moderate priority
Above 7	High Priority

When the symptom burden of the EFA section approaches 7 or higher, then there is a need for further assessment and treatment. This signifies that there is significant distress in the systems that help regulate essential fatty acids in the body. This may be caused by increased consumption of hydrogenated oil, gallbladder insufficiency, which decreases the emulsification and absorption of all fats, a low fat diet, and a diet low in essential fatty acids in general.

Refer to the explanation on each individual question in this book and follow the general guidelines below to further assess for essential fatty acid insufficiency in your clients.

Assessing Essential fatty acid deficiency.

Further assessment	1. Oral pH less than 7.2 indicates essential fatty acid deficiency 2. Repeated muscle challenge. This challenge involves a simple, normal muscle test repeated once per second, 20 times with regular intensity. As in a standard muscle test, the joint is positioned in such a way that the muscle to be tested is shortened. The practitioner applies pressure to the joint to lengthen the muscle, until a "locking" is noted. A positive result occurs when "locking" of the muscle and joint does not occur, indicating deficient free fatty acids. 3. Fatty acid profile via laboratory testing of blood.

Supplemental Support

1. Flax seed oil
2. Blackcurrant seed oil
3. EPA and DHA from fish oil
4. Mixed fatty acids (walnut, hazelnut, sesame, and apricot)
5. Phosphatidylcholine
6. Beet juice, taurine, vitamin C and pancreolipase with or without bile salts

NOTES:

7. Sugar Handling Section

Blood sugar dysregulation is reaching almost epidemic proportions in the Western world, and the west is intent on exporting this curse to many developing countries too, which are seeing unprecedented explosions in obesity over the last 10 years.

Blood sugar dysregulation does not suddenly emerge. You cannot wake up one day with Type II diabetes and not have a clue that something is going wrong. Type II diabetes follows an insidious pattern of development and involves, to some extent, dysregulation in the three organs of sugar regulation: the endocrine pancreas, the liver, and the adrenal glands. These three organs work in harmony to regulate and normalize blood glucose levels across the day and night.

As you consume a carbohydrate meal the pancreas releases the hormone insulin and opens the cells to accept glucose, thus lowering total blood glucose levels. In between meals and at night the adrenal glands release small amounts of glucocorticoid hormones that stimulate the liver to release glycogen, the storage form of glucose.

This is how the body evolved to deal with carbohydrates. Unfortunately, problems begin to emerge when stress levels are high and constant and you consume large amounts of carbohydrates at every meal. In this situation the insulin is released, blood glucose begins to drop but unfortunately the amount of insulin released causes the blood glucose level to drop below the normal fasting level. This leads to a condition called reactive hypoglycemia and to many of the symptoms you will find in the sugar handling section of the NAQ.

As the blood glucose levels drop with the reactive hypoglycemia, the adrenals and the liver come to the rescue. Glucorcorticoids are released and the liver normalizes blood glucose levels by releasing stored glycogen. Unfortunately this leads to adrenal fatigue and a condition called insulin resistance. As the cells become exposed to more and more insulin they begin to become resistant to its action. This causes the blood glucose levels to begin to rise and it is very hard for the body to lower them. Type II diabetes and obesity are the likely consequence of untreated sugar regulation, along with the many complications associated with uncontrolled blood glucose levels.

Hypoglycemia, or low blood sugar, can cause fatigue, depression and sugar cravings. Hypoglycemia is both a cause of certain health problems and the effect of other health problems. It can cause fatigue, depression, dizziness, sugar cravings, obesity, and headaches. It can be caused by dysbiosis, digestive problems, stress and adrenal problems, nutrient deficiency, allergies, and poor eating habits. Getting your clients' blood sugar under control will help them to feel a whole lot better. Handouts in the back of the book are very helpful to normalize your clients' blood sugar.

Assessing the symptom burden of the Sugar Handling Section:

Symptom count	Significance
5 – 6	Low priority
7 – 10	Moderate priority
Above 11	High Priority

When the symptom burden of the sugar handling section approaches 11 or higher, then there is a need for further assessment and treatment. This signifies that there is significant distress in the systems that help regulate blood sugar in the body. This may be caused by increased consumption of refined sugars in the diet, adrenal insufficiency, increased hydrogenated oil consumption, obesity, lack of exercise,

Refer to the explanation on each individual question in this book and follow the general guidelines below to further assess the sugar handling in your clients.

Assessing Blood Sugar Dysregulation

Further assessment	1. Check for tenderness in the Chapman reflex for the liver-gallbladder located over the 6th intercostal space on the right side 2. Check for tenderness in the Liver point located on the 3rd rib, 3" to the right of the sternum, at the costochondral junction. 3. Check for tenderness underneath the right rib cage 4. Check for tenderness or nodularity in the right thenar pad, which is a pancreas indicator if tender 5. Check for tenderness in the Chapman reflex for the pancreas located in the 7th intercostal space on the left 6. Check for tenderness or guarding at the head of the pancreas located in the upper left quadrant of the abdominal region 1/2 to 2/3 of the way between the umbilicus and the angel of the ribs 7. Check for tenderness in the inguinal ligament bilaterally, an adrenal indicator 8. Check for tenderness at the medial knee bilaterally, at the insertion of the sartorius muscle at the Pes Anserine. This is an adrenal indicator. 9. Check for a paradoxical pupillary reflex by shining a light into a client's eye and grading the reaction of the pupil. A pupil that fails to constrict indicates adrenal exhaustion 10. Check for the presence of postural hypotension. A drop of more than 10 points is an indication of adrenal insufficiency. 11. Check for a chronic short leg due to a posterior-inferior ilium. An adrenal indicator when confirmed with postural hypotension and a paradoxical pupillary response. 12. Check fasting blood glucose 13. Run a six-hour glucose-insulin tolerance test.

Supplemental Support

1. Multiple nutrients to support sugar handling problems 2. Adaptogenic herbs to support adrenal function 3. Adrenal tissue (neonatal bovine) 4. Beet juice, taurine, vitamin C and pancreolipase 5. Broad spectrum anti-oxidants 6. Nutrients to normalize cholesterol and triglycerides 7. Pancreatic tissue (neonatal bovine)

8. Herbs that cleanse the liver
9. L-Carnitine
10. Chromium
11. Nutrients to support eye function
12. Buffered vitamin C with bioflavanoids
13. Multiple nutrients for supporting renal function

NOTES:

8. Vitamin Need Section

When assessing clients' nutritional needs you should ask yourself the following question: does this client's typical diet provide enough vitamins and minerals?

According to nutrition experts, the average Western diet contains too many refined carbohydrates, not enough essential fatty acids, and too little fiber. The combination of low fiber and highly refined carbohydrates and fat contributes to an increased risk of heart disease, cancer, and diabetes. Even conventional medical authorities believe that the average Western diet is not ideal, since it is linked to poor health. A good diet should consist of fresh fruits and vegetables, whole grains, legumes, nuts and seeds, and (for nonvegetarians) nonfat dairy products, and fish.

People do not eat the same foods their great-grandparents ate, and these dietary changes might affect nutrient requirements. Some foods were not available in Europe or Asia until the discovery of the New World. Before 1492, there were no potatoes in Ireland, no tomatoes in Italy, and no eggplant or green peppers in England. All these foods are New World crops. Other foods, such as rice and soy, are also relatively new to Europeans.

Another recent phenomenon is that modern foods are generally picked before they are ripe. Ripening increases the nutrient content of the food, so diets based on unripened foods may be lacking in some nutrients.

Many of today's foods are processed with extra ingredients compared to food in the past. An example is a loaf of bread, which 100 years ago was prepared with only wheat, water, butter, baker's yeast, and a sweetener to help the yeast rise. Today, a modern loaf of bread may contain more than 100 ingredients, including preservatives, coloring agents, insecticides, herbicides, fungicides, and chemical residues from various packaging and cleaning procedures. These multiple ingredients may complicate digestion and increase the risk of allergic reaction.

Certain additives to the food chain have increased the need for certain vitamins and minerals. An example of this is the hydrazine residues in foods resulting from the fungicides used by farmers. The fungicides, along with nutrients from the soil, are absorbed by plants. Hydrazine compounds compete with and increase the body's need for vitamin B6.

Plants do not always need the same nutrients as people. For example, plants do not require selenium, iodine, or chromium to thrive. But if people are deprived of selenium, they can develop certain heart muscle problems and have an increased risk of cancer; if deprived of iodine, people can develop goiters; and if deprived of chromium, they can develop blood sugar problems.

People today do not eat the same quantities of quality food their ancestors ate (and in general, people do not do as much work). For example, if people require the amount of beta-carotene available in two pounds of carotene-containing food, but now only eat two single carrots, then they are risking getting less than optimal amounts of beta-carotene.

The following section will give some basic information on the different vitamins and their role in physiology:

B Vitamins

B vitamins are necessary for energy production, carbohydrate metabolism, blood cell production, enzyme function and many other uses. Deficiency, or "poor vitamin status," perhaps a better term, is fairly common because of the amount of refined foods people eat and the preponderance of digestive problems. Let's consider each of the B vitamins individually to give you some insight into your client's health.

Thiamin: Deficiency of thiamin makes it difficult for a person to digest carbohydrates. It also leaves too much pyruvic acid in the blood, causing loss of mental alertness, labored breathing, and cardiac damage. Early signs of deficiency include easy fatigue, loss of appetite, irritability and emotional instability. Confusion and loss of memory will appear if the deficiency persists.

Beriberi is the disease of thiamin deficiency. The most advanced neural changes occur in the peripheral nerves, particularly the legs. The distal segments are involved earliest and most severely.

Early deficiency produces fatigue, irritation, poor memory, sleep disturbances, precordial pain, anorexia, abdominal discomfort and constipation. Peripheral neurologic changes are bilateral and symmetric, usually in the lower extremities. Paresthesias of the toes, burning of the feet (especially at night), calf muscle cramps, pain in the legs, loss of vibratory sense in the toes and difficulty in rising from a squatting position are early signs. Later signs include loss of ankle jerk, then knee jerk and loss of vibratory and position sensation in the toes, atrophy of the calf and thigh muscles and finally foot drop and toe drop. The arms may become involved after the leg signs are well-established.

Cerebral beriberi or Wernicke-Korsakoff syndrome is a state of mental confusion commonly seen in alcoholics.

Vitamin B_1 is necessary for hydrochloric acid (HCl) production. One possible way to check for thiamin need is to use neurolingual testing and see if the Chapman Reflex for the stomach is less tender while the client is holding thiamin in his or her mouth. You can use **(Bio-3G-B)** as a thiamin source.

Riboflavin: Riboflavin is water soluble. It is stable to heat, oxidation, and acid. It disintegrates in the presence of alkali or UV light. Riboflavin is necessary for cell respiration because it works with enzymes in the utilization of cell oxygen. It functions as part of a group of enzymes that are involved in the breakdown and utilization of carbohydrates, fats, and proteins.

Riboflavin is not known to have any toxic reactions. An early sign of deficiency is the appearance of cracks and sores in the corners of the mouth; a red, sore tongue; a feeling of grit and sand on the insides of the eyelids; burning of the eyes; changes in the cornea; sensitivity to light; lesions of the lips; scaling around the nose, mouth, forehead and ears; trembling; sluggishness; dizziness, and a lack of stamina. You can use Riboflavin and the associated B vitamins.

Niacin: Niacin is water soluble and is more stable than thiamin or riboflavin. Niacin is available in three synthetic forms: Niacinamide, nicotinic acid, and nicotinamide. As a coenzyme, it assists enzymes in the breakdown and utilization of proteins, fats, and carbohydrates.

Niacin has been used to improve circulation and to reduce cholesterol. Tryptophan can be converted into niacin by the body. Excessive consumption of sugar and starches will deplete the body's supply of niacin.

Niacin, in doses of 100 mg or more, can cause an unpleasant flush. Taking Niacinamide does not cause the flush. In doses of 2 g/day or more, it can cause liver damage. High doses may also precipitate a gout attack, or make a case of gout worse by competing with the excretion of uric acid. Niacin is involved with the release of stomach acid and should, therefore, be taken on a full stomach. High doses of niacin are capable of bringing down cholesterol. One way to get around the liver damage caused by high doses of niacin is to bind the niacin to an inositol molecule. Inositol hexaniacinate is a form of niacin that is safe for the liver at high doses. (It is found in **Nutrients to normalize cholesterol and triglycerides**.)

Niacin deficiency, in the early stages, leads to muscular weakness, general fatigue, loss of appetite, indigestion, and various skin eruptions. It can also cause bad breath, small ulcers, canker sores, insomnia, irritability, nausea, vomiting, recurring headaches, tender gums, and depression.

Severe deficiency leads to pellagra, which is characterized by the three Ds—dermatitis, dementia and diarrhea. Primary deficiency usually occurs in areas where maize (Indian corn) is a major part of the diet. Bound niacin, found in maize, is not assimilated in the intestinal tract (unless treated with alkali—as in making of tortillas). Corn protein is also deficient in tryptophan. Amino acid imbalance may also play a part. Pellagra is common in India among those who eat a lot of millet (which has a high leucine content). It can also be seen in diarrheal disease, cirrhosis of the liver, and alcoholism.

Pellagra is characterized by cutaneous, mucous membrane, central nervous system (CNS) and gastrointestinal (GI) symptoms. The complete syndrome of advanced deficiency includes scarlet stomatitis and glossitis, diarrhea, dermatitis, and mental aberrations. Symptoms may occur alone or in combination.

Pantothenic Acid: Pantothenic acid is water soluble. There is a close correlation between pantothenic acid tissue levels and functioning of the adrenal cortex. It stimulates the adrenal glands and increases production of cortisone and other adrenal hormones. It plays a vital role in cellular metabolism. As a coenzyme it helps with the release of energy from carbohydrates, fats, and proteins. It also helps with the utilization of other vitamins, especially riboflavin. It is an essential constituent of coenzyme A.

Pantothenic acid is essential for the synthesis of cholesterol, steroids, and fatty acids. It can improve the body's ability to withstand stressful conditions. Deficiency is rare, but symptoms can include vomiting, restlessness, abdominal pains, burning feet, muscle cramps, gas and abdominal distention.

Because pantothenic acid is so vital to adrenal function, you can use neurolingual testing. Have the client place pantothenic acid in his or her mouth and see if it diminishes the tenderness of the Chapman adrenal reflex (the reflex is located 1 inch lateral and 1 inch superior to the navel).

Pyridoxine: B_6 is required for the proper absorption of B_{12} and the production of HCl. It plays an important role in fat metabolism. It acts as a coenzyme in the breakdown and utilization of carbohydrates, fats, and proteins. It must be present for the production of antibodies and red blood cells. The release of glycogen for energy from the liver and muscles is facilitated by B_6. It also aids in the conversion of tryptophan to niacin.

Deficiency can lead to low blood sugar and poor glucose tolerance. It can also cause water retention during pregnancy, cracks around the mouth and eyes, numbness and cramps in the arms and legs, slow learning, visual disturbance, neuritis, arthritis, and an increase in urination. Gestational diabetes is frequently resolved by simply taking 50 mg of B_6 per day. People who are sensitive to monosodium glutamate (MSG) have their symptoms resolved by taking B_6 supplements. Excess estrogen depletes B_6; menstrual problems are often helped by B_6 supplementation.

Vitamin B_6 is necessary for transamination. In other words, it moves amine molecules. One easy way to find a B_6 need is when alanine aminotransferase (ALT) or aspartate aminotransferase (AST) levels (previously called SGOT and SGPT, respectively) are in the low teens or lower. Normal laboratory values can be as low as 0, but levels much lower than 20 may indicate a need for B_6. Vitamin B_6 is also a necessary cofactor for essential fatty acid metabolism. You can perform the essential fatty acid test—do a multiple muscle test rhythmically; the chosen muscle should endure 20 successive challenges. If it does not, see if the number increases while the client holds a B_6 tablet in his or her mouth.

Folic Acid: Folic acid functions as a coenzyme, together with vitamins B_{12} and C, in the breakdown and utilization of proteins. Folic acid performs its basic role as a carbon carrier in the formation of heme. It is also needed for the formation of nucleic acid.

Folic acid is necessary for proper brain function. It is concentrated in the spinal and extracellular fluids. It is essential for mental and emotional health. Folic acid increases the appetite and stimulates the production of hydrochloric acid. It also aids in liver function.

Folic acid is easily destroyed by high temperature, by light and by being left at room temperature for long periods. It is one of the nutrients most often deficient in our diets. Deficiency can lead to glossitis, GI disturbances, poor growth, skin problems, obstetric disorders such as toxemia of pregnancy, neuropathy and psychiatric disorders. It can cause a megaloblastic anemia.

The need for the vitamin is especially increased during pregnancy. The fetus needs folic acid for its rapid growth and quickly depletes the mother's reserves. The World Health Organization reports that one-third to one-half of pregnant women are folic acid deficient. Spina bifida is associated with low levels of folic acid in the mother at the time of conception. Almost any interference with the metabolism of folic acid in the fetus can contribute to deformities like cleft palate or brain damage. It can cause slow development and poor learning ability in the child.

Folic acid is necessary for all cells that multiply rapidly. One sure sign of a folic acid deficiency is a woman who has an “irregular” Pap smear, when no cancer is present, but the cells are irregular, causing the physician concern. This is an almost sure sign of folic acid deficiency. Giving 5 mg/day of folic acid will frequently resolve the problem. Polyps may also be a sign of folic acid need.

Deficiency of folic acid in pregnancy can lead to toxemia, premature birth, afterbirth hemorrhaging, and megaloblastic anemia (in both mother and child).

In the United States, folic acid supplements must be less than 800 μg because taking folic acid can mask a B_{12} deficiency. It is a good idea to give these two nutrients together.

One way to test for folic acid is to check for segmented neutrophils. This is a test that can be added to a complete blood count (CBC). Segmented neutrophils are immature cells. Levels higher than 15 are cause for concern (especially in women desiring to get pregnant). In ideal health, the number should be close to zero.

In a routine CBC, certain "normal" values may reflect a folic acid or a B_{12} need (these values are the same for both folic acid and for B_{12}). The RBC count will be low or low normal, the white blood cell (WBC) count will be low or low normal (possibly with fewer polymorphonuclear leukocytes [PMNs] and more lymphocytes) and the mean corpuscular volume (MCV) will be greater than 90 or the mean corpuscular hemoglobin (MCH) will be above 32).

***Vitamin B₁₂*:** B_{12} is unique in that it is the first cobalt-containing substance found to be an essential nutrient. It is the only vitamin that contains essential mineral elements. Animal protein is almost the only place that contains B_{12}, although vegetarians can get it from microbial synthesis and from legume nodules where it is synthesized by microbes.

Vitamin B_{12} is necessary for normal metabolism of nerve tissue and is involved in protein, fat and carbohydrate metabolism. B_{12} aids folic acid in the synthesis of choline. It helps the placement of vitamin A into body tissues.

Vitamin B_{12} deficiency is the most common cause of depression in the elderly (also consider it for elderly clients who are becoming forgetful). In severe cases it can cause symptoms that will mimic Alzheimer's disease. Testing serum B_{12} often yields normal results, yet the client will respond to B_{12} therapy.

B_{12} is poorly absorbed unless intrinsic factor, a mucoprotein secreted in the stomach, is present. Autoimmune reactions in the body can bind intrinsic factor or can affect the cells that produce it. Absorption of B_{12} appears to decrease with age, and with iron, calcium and B_6 deficiencies. Absorption increases during pregnancy.

Generally, B_{12} is given as an injection, but it is well established that high doses (in the 2-4 mg/day range) will yield satisfactory results.

Pernicious anemia develops insidiously and progressively as the large hepatic stores of B_{12} are depleted. It may take 5 or 6 years to develop. Usually the problem is more profound than that expected based on the symptoms. This is due to physiologic adaptation. Splenomegaly and hepatomegaly may occasionally be seen. GI problems may be present, including anorexia, intermittent constipation and diarrhea and poorly localized abdominal pain. Considerable weight loss is common. Peripheral nerves are commonly involved, even in the absence of anemia. Second to this is spinal cord involvement beginning in the dorsal column with loss of vibratory sensation in the lower extremities, loss of position sense and ataxia. Lateral column involvement follows with spasticity and hyperactive reflexes and a Babinski's sign. Some clients have irritability, mild depression or actual paranoia. Occasionally yellow-blue color blindness occurs.

Rare signs are fever of unknown origin that responds promptly to B_{12} therapy. Endocrine deficiencies, especially of the thyroid and adrenal glands, if they are associated with pernicious anemia, suggest an autoimmune basis for gastric mucosal atrophy. Hypogammaglobulinemia may be present.

Anemia is macrocytic with an MCV higher than 100. An MCV above 90 though is a sign that the client is becoming low in B12. There is a serum test for B_{12} levels, but it may not be reliable. The Schilling test measures the absorption of radioactive B_{12} with and without intrinsic factor.

A test for B_{12} need developed by George Goodheart, MD, involves testing a muscle, suddenly stretching it and retesting it. If the muscle weakens, it is a sign that the client needs B_{12}.

In a routine CBC, certain "normal" values may reflect a folic acid or a B_{12} need (these values are the same for both folic acid and B_{12}). The RBC count will be low or low-normal, the WBC count will be low or low-normal (possibly with fewer PMNs and more lymphocytes) and the MCV will be greater than 90 or the MCH will be above 32).

Choline and Inositol: Choline is considered one of the B-complex vitamins. Together with inositol it forms a basic constituent of lecithin. It is found in egg yolk, liver, brewer's yeast and wheat germ. It is associated with the utilization of fats and cholesterol in the body. It prevents fats from accumulating in the liver and facilitates the movement of fats into the cells. Choline is also essential for the health of the myelin sheaths of the nerves. It also helps to regulate and improve liver and gallbladder functioning and aids in the prevention of gallstones.

Choline deficiency is associated with fatty deposits in the liver and may be related to cirrhosis of the liver, atherosclerosis, and high blood pressure.

Inositol is recognized as part of the vitamin B complex and is closely associated with choline and biotin. It is found in high concentrations in lecithin. It is found in animal and plant tissues. In animal tissues it occurs as a component of phospholipids; in plant cells it is found in phytic acid.

Inositol is a component of lecithin, along with choline. In combination with choline it prevents the fatty hardening of arteries and protects the liver. Large quantities of inositol are found in the spinal cord nerves and in the brain and cerebrospinal fluid. It is thought to be helpful in brain cell nutrition. It is needed for the growth and survival of cells in bone marrow, eye membranes, and the intestines.

Inositol works in some cases of pesticide poisoning. It is lipotropic and helps to free the pesticide from adipose tissue. High doses of inositol often work for neuralgia like pain.

Vitamin A: Vitamin A helps cells reproduce normally—a process called differentiation. Cells that have not properly differentiated are more likely to undergo precancerous changes. Vitamin A, by maintaining healthy cell membranes, helps prevent invasion by disease-causing micro-organisms. Vitamin A also stimulates immunity and is needed for formation of bone, protein, and growth hormone. Beta-carotene, a substance from plants that the body can convert into vitamin A, also acts as an antioxidant and immune system booster. Other members of the antioxidant carotene family include cryptoxanthin, alpha-carotene, zeaxanthin, lutein, and lycopene, but most of them do not convert to significant amounts of vitamin A.

Vitamin A is found in dark green and orange-yellow vegetables are good sources of beta-carotene. Liver, dairy, and cod liver oil provide vitamin A. Vitamin A can also be found in vegetarian supplements.

Individuals who limit their consumption of liver, dairy foods, and vegetables can develop a vitamin A deficiency. The earliest deficiency sign is poor night vision. Deficiency symptoms can also include dry skin, increased risk of infections, and metaplasia (a precancerous condition).

How much Vitamin A to recommend clients is often a question I get asked a lot. In males and postmenopausal women, up to 25,000 IU (7,500 mcg) of vitamin A per day is considered safe. In women who could become pregnant, the safest intake level is being re-evaluated; less than 10,000 IU (3,000 mcg) per day is widely accepted as safe.

Women who are or could become pregnant should take less than 10,000 IU (3,000 mcg) per day of vitamin A to avoid the rare risk of birth defects. For other adults, intake above 25,000 IU (7,500 mcg) per day can—in rare cases—cause headaches, dry skin, hair loss, fatigue, bone problems, and liver damage. Beta-carotene, however, does not cause any side effects, aside from excessive intake (more than 100,000 IU, or 60 mg per day) sometimes giving the skin a yellow-orange hue.

Individuals taking beta-carotene for long periods of time should also supplement with vitamin E, as beta-carotene may reduce vitamin E levels. Taking vitamin A and iron together helps overcome iron deficiency more effectively than iron supplements alone.

Antioxidants: Antioxidants function to deal with free radicals, which are created in times of high oxidative stress. Free radicals are inherently unstable, since they contain "extra" energy. To reduce their energy load, free radicals react with certain cells in the body, interfering with the cells' ability to function normally. Fortunately there are many natural antioxidants that interfere with free radicals before they can damage the body. Antioxidants work in several ways: they may reduce the energy of the free radical, stop the free radical from forming in the first place, or interrupt an oxidizing chain reaction to minimize the damage of free radicals.

Superoxide dismutase (SOD), catalase, and glutathione peroxidase are enzymes produced by the body itself to defuse many types of free radicals. Supplements of these compounds are also available to augment the body's supply and are richly supplied in the Biotic's products tableting base.

In addition to enzymes, many vitamins and minerals act as antioxidants in their own right, such as vitamin C, vitamin E, beta carotene, lutein, lycopene, vitamin B3 in the form of niacin, vitamin B2, vitamin B6, coenzyme Q10, and cysteine (an amino acid). Herbs, such as bilberry, turmeric (curcumin), grape seed or pine bark extracts, and ginkgo biloba can also provide powerful antioxidant protection for the body. A wide variety of antioxidant enzymes, vitamins, minerals, and herbs may be the best way to provide the body with the most complete protection against free radical damage.

Assess Vitamin insufficiencies

Further assessment	1. An excellent way to assess for Thiamine (vitamin B1) deficiency is with the Acoustic Cardiogram (ACG), which will show a depressed S1 heart sound reading. There will not be enough amplitude in the graph. 2. An increased Anion gap and a decreased CO_2 on a chem. Screen is indicative of low thiamine levels. 3. An excellent way to assess for B vitamin need is with the Acoustic Cardiogram (ACG). By analyzing the graphical output of the heart sounds one can determine the type of B vitamins that are deficient. For instance thiamine (vitamin B1) deficiency will show a depressed S1 heart sound reading. There will not be enough amplitude in the graph. Riboflavin (vitamin B2) will show an elongated S1 heart sound reading due to weak aortic and pulmonic valve closure. 4. Check the CBC for signs of B12 and folic acid deficiency: MCV > 90, ↓ RBCs 5. Hyper segmented neutrophils seen on a peripheral blood smear is a microscopic sign for folate deficiency 6. An excellent way to assess for Riboflavin (vitamin B2) deficiency is with the Acoustic Cardiogram (ACG), which will show an elongated S1 heart sound reading due to weak aortic and pulmonic valve closure. 7. B6 levels can be assessed by running a serum homocysteine or a B6 EGOT (Erythrocyte Glutamine-Oxaloacetate Transaminase) test. 8. Vitamin C levels can be assessed with the lingual or urinary vitamin C test. 9. Check MCV, MCH, LDH and MCHC levels on a CBC and Chem. Screen to assess Vitamin B12 insufficiency.

Supplemental Support

1. Low dose naturally occurring B Vitamin Complex
2. B12
3. Folic acid
4. Emulsified Vitamin E drops
5. Broad spectrum anti-oxidants
6. Chlorophyllins
7. Naturally occurring riboflavin
8. Naturally occurring thiamine
9. Pyridoxal-5-phosphate
10. Broad spectrum bioflavanoids, vitamin C, thymus and spleen
11. Buffered Vitamin C with bioflavanoids
12. Emulsified Vitamin A drops

9. Adrenal Section

Stress can undermine the health of you and your clients. The connection between stress and high blood pressure, heart disease, and many digestive problems is well-established in the medical literature. Stress creates hormonal and blood sugar changes, causes the body to excrete nutrients and adversely affects the immune system.

The adrenal glands are directly affected by stress. They are responsible for the "fight or flight" response. Hans Selye, MD, conducted some experiments creating stress in rats. The rats were made to tread water with their legs tied until they became exhausted and died.

Dr. Selye took the rats at various stages of their ordeal and dissected out their adrenal glands. He found that the adrenal glands responded to stress in three distinct stages. In the initial stage, the adrenal glands enlarge and the blood supply to them increases. As the stress continues, the glands begin to shrink. Eventually, if the stress continues, the glands reach the third stage, which is adrenal exhaustion.

The adrenal glands produce certain hormones in response to stress. They are responsible for the fight or flight response. In a stressful situation, they raise blood pressure, transfer blood from the intestines to the extremities, increase the heart rate, suppress the immune system and increase the blood's clotting ability.

This response is meant to be short-lived. When primitive man walked through the forest, he'd see a wild animal. His heart rate would increase, his pupils would dilate, his blood would go out of his digestive system and into his arms and legs, his blood clotting ability would improve, he would become more aware and his blood pressure would rise. At that point he'd either pick up a stick and try to fight the animal or run. The physiological changes brought on by the adrenal glands would make the body more efficient at doing either of those things. It is called the fight or flight response.

If he survived the ordeal, chances are it would be a while before such a strain was put on the adrenal glands and the rest of his body. He would have an opportunity to relax, eat nuts and berries (and a little meat from the wild animal, if he was lucky.) His adrenal glands would have a chance to recover.

Many people in modern society do not have the luxury of a recovery period for their overworked adrenal glands. The changes caused by the overproduction of adrenal hormones stay with them. The stimulation of the adrenal glands causes a decrease in the immune system function, so an individual under constant stress will tend to catch colds and have other immune system problems, including allergies. Blood flow to the digestive tract is decreased. Stress causes many digestive problems such as indigestion, colitis and irritable bowel. Adrenal hormones cause an increase in the blood clotting ability, so prolonged stress can lead to formation of arterial plaque and heart disease.

Worrying makes the adrenal glands work. Relaxing and thinking peaceful thoughts enables them to rest and heal. That is why Yoga and meditation are so good for you. You go a long way in preserving your health and energy if you do not fret about things over which you have no control. It's the amount of worry and not necessarily the size of the problem that stresses your adrenal glands. If you worry a lot about little problems, you do as much damage to your adrenal glands as someone who really has a lot of stress. If you can control your worrying when under stress, you minimize the damage stress does to your health. A wise man once said that worry is interest paid in advance on money you haven't even borrowed yet.

Selye described the progression of stress on the adrenal glands as the general adaptation syndrome. The first stage is called the alarm reaction. This is when someone (with healthy adrenal glands) can perform amazingly well when the need arises. The primitive man, seeing the saber tooth tiger, was able to run faster than he ever dreamed possible during the alarm reaction. If the stress continues, the body moves into the resistance stage, during which the adrenal glands become enlarged. The individual is responding to the stress and handling it. He or she may feel keyed up. The person may have cold, clammy hands; a rapid pulse or reduced appetite, but hasn't begun to feel any of the more serious symptoms of the next stage. During the exhaustion stage the adrenal glands begin to fail to meet the demands placed upon them. During this stage, the individual begins to have a variety of symptoms including fatigue, digestive problems, obesity, depression, dizziness, fainting, allergies and many other problems.

People with weak adrenal glands frequently crave coffee and sugar, as well as salt. Sugar and caffeine stimulate the adrenal glands. It's as if your adrenal glands are two horses towing a wagon load of bricks up a mountain. Sugar or caffeine is the whip you use to get the horses to keep trying. What they need to get to the top of the mountain is nourishment and a rest period.

To effectively treat the adrenal glands, you must eliminate as much stress from your life as possible. Emotional stress is the kind of stress most people think of when stress is mentioned, but there are many different kinds of stress. Thermal stress results from being exposed to extremes of temperature; physical stress from heavy physical work, poor posture, structural misalignments, lack of sleep and being overweight; and chemical stress from ingestion of food additives, exposure to pollutants and consumption of sugar and alcohol. Changes in blood sugar are also a form of chemical stress. Eating frequent, small meals is often very helpful, since people suffering from hypoadrenia are often hypoglycemic (having low blood sugar).

Situations are not always controllable, but stress is. Stress is cumulative. Emotional, structural and chemical stress all affect the body the same way. Your adrenal glands do not know the difference between an IRS audit, treading water or excessive sugar consumption; excess sugar consumption will add to the stress of the IRS audit.

If you reduce the stress that you can control, stressful situations will not have as much of a physical effect on you. For instance, eating frequent meals and avoiding sugar will reduce stress on the adrenal glands. So even if you can't do anything about Aunt Millie and Uncle Edgar coming to spend the summer, you can reduce your stress by controlling your diet. Also, how you think of the stress will make a difference in the health of your adrenal glands. Aunt Millie's handy tips on how you should raise your kids or clean your house, or Uncle Edgar's penchant for eating everything that isn't nailed down (without offering to pay for groceries) won't stress your adrenal glands if you don't focus on it.

If you can't change your work situation, then improve your diet and get plenty of rest. Change how you think about your job situation. Focus on the positive: You do have a job, you do eat regular meals. (Much of the world doesn't.) Just do the best you can and think of the things you can't control in positive terms. Jesus says in Luke 12:25, "And which of you with taking thought can add to his stature one cubit?" Or, to quote the great teacher and spiritual advisor, Yogi Babaganoush, "Chill out man." Think to yourself, "What could be good about this situation?" Then take a minute to really look for positive answers.

Hanging on to anxiety over past situations is stressful. Thought has power. Worry gives you all of the physiologic responses of Selye's rats or the caveman facing the wild animal. It's a waste of energy and it undermines your health.

Your adrenal glands simply don't know the difference between imagined danger and real danger. Think about it; if you hear a noise at night and think it's the wind, you can go back to sleep. If you think it's an intruder you can't get back to sleep even after you get up to investigate. The thought of facing an intruder made the adrenal glands start producing their hormones.

Meditation and biofeedback have been of such value in controlling stress. They don't help with the situation, just how you perceive it and your body's response to the stress. Doctors are beginning to find that laughter helps the prognosis of cancer clients. They even have clients watch sitcoms in the hospital: "Mr. Smith, it's time for your chemotherapy and 'Lucy' reruns."

Minimizing chemical stress is also important. We have plenty of chemical stress today. Environmental pollution, food additives, sugar, alcohol and caffeine contribute stress to your adrenal glands. You must remove chemical stresses from your diet—effortlessly and without putting yourself under pressure. Gradually improve your diet by removing chemical additives. Move toward a more organic way of eating. Enjoy the change without fretting over how your diet isn't perfect yet.

Ironically, stress often makes you crave the foods that are bad for you. While under stress, it is hard to be diligent in keeping additives and refined sugar out of the diet. Clients often complain that they have no time and can't eat properly. Lack of time really isn't the problem because raw nuts, fruits and vegetables take no time to prepare. Lack of time is usually used as an excuse to give in to craving the wrong foods. Once you understand that, you can eat healthily with little effort

Eating sugar and skipping meals are two things that are especially stressful to the adrenal glands, which work to maintain your blood sugar level. Eating sugar causes a temporary increase in blood sugar, which soon drops. Skipping meals also causes the blood sugar to drop. The adrenal glands then have to work to increase the blood sugar. Hypoadrenia and hypoglycemia (low blood sugar) usually exist together.

Assessing the symptom burden of the Adrenal Section:

Symptom count	Significance
8 – 12	Low priority
13 – 20	Moderate priority
Above 21	High Priority

When the symptom burden of the adrenal section approaches 21 or higher, then there is a need for further assessment and treatment. This signifies that there is significant distress in the systems that help regulate the adrenals in the body. This may be caused by increased consumption of refined carbohydrates and sugar in the diet, high levels of stress, over exercise, lack of sleep, pain, inflammation, worry, anxiety etc.

Refer to the explanation on each individual question in this book and follow the general guidelines below to further assess for adrenal imbalance in your clients.

Assessing for adrenal dysfunction

Further assessment	1. Check for tenderness in the inguinal ligament bilaterally, an adrenal indicator 2. Check for tenderness at the medial knee bilaterally, at the insertion of the sartorius muscle at the Pes Anserine. This is an adrenal indicator. 3. Check for a paradoxical pupillary reflex by shining a light into a client's eye and grading the reaction of the pupil. A pupil that fails to constrict indicates adrenal exhaustion 4. Check for the presence of postural hypotension. A drop of more than 10 points is an indication of adrenal insufficiency. 5. Check for a chronic short leg due to a posterior-inferior ilium. An adrenal indicator when confirmed with postural hypotension and a paradoxical pupillary response. 6. Check the cortisol/DHEA rhythm with a salivary adrenal stress profile 7. Increased chloride in the urine is a sign of hypoadrenal function 8. Assess for adrenal insufficiency with the Acoustic Cardiogram (ACG), which will show static in both the systolic and diastolic rest phases. You will also see an elevated S2 sound.

Supplemental Support

1. Adrenal tissue (neonatal bovine)
2. Adaptogenic herbs to support adrenal function
3. Multiple nutrients for blood sugar handling problems
4. Naturally occurring thiamine

NOTES:

10. Pituitary

The anterior pituitary is a gland located deep in the brain. It produces a number of very important hormones that help in the regulation of many of the major glands in the body including the thyroid, the ovaries, the testes, and the adrenals. The hormones released from the pituitary gland are themselves ultimately under the control of the hypothalamus, another important gland in the brain. The hypothalamus is able to sense how much circulating hormone there is in the body. When levels of circulating hormone begin to drop the hypothalamus releases stimulating factors that stimulate the pituitary to secrete releasing hormones. This biofeedback system ensures a healthy level of circulating hormone from the major glands. Unfortunately this system is often dysfunctional.

Symptoms for hypothalamus and pituitary dysfunction are vague and can easily mean other things. Think of this as an area to consider if you are not getting the kind of results you would hope for when treating adrenal, thyroid, or sex hormone issues. I have found that adrenal, thyroid or other endocrine problems respond well to glandular therapy using specific glandulars for the pituitary and hypothalamus.

Assessing the symptom burden of the Pituitary Section:

Symptom count	Significance
3 – 4	Low priority
5 – 8	Moderate priority
Above 8	High Priority

When the symptom burden of the pituitary section approaches 8 or higher, this is a sign that you should consider pituitary involvement in your client. It is hard to specify individual assessment methods for the pituitary. Consider that the cause of the pituitary dysfunction lies within one of the other hormonal systems or with blood sugar dysregulation, and check those systems out accordingly.

Supplemental Support

1. Pituitary/hypothalamus tissue (neonatal bovine)

NOTES:

11. Thyroid

Many physicians believe that hypothyroidism is under diagnosed and that many people who have had blood tests indicating normal thyroid function may actually suffer from hypothyroidism. These physicians believe that many clients with normal test results have some thyroid hormone that isn't active. In other words there is enough hormone to make the test appear normal even if the person is actually deficient in active hormone.

It has been shown that reverse thyroid hormone, which is a molecule of thyroid hormone that has the mirror image of the active hormone, gets produced in large quantities and is grossly under-valued in terms of its negative effects on thyroid hormone metabolism. The presence of large amounts of reverse thyroid hormone comes about with high levels of stress, adrenal insufficiency, selenium and iodine deficiency, liver and kidney dysfunction, and yo-yo dieting. Its effect is to cause the symptoms of an under functioning thyroid gland.

Broda Barnes, MD, was perhaps the first physician to come to the conclusion that many people suffering from chronic illness had under functioning thyroids. In his book, *Hypothyroidism, the Unsuspected Illness* (Broda Barnes and Lawrence Galton, Harper Collins Publishers, Inc., 1976), he states that hidden hypothyroidism is responsible for many chronic health problems including heart disease, immune system problems and chronic fatigue. He also felt that laboratory tests don't diagnose many cases of hypothyroidism.

Barnes developed a way to screen for hypothyroidism by taking a basal body temperature. Basal body temperature is taken the very first thing in the morning, before there is any movement or activity. The thyroid is the body's thermostat, controlling metabolism. Body temperature is a reflection of that metabolic activity and people with under functioning thyroids tend to have low basal body temperatures. You can get your clients to record their basal body temperature and bring it into the office for interpretation. A basal underarm body temperature consistently below 97.8 is a sign of an under active thyroid.

Combining the basal body temperature and information in a health history can give valuable information about how well the thyroid is functioning. The symptoms listed in the thyroid section of the NAQ are evidence of poor thyroid function. The more symptoms present, the more likely it is that there is a thyroid problem.

Barnes states in his book that hypothyroidism is very common for a variety of reasons. Iodine deficiency is common, especially in the world's "goiter belts," or areas that are removed from the seashore (like the American Midwest). Adding iodine to salt has virtually eliminated the occurrence of goiters, but Barnes says the additional iodine is not enough to bring the other symptoms of hypothyroidism under control. Other nutrients, like vitamin B_{12}, vitamin A and tyrosine are also necessary for proper thyroid function. Chemical pollution and heavy metal toxicity can also adversely affect the thyroid. This is one reason why dealing with liver function and improving the body's ability to remove toxins is so important. Nitrites added to packaged meats, certain sulfa drugs given to farm animals and even certain soft plastics used to hold drinks could be a source of chemicals that harm the thyroid. Poor digestion, especially poor protein digestion may also be a source of this problem.

Barnes recommends the use of natural thyroid extract (also called Armor thyroid). He preferred the natural product to the usually prescribed synthetic hormone (called Synthroid) because Armor thyroid is a whole product and contains all of the components of thyroid hormone. Some clients can improve thyroid function with nutrient supplementation, exercise, dietary changes, and by addressing some of the other core health issues.

There is also a condition called hyperthyroidism, which is less common. A number of symptoms on the NAQ help identify this condition. Please refer to the individual question explanations for a discussion of what to do with symptoms of hyperthyroidism.

Assessing the symptom burden of the Thyroid Section:

Symptom count	Significance
5 – 7	Low priority
8 – 12	Moderate priority
Above 12	High Priority

When the symptom burden of the thyroid section approaches 12 or higher, then there is a need for further assessment and treatment. This signifies that there is significant distress in the systems that help regulate the thyroid gland in the body. This may be caused by increased levels of stress, adrenal insufficiency, iodine and/or selenium deficiency, liver dysfunction, kidney insufficiency, a low calorie diet etc.

Refer to the explanation on each individual question in this book and follow the general guidelines below to further assess for thyroid dysfunction in your clients.

Assessing thyroid dysfunction

Further assessment	1. Check for tenderness in the Chapman reflex for the thyroid located in the second intercostal space near the sternum on the right 2. Check for a delayed Achilles return reflex, which is a strong sign of a hypo-functioning thyroid 3. Check for general costochondral tenderness, which is a thyroid indicator 4. Check for pre-tibial edema, which is a sign of a hypo-functioning thyroid 5. Iodine test: Use a tincture of 2% iodine solution, and paint a 3” by 3” square on the client’s abdomen. The client is to leave the patch unwashed until it disappears. The square should still be there in 24 hours. If it has disappeared, there is an indication of iodine need 6. Have client assess their basal metabolic temperature by taking their axillary temperature first thing in the morning for 5 straight days. An average temperature below 36.5°C is an indication of hypo-thyroidism

Supplemental Support

1. Multiple nutrients to support thyroid function with pituitary glandular
2. Potassium iodide
3. Pituitary/hypothalamus tissue (neonatal bovine)
4. Thyroid glandular
5. Nutrients to support thyroid function
6. Flax seed oil
7. Naturally occurring thiamine

NOTES:

12. Men Only

The majority of the questions in this section deal with problems with the prostate or other male health issue. In dealing with the prostate, there are two issues. One is to rule out cancer or other pathology, which can be accomplished with laboratory tests and physical examination. The second is to treat the problem naturally if there is no pathology.

Benign prostatic hypertrophy (BPH) is an enlargement of the prostate, causing it to exert pressure on the urethra. Resulting symptoms include interruption of urinary flow, a feeling of incomplete evacuation after urinating, a feeling of urgency before urinating, pain, burning, and even impotence. If you are not trained to perform a digital exam of the prostate and you suspect an enlarged prostate please refer to a trained physician for this examination. Early detection of BPH can save your clients from considerable discomfort and also alert them to lifestyle and dietary changes that could significantly reduce their chances of developing cancer of the prostate, one of the leading killers in men.

One of the other areas on men only section deals with impotence, which can be caused by a number of factors including drug therapy, circulatory problems or nutrient deficiency. Low sperm counts can be the result of nutrient deficiency or other problems.

Assessing the symptom burden of the Men Only Section:

Symptom count	Significance
4 – 5	Low priority
6 – 7	Moderate priority
Above 7	High Priority

When the symptom burden of the Men Only section approaches 7 or higher, then there is a need for further assessment and treatment. This signifies that there is significant distress in the systems that help regulate the male hormonal system in the body. The majority of the questions in the Men Only section of the NAQ have to do with prostatic health. A high symptom burden may be caused by enlarged prostate, zinc deficiency, andropause (a condition of decreasing testosterone), and impotence.

Refer to the explanation on each individual question in this book and follow the general guidelines below to further assess prostate and male hormonal system in your clients.

Assessing dysregulation in the Male reproductive system

Further assessment	1. Check for tenderness in the Chapman's reflex for the prostate and testes located lateral to the pubic symphisis on the rami 2. Check for tenderness in the middle portion of the illio-tibial band, an indicator for the prostate 3. Check creatinine levels on a blood chemistry screen. If the client has a creatinine 1.2 or > they have a developing prostate problem e.g. BPH. PSA will only show prostatic problem when it's too late. 4. Check client's PSA and PAP levels to follow course of therapy 5. Check client's zinc levels with a zinc test.

Supplemental Support

1. Saw palmetto and other nutrients to support prostate health
2. EPA and DHA from fish oil
3. Aqueous zinc
4. Nutritional zinc
5. Flax seed oil
6. Potassium iodide
7. Peruvian Maca and deer antler velvet

NOTES:

13. Women Only

The majority of the questions in the Female only section of the NAQ deal with issues of PMS, menopause, menstrual irregularity, and problems with fertility. All of these conditions have a variety of causes. Many times taking care of general health issues solves them. This is an example of the principles of the foundations of health coming into play. You can resolve a large number of the problems in the female reproductive system by resolving issues further upstream. For instance, mood swings during the menstrual cycle can be the result of poor thyroid function. Poor liver function or dysbiosis can cause imbalance between progesterone and estrogen. Menopausal hot flashes can be the result of poor adrenal function or EFA deficiency. It is best to treat root causes of health problems, but sometimes symptom management is necessary. You will need to decide on an effective and natural approach to this issue.

Helping clients improve their diet is a good first step in improving health in relation to their menstrual cycle. The average American eats 150 pounds of sugar and ten pounds of chemical food additives every year. Most Americans get half of their calories from refined carbohydrates. People consume hydrogenated oils at an alarming rate. The resulting vitamin deficiencies and detrimental effects on all organs and systems of the body are the beginning of many health problems, including menstrual irregularities. Getting adequate exercise is also very important. Based on the results of this questionnaire, and other findings, you will be able to find the best way to fix the root causes of problems with your clients' menstrual cycle and other women's health issues.

Assessing the symptom burden of the Women Only Section:

Symptom count	Significance
6 – 9	Low priority
10 – 15	Moderate priority
Above 15	High Priority

When the symptom burden of the EFA section approaches 15 or higher, then there is a need for further assessment and treatment. This signifies that there is significant distress in the systems that help regulate the female hormonal system. This may be caused by increased consumption of hydrogenated oil, gallbladder insufficiency, which decreases the emulsification and absorption of all fats, a low fat diet, and a diet low in essential fatty acids in general.

Refer to the explanation on each individual question in this book and follow the general guidelines below to further assess the female reproductive in your clients.

Assessing dysregulation in the Female reproductive system

Further assessment	1. Check for tenderness in the Chapman reflex for the ovaries and uterus located lateral to the pubic symphisis on the rami attachment of the Rectus abdominus muscle. 2. Assess client's hormonal status across the menstrual cycle with a cycling female salivary hormone assessment. 3. Assess pituitary hormonal influences by running serum FSH and LH levels.

Supplemental Support

1. Multi nutrients supporting female endocrine health
2. Flax Seed Oil
3. Adrenal tissue (neonatal bovine)
4. Black Currant Seed Oil
5. Pituitary/hypothalamus tissue (neonatal bovine)
6. Ovary tissue (neonatal bovine)

NOTES:

14. Cardiovascular System

Cardiovascular disease is one of the major killers in the western world. It is important to decide whether the cardiovascular dysfunction in your clients is actually due to pathology in the heart itself or due to other conditions that put a significant burden on the heart. For instance there are over 12 different causes of hypertension and the majority of them have nothing to do with the heart itself. Nutritional support can coincide with traditional methods. The important thing, when you look at cardiovascular disease is to protect the life of the client. Nutritional and other natural therapies take time to work and are best for chronic problems. Traditional medical practitioners best treat acute medical emergencies.

Everyone is concerned with cholesterol and the amounts of fat clients eat. This is a one-dimensional idea and the dietary issues here are much more complex than simply avoiding fat. The issue may not be the amount of fat or oil, but the quality of the fats eaten; Omega 3 essential fatty acids may actually be cardioprotective. Consuming hydrogenated oil is dangerous to the heart (among other things). Avoid margarine. Many people consume margarine, thinking that it is good for the heart. The truth is that margarine is full of hydrogenated oil and is worse for your heart than butter is.

Not many people pay attention to sugar and refined foods. Refined sugar and flour may play an important role in increasing cholesterol. Anti-cholesterol medications work by suppressing a liver enzyme, HMG CoA reductase. Increasing insulin increases the activity of this enzyme, so eating sugar can have an unfavorable effect on cholesterol. Sugar and refined grains also increase the growth of yeast and other dysbiotic organisms in the gut. Bile salts can be deconjugated by these organisms and turned into bile acids; this may trigger production of cholesterol by the liver. Epidemiologic studies show that native populations have increased heart disease when exposed to the Western diet, but their fat consumption doesn't actually go up; their consumption of refined carbohydrates does.

A refined, vitamin-deficient diet does not provide enough vitamin B_6, B_{12} or folic acid. These nutrients are necessary to keep homocysteine levels low. High homocysteine levels increase cardiac risk.

Assessing the symptom burden of the Cardiovascular Section:

Symptom count	Significance
3 – 4	Low priority
5 – 8	Moderate priority
Above 8	High Priority

When the symptom burden of the cardiovascular section approaches 8 or higher, then there is a need for further assessment and treatment. This signifies that there is significant distress in the systems that help regulate the cardiovascular system in the body. This may be caused by increased consumption of hydrogenated oil, digestive dysfunction, EFA insufficiency and a diet low in essential fatty acids in general, increased levels of homocysteine, nutrient deficiencies, increased refined carbohydrates, kidney insufficiency, and biliary insufficiency, to name a few.

Refer to the explanation on each individual question in this book and follow the general guidelines below to further assess for cardiovascular dysfunction in your clients.

Assessing the Cardiovascular system

Further assessment	1. Check for tenderness in the Chapman reflex for the heart located in the left second intercostal space near the sternum 2. Check for tenderness in the Chapman reflex for the kidney located 1" lateral and 1" superior from the umbilicus on the medial margin of the Rectus abdominus muscle (have client tighten stomach muscle to palpate. 3. Assess for tenderness over the transverse processes at T1 for the MI type, and T2 for the myocardium and the congestive type, 4. Assess blood pressure 5. An excellent way to assess the heart from a functional perspective is with the Acoustic Cardiogram (ACG). By analyzing the graphical output of the heart sounds one can determine many functional disturbances that can be assessed and corrected using nutrition.

Supplemental Support

1. Nutrients to support cardiovascular health
2. CoQ10
3. Naturally occurring thiamine
4. Riboflavin and the associated B vitamins
5. EPA and DHA from fish oil
6. Naturally occurring thiamine
7. Multiple nutrients for supporting renal function

NOTES:

15. Kidney and Bladder

The majority of the questions in this section of the NAQ is concerned with problems with the kidney itself and with symptoms associated with advancing kidney disease or infection. It is important to refer the client to a physician who can diagnose and treat kidney disease.

Assessing the symptom burden of the Kidney and the Bladder Section:

Symptom count	Significance
3	Low priority
4	Moderate priority
Above 4	High Priority

When the symptom burden of the kidney and bladder section approaches 4 or higher, then there is a need for further assessment and treatment. This signifies that there is significant distress in the systems that help regulate the kidney.

Refer to the explanation on each individual question in this book and follow the general guidelines below to further assess for kidney insufficiency in your clients.

Assessing Kidney and Bladder dysfunction

Further assessment	1. Check for tenderness in the Chapman reflex for the kidneys located 1" lateral and 1" superior from the umbilicus on the medial margin of the Rectus abdominus muscle. Have clients tighten stomach muscles to palpate. 2. Check for an increase in blood pressure when the client goes from standing to supine 3. Routine and functional urinalysis panel 4. Blood chemistry renal function panel 5. Check for nitrites, lymphocytes and RBCs in the urine. If necessary order or perform urine culture and microscopy. 6. Check for tenderness with Murphy's punch to the kidneys on the lower back. 7. Check urine pH. Extremes of pH on the acid and alkaline side can determine whether or not certain stones will form 8. X-ray or intravenous pyelogram may be necessary

Supplemental Support

1. Multiple nutrients for supporting renal function
2. Flax Seed Oil
3. Pyridoxal-5-phosphate
4. Magnesium
5. Emulsified vitamin A drops
6. Buffered vitamin C plus bioflavanoids
7. Larch arabinogalactans

16. Immune System

We live in toxic times, and it is becoming clear that our bodies are getting less able to deal with such levels of toxicity. We only have to look at the increasing levels of cancer to know that something is not right with our immune systems. And as these increasing levels of cancer are occurring in younger and younger people we know that something has to be done about the decrease in our immune response. The immune system is constantly being challenged. Theron Randolph, MD, firmly believed that the pollution of the environment and our constant exposure to chemicals is responsible for allergies and other immune system problems.

Another problem is the highly refined diet that many people eat. Consumption of refined sugar and refined carbohydrates can actually decrease the efficacy of white blood cells. Trans fats from hydrogenated oils and partially hydrogenated oils become incorporated into our cells, compromising their integrity, making it easier for bacteria and viruses to invade.

Dysbiosis, heavy metals and increased intestinal permeability can all place demands on the immune system. The old saying an ounce of prevention is worth a pound of cure is an important one when looking at the immune system. I am not a big fan of vaccinations in general because I feel the best way to deal with infections is to boost the body's natural and inherent ability to deal with infectious organisms in our environment. So, what are the best ways to do this?

One of the best ways is to avoid suppressing the immune system. Unfortunately one of the things about living in the 21st century is the constant exposure to foods, such as refined carbohydrates and hydrogenated oils, metabolic toxins, and xenoestrogens, which are "fake" hormones that block the natural function of our hormonal systems. These all reduce the natural immunity and burden the already burdened detoxification systems in the liver. It has been demonstrated that even a small amount of sugar will suppress the immune system for up to 8 hours. Alcohol and stress will also suppress normal immune function and slow down the detoxification process.

One of the other ways to boost the immune system and support the detoxification processes is to increase the body's natural immune response. In the past people have relied on immune staples such as the herbs Echinacea and goldenseal, perhaps boosted with some elderberry and high doses of vitamin C. Unfortunately I don't think these staples are often enough to strengthen and boost the immune system to deal with the levels of toxins in our environment.

Fortunately, you can do things to support your clients' immune system. There are nutrients and herbs that will improve immune function. For many people, simple changes in diet work wonders in improving immune function.

Calcium d-glucarate is a nontoxic, natural substance found in high concentrations in fruits and vegetables. The benefits of d-glucarate were first discovered by researchers at the M.D. Anderson Cancer Center. Many studies have shown it to be highly protective against cancer due to properties that increase the ability of the body to detoxify and eliminate toxins and other harmful substances. Calcium d-glucarate is also an effective product for removing excess hormones and foreign chemicals that have negative hormonal activity in the body.

This may be one of the reasons that d-glucarate is important in protecting against breast cancer and controlling postmenopausal symptoms. I feel that d-glucarate's role in improving your body's immunity lies in its ability to process and eliminate harmful toxins and carcinogens that tax the immune system, and also in its ability to bind to and remove toxic cellular waste. By increasing the levels of d-glucarate your clients will have to spend less energy eliminating harmful substances. Energy that can be better used to fight incoming infections. There is also increasing evidence that d-glucarate has antibacterial and antiviral properties.

Assessing the symptom burden of the Immune Section:

Symptom count	Significance
3 – 4	Low priority
5 – 8	Moderate priority
Above 8	High Priority

When the symptom burden of the immune section approaches 8 or higher, then there is a need for further assessment and treatment. This signifies that there is significant distress in the immune system. This may be caused by increased consumption of hydrogenated oil, digestive dysfunction, dysbiosis in the digestive tract, bowel toxemia, EFA insufficiency and a diet low in essential fatty acids in general, nutrient deficiencies, and increased refined carbohydrates in the diet.

Assessing Immune Insufficiency

Further assessment	1. Check for tenderness in the Chapman reflex for the thymus located in the 5th intercostal space on the right near the sternum 2. Check for tenderness in the Chapman reflex for the lungs located bilaterally in the 3rd and 4th intercostal space near the sternum 3. Check for tenderness in the histamine point located at five o'clock on the pectoralis muscle in the intercostal space between the 5th and 6th rib on the right side only 4. Assess the client for allergic tension. Take a full one-minute pulse sitting, then stand, wait 15 seconds and take another full minute pulse. If the standing pulse goes up by more than six beats, this is an indication of "allergic tension" 5. Assess the client's vitamin C status with the lingual and urinary ascorbic acid tests

Supplemental Support

1. Calcium d-glucarate
2. Multiple nutrients that support the immune system
3. Thymus tissue (neonatal bovine)
4. Herbal support against viruses
5. Nutrients that support against bacteria
6. Lung tissue (neonatal bovine) and other nutrients to support lung function
7. Multiple herbal anti-histamines

Nutritional Assessment Questionnaire- Symptom Burden Analysis

NAME:________________ DATE:________________

								Score
Immune System	11+	9	8	6	4	3	2	
Kidney & Bladder	5		4		3		2	
Cardiovascular	11+	9	8	6	4	3	2	
Women Only	21+	18	15	12	9	6	4	
Men Only	10+	8	7	6	5	4	2	
Thyroid	17+	15	12	10	7	5	3	
Pituitary	10+	9	8	6	4	3	2	
Adrenal	28+	24	20	16	12	8	4	
Vitamin Need	28+	24	20	16	12	8	4	
Sugar Handling	14+	12	10	8	6	5	3	
Essential Fatty Acids	8+	7	6	5	4	3	2	
Mineral Needs	25+	23	19	15	12	8	5	
Large Intestine	20+	18	15	12	9	6	3	
Small Intestine	16+	14	12	10	7	5	2	
Liver & GB	22+	19	17	14	11	7	4	
Upper GI	19+	17	14	11	9	6	3	
	HIGH PRIORITY			MODERATE PRIORITY		LOW PRIORITY		

DIET

1. Alcohol
2. Artificial sweeteners
3. Candy, sweets, sugary snacks, deserts, refined sugar
4. Carbonated beverages
5. Chewing tobacco
6. Cigarettes
7. Cigars/pipes
8. Coffee and caffeine containing foods and beverages
9. Eat fast food regularly
10. Fried foods
11. Luncheon meats
12. Margarine
13. Milk products
14. Radiation exposure
15. Refined flour/ Baked goods
16. Vitamins and minerals
17. Water, distilled
18. Water, tap
19. Water, well
20. Diet often for weight control

1. Alcohol

Alcohol is a metabolic toxin that carries with it some health risks. Its impact on the body is far reaching causing irritation to the lining of the gastrointestinal tract, leading to increased intestinal permeability (Leaky gut syndrome), a condition that allows unwanted substances to move from the digestive tract into the bloodstream. A leaky gut can cause allergies because the unwanted material that is absorbed through the hyper-permeable digestive tract stimulates the immune system.

The regular use of alcohol can have a strong impact on your brain chemistry. Alcohol, and other substances such as refined sugars and flours and certain drugs, will interfere with the receptors in the brain for neurotransmitters. The brain identifies that the receptor for a certain neurotransmitter is already filled, so it reduces the amount of neurotransmitters it produces. As the levels of neurotransmitters drop you begin to crave alcohol or refined sugars to fill newly emptied receptors in the brain. At some point you will no longer be able to fill the receptors with these "empty" foods and substances. At this point you will begin to experience mood swings and an even more intense craving for alcohol or refined sugars. To correct these imbalances you may require amino acid therapy. Ask your doctor about using L-Tyrosine, GABA, L-Taurine, L-Glutamine, and DL-Phenylalanine to help correct the imbalance in brain chemistry caused by constant alcohol use.

The liver is also affected by alcohol. It takes the liver eight hours to detoxify one "measure of alcohol" i.e. one drink. During this time the other items that need detoxification are put on hold. Drinking daily may have long-term health repercussions. Excessive drinking varies from person to person, but it has long been recognized that the consumption of more than two drinks/day (two glasses of wine, two 12-ounces of beer, or two shots of spirits) can contribute to significant health problems: Intestinal Dysbiosis, leaky gut, blood sugar abnormalities, reactive hypoglycemia, multiple mineral-vitamin deficiency, sub clinical liver dysfunction, obesity, heart disease, liver disease and damage, and fetal alcohol syndrome if consumed even in low amounts during pregnancy. Alcohol is very high in calories and has virtually no nutritional value. The exact amount that will cause problems will vary from person to person. The occasional glass of wine or beer is unlikely to be a problem, it has been noted in some research that the occasional alcoholic beverage may actually have some benefits to human physiology. It is clear that the overuse or alcohol abuse does not.

NOTES:

2. Artificial sweeteners

Most people use artificial sweeteners to avoid the high-calorie sweeteners such as honey and table sugar. Artificial sweeteners come in many forms including Aspartame (NutraSweet), saccharine, Sucralose and Acesulfame-K. They appear in many foods and soft drinks. H.J. Roberts M.D. in his book *Aspartame (NutraSweet): Is It Safe?* [1], points out that people will have increased craving for sweet and fatty foods along with their regular consumption of aspartame. Artificial sweeteners can also make you feel bloated and fat, which can cause you to shun real and whole foods. The following sections detail the problems associated with each form of artificial sweetener.

Aspartame

Aspartame is a low-calorie sweetener used in foods and beverages and as a tabletop sweetener. It is sold under the name NutraSweet and is about 200 times sweeter than sugar. It is made by joining two amino acids, aspartic acid and phenylalanine and a small amount of methanol. Phenylalanine, as an amino acid, is quite stimulating to the body, especially when combined with caffeine. The ingredients of aspartame also interfere and compete with the essential amino acid L-tryptophan, which is essential for the synthesis of the neurotransmitter serotonin. Aspartame is used in many products including major brands of beverages, foods and other products such as cold cereals; drink mixes, gelatin, puddings, dairy products, and toppings. It loses its sweetness during long periods of storage and is not suitable for baking since heat causes the loss of sweetness. It is our recommendation that you discontinue use of this product. While there have been numerous studies, which argue its safety, many people have some very uncomfortable reactions from its use. Clients with phenylketonuria must not use it because of the release of phenylalanine during its metabolism.

H. J. Roberts, M. D., in his book *Aspartame (NutraSweet): Is It Safe?*, alerts us to the potential hazard of this sweetener. The book reports that aspartame may produce a wide variety of physical and mental symptoms. These may include convulsions, headaches, behavioral disorders and gastrointestinal problems.

In the United States the Aspartame Consumer Safety Network (ACSN) serves as a support group and clearinghouse for information. can write to them at PO Box 780634, Dallas, TX 75378. They produce a booklet called "The Deadly Deception," which reports such things as "85% of all complaints registered with the Food and Drug Administration (FDA), the US government agency that overseas food and drug safety, concerns aspartame's adverse reactions." Five deaths and at least seventy different symptoms have resulted from its use. Julia Ross, in her book "Diet Cure" reports that "so far, more than 10 thousand aspartame users have reported over 100 adverse symptoms, compiled by the Food and Drug Administration (FDA). They include everything from menstrual changes, weight gain, and headaches to severe depression, insomnia, and anxiety attacks."[2]

---

[1] H.J. Roberts, M.D., Aspartame, is it safe? (The Charles press, 1990)

[2] Julia Ross, MA *The Diet Cure* (New York, NY: Penguin books , 1999), p.36-37

Saccharin
This non-nutritive sweetener passes through the body unchanged and is excreted in the urine. A few studies have suggested it as being a suspected cancer-causing agent. It is widely used in beverages, jams, jellies, gelatin desserts, puddings, and salad dressings. Saccharine use can lead to an increase consumption of refined sugars and increase the craving for sweet foods[3]. Like NutraSweet, you should discontinue the use of this product.

Sucralose

Acesulfame-K
This product is used primarily in packet or tablet form, but appears as a sweetener in sugar-free chewing gum. Like saccharin, laboratory tests have shown this product causes cancer in animals.

The manufacturer is seeking approval for use in soft drinks and baked goods but like the other artificial products, it has no place on the tables or in the foods of humans.

Alternatives to Artificial Sweeteners
As with all your dietary choices, we recommend whole food, and not foods that have been "manufactured" by companies. An extract of the herb Stevia rebaudiana is a safe and effective sweetener that has no calories. Try making lemonade with fresh squeezed lemon juice, water and a little stevia. If you crave carbonated drinks try making the lemonade with sparkling water.

---

[3] Dennis Remington, MD., and Barbara Higard. *The Bitter Truth about Artificial Sweeteners* (Vitality House International, 1987), p.29

3. Candy, sweets, sugary snacks, deserts, refined sugar

Regular candy and refined sugar consumption can be a strong indicator of blood sugar dysregulation, B vitamin need, mineral need, yeast overgrowth in the intestines and adrenal stress. Many people eat a candy bar every day, as a snack, on their breaks or on their way back home from work or school. Refined sugar is a source of calories without any nutritional value. The processed nature of candy and other sweets removes any minerals or vitamins. The body has to deal with a large intake of sugar by using nutrients from other foods to get the energy out. Glucose is broken down into energy in a biochemical process called glycolosis. This process requires large amounts of essential B vitamins to proceed smoothly. A diet that is high in refined sugars is often severely deficient in B vitamins, which are found in dark leafy green vegetables. The body has to use B vitamins from other areas of the body to process glucose through glycolosis.

People often eat candy or other sweets as a way to cope with sugar cravings. Many things can cause sugar or refined carbohydrate cravings e.g. a yeast overgrowth in the intestines, low stomach acid or digestive enzymes, and food allergies or sensitivities. The more sugar you eat, the more you crave it. Sugar is very addictive.

Another of the major problems with candy and other sweets is the large amount of calories present in a relatively small amount of food. The average candy bar has about 150 calories. If you eat one serving per day you will be adding an extra pound of fat every 3-4 weeks; 12-15 pounds per year. This type of consumption will have long term effects on health: tooth decay, obesity, diabetes, heart disease, high blood pressure, PMS, and numerous other health problems.

The regular use of candy, refined sugar and other sweets can have a strong impact on your brain chemistry. Candy, and other substances such as refined sugars, flours, alcohol and certain drugs, will interfere with the receptors in the brain for neurotransmitters. The brain identifies that the receptor for a certain neurotransmitter is already filled, so it reduces the amount of neurotransmitters it produces. As the levels of neurotransmitters drop you begin to crave alcohol or refined sugars to fill newly emptied receptors in the brain. At some point you will no longer be able to fill the receptors with these "empty" foods and substances. At this point you will begin to experience mood swings and an even more intense craving for alcohol or refined sugars. To correct these imbalances you may require amino acid therapy. Ask your doctor about using L-Tyrosine, GABA, L-Taurine, L-Glutamine, and DL-Phenylalanine to help correct the imbalance in brain chemistry caused by regular candy bar or refined sugar consumption.

Candy and sweets not only have no nutritional value, they rob nutrients from the body's stores and from other foods. It is best to cut them out of your diet and choose fruit or nuts as a healthier snack.

4. Carbonated beverages

Regular consumption of carbonated beverages can be extremely costly to your health. Most carbonated soft drinks are high in phosphoric acid, which provides a large amount of inorganic phosphorous in the diet, a nutrient that the body needs in only small amounts. A high consumption of phosphorous has been linked to increased bone loss, as it disrupts the finely regulated calcium:phosphorous ratio, which should ideally be kept in a ratio of 10:4. If the ratio drifts from this optimal range you begin to lose calcium from the bones. So any type of carbonated beverage can increase the risk of developing osteoporosis. This is important information for anyone, but especially women, who are at a higher risk of osteoporosis.

Carbonated beverages are also extremely acidic. It takes about 4-5 cups of water to bring the pH of one can of a soft drink close to the optimum pH of the body! The body uses up a large amount of energy and resources to bring the can of soft drink back to a normal pH in the body.

Soft drinks also contribute to a high caloric intake. One 12 ounce can of non-diet soft drink contains around 100 calories. If you have one can per day you will be adding an extra pound of fat every 3-4 weeks. In a year you will have gained nearly 14 pounds! Diet sodas are as bad, if not worse than regular soft drinks. They contain aspartame (NutraSweet), a product linked to convulsions, headaches, behavioral disorders, gastrointestinal problems and other health problems. The one difference between diet drinks and regular soft drinks is that regular drinks have at least something the body can use, namely the sugar content. Diet sodas have nothing but poison for the body to deal with. It is my advice that they should not be consumed, period.

Lastly, most soft drinks contain caffeine, which is a nervous system stimulant that causes stress on the adrenal glands and other areas of your body, contributing to nervous stomach, anxiety, depression, high blood pressure, increased mineral loss from the body and other health problems.

Carbonated soft drinks have no place in a well balanced diet. Choose water instead. We should be drinking at least 5 eight-ounce glasses of filtered or bottled water per day to stay adequately hydrated. Put a little lemon or lime in the water for added flavor. Water is the perfect beverage: it contains no calories, no preservatives, no additives, and is essential for life. Try making lemonade with fresh squeezed lemon juice, water and a little stevia. If you crave carbonated drinks try making the lemonade with sparkling water.

NOTES:

5. Chewing tobacco

Most of the emphasis on the harmful effects of tobacco has been centered on cigarettes, but much less on chewing or "smokeless" tobacco. It has been proved beyond a doubt that smoking causes lung cancer and other fatal diseases. Chewing tobacco has been linked with throat and mouth cancer, a major concern. Chewing tobacco is also a source of nicotine, an addictive substance. Nicotine acts like an injection of adrenaline, increasing pulse rate and blood pressure, which makes the heart work faster and harder, so that the heart actually needs more oxygen. Chewing tobacco will result in increased levels of nicotine in the blood and the problems associated with its addictive qualities. Research on addiction indicated that nicotine works much like heroin, cocaine, and alcohol. When nicotine was given to volunteers intravenously (into veins), many of them could not tell the difference between the effects of nicotine and that of cocaine. Nicotine produces pleasurable sensations and physical dependency by affecting the brain and spinal cord.
It is important to remember that tobacco use (both smoking and chewing) has associated health risks and its use will prevent you from attaining your highest health potential.

NOTES:

6. Cigarettes

It has been proved beyond a doubt that smoking causes lung cancer, heart disease, stroke and other fatal diseases. Carbon monoxide in cigarette smoke reduces the capacity of the blood to carry oxygen to the heart and other body tissues. Also, it speeds the accumulation of fatty deposits (cholesterol) in arterial walls, contributing to hardening of the arteries (arteriosclerosis).

Nicotine acts like an injection of adrenaline, increasing pulse rate and blood pressure, which makes the heart work faster and harder, so that the heart actually needs more oxygen. However, carbon monoxide takes the place of oxygen in the oxygen-carrying molecule (hemoglobin) in red blood cells, making *less* oxygen available. Smoking also puts tremendous strain on the adrenal glands.

The above 2 factors increase the risk of heart disease and heart attacks. Low-tar cigarettes make no difference. Smokers are twice as likely to have heart problems as non-smokers. The increased risk disappears within 5 years of stopping smoking.

Smoking causes chronic bronchitis. Even children of heavy smokers may get bronchitis from breathing in smoke-filled rooms. Hydrogen cyanide, a chemical in cigarette smoke, inflames the lining of the bronchial tubes.

Cigarette smoke paralyzes the millions of cilia lining the airways. Their function is to move in waves, sweeping mucus and particles out of the lungs and airway, cleaning out the lungs. Cigarette smoke also contains particles, which the lungs cannot get rid of, so they build up, causing the lungs to turn black. Carcinogens in smoke irritate lung tissue over time, significantly increasing the risk of lung cancer. Lung cancer is difficult to detect until it is incurable, and lung cancer is not a pleasant way to die.

Research on addiction indicated that nicotine works much like heroin, cocaine, and alcohol. When nicotine was given to volunteers intravenously (into veins), many of them could not tell the difference between the effects of nicotine and that of cocaine. Nicotine produces pleasurable sensations and physical dependency by affecting the brain and spinal cord.
Given the above information it is important to remember that tobacco use (both smoking and chewing) has associated health risks and its use will prevent you from attaining your highest health potential. It is strongly suggested that you take a good antioxidant and extra vitamin C to help reduce the cellular damage.

NOTES:

7. Cigars/pipes

Most of the emphasis on the harmful effects of tobacco have centered on cigarettes, but much less on cigars and pipes. It has been proved beyond a doubt that smoking causes lung cancer, heart disease, strokes and other fatal diseases. Cigars and pipes can also cause the above diseases but they are especially linked with throat and mouth cancer, a major concern. Cigars and pipes are also a source of nicotine, an addictive substance. Nicotine acts like an injection of adrenaline, increasing pulse rate and blood pressure, which makes the heart work faster and harder, so that the heart actually needs more oxygen. Smoking cigars or a pipe will result in increased levels of nicotine in the blood and the problems associated with its addictive qualities. Research on addiction indicated that nicotine works much like heroin, cocaine, and alcohol. When nicotine was given to volunteers intravenously (into veins), many of them could not tell the difference between the effects of nicotine and that of cocaine. Nicotine produces pleasurable sensations and physical dependency by affecting the brain and spinal cord.

It is important to remember that tobacco use (both smoking and chewing) has associated health risks and its use will prevent you from attaining your highest health potential.

NOTES:

8. Caffeinated beverages

Caffeine has no nutritional value, but caffeinated beverages have been drunk for its stimulating effects. Coffee and caffeine containing foods and beverages are stimulating to the nervous system. For a long time, the popularity of coffee and other caffeine containing foods and beverages has led people to ignore the initial discoveries of caffeine's harmful effects on health. Caffeine is rapidly absorbed from the intestine and within a few minutes enters all organs and tissues. The effect remains for about 3 hours and it almost completely disappears from the body overnight.

In amounts typically consumed, caffeine acts as a drug. Many people develop a dependence on it. When the caffeine is withdrawn, it may cause withdrawal symptoms, such as headaches, irritability, restlessness, or fatigue.

Caffeine is now implicated in many different health problems. These include:

1. Over-stimulation of the adrenal glands leading to adrenal hypo-function and fatigue.
2. It stimulates acid secretion in the stomach. Two cups may increase stomach acid for more than 1 hour. This may aggravate an existing ulcer, promote an ulcer or interfere with healing.
3. It has been implicated in cancer. While it has not been shown to directly cause cancer, it has been shown to interfere with repair of chromosomes in cells. Further research should help disclose its relationship to bladder and pancreas cancer.
4. It crosses the placenta and in animal studies has been implicated in birth defects. It should not be used during pregnancy.
5. It raises blood pressure in sensitive people.
6. It increases blood coagulation and so may increase the risk of coronary thrombosis.
7. It increases mental speed (arithmetic, typing) but impairs motor co-ordination (target shooting, writing, driving). The improvement in mental efficiency fell off below normal from 1-3 hours after the coffee.
8. It increases blood sugar and aggravates hypoglycemia and diabetes.
9. It has also been linked to fibrocystic breast disease and has been identified as a contributing factor in PMS
10. It increases the consumption of alcohol. In animal experiments, when coffee was added to the diet, the animals voluntarily drank 2-4 times more alcohol than the amount consumed without alcohol.
11. Caffeine's diuretic effect causes loss of potassium, calcium, magnesium, zinc and other minerals, the B Vitamins, especially thiamine, B1, and Vitamin C.
12. Caffeine, and particularly coffee, reduces absorption of iron and calcium, especially when it is drunk around mealtime. These minerals are extremely important for women.

High amounts of caffeine can cause insomnia, restlessness, excitement, trembling, rapid heart beat, increased breathing, desire to urinate, ringing in the ears, and heartburn.
If you drink coffee or other caffeine containing beverages regularly you may find it hard to quit or cut back. Please consult with your clinician to discuss effective ways to quit caffeine containing foods and beverages.

9. Eat fast food regularly

We live in a fast paced society with many demands on our time. Unfortunately choices we make with our time have long term impacts on our health. The choice to use fast food on a regular basis is one of these.

One of the major concerns of fast food is the type of oils and fats used to prepare and cook the food. Deep-fried foods and hydrogenated fats are the mainstay of fast food. Both of these will have long-term repercussions on health. Hydrogenated fats are a source of trans fatty acids. A type of unnatural, man-made fat that has been linked with the following health problems:

1. Cancer: high levels of trans fats have been associated with an increased risk of breast cancer
2. Trans fats have been linked with increased platelet stickiness, which is associated with coronary heart disease
3. Pain and inflammation becomes much worse for people who eat hydrogenated fats.
4. Trans fatty acids block the body's production of naturally occurring anti-inflammatories.
5. Trans fats are a source of immune system problems. They are incorporated into the cell membrane, where they increase cell membrane permeability making them more susceptible to infection.
6. Trans fats block the body's ability to metabolize and use the essential fatty acids, causing muscle fatigue and skin problems.

The problem with fast food does not stop there. It is also high in calories, and refined sugars, but low in active vitamins and minerals. The body has to metabolize the meal by robbing its stores of nutrients, leading to low energy, and nutrient deficiencies. A relatively high refined carbohydrate meal will play havoc on your blood sugar regulation, causing a reactive hypoglycemia, which is marked by fatigue a few hours after your meal and a craving for carbohydrate.

Eating food that is high in calories, refined sugars and trans fats will increase the risk of developing serious health problems. If you choose to eat in fast food restaurants please read the "Life in the fast lane" narrative, which will help you choose foods that can contribute to good health.

NOTES:

10. Fried foods

Fried foods refer to the regular consumption of commercially prepared fried or deep-fried foods. Sautéing or stir-frying food in a little olive oil is not a problem. The problem for our health is the nature of the oil that is used for commercial frying. It is usually hydrogenated oil that sits around for a long time, is changed infrequently and is a source of oxidized fats. Any fat that is subjected to high heat for long periods of time will become oxidized or rancid, forming free radicals, which are then consumed.

The body not only has to deal with the intake of free radicals but also large amounts of hydrogenated fats, which are a source of trans fatty acids. A type of unnatural, man-made fat that has been linked with the following health problems:

1. Cancer: high levels of trans fats have been associated with an increased risk of breast cancer
2. Trans fats have been linked with increased platelet stickiness, which is associated with coronary heart disease
3. Pain and inflammation becomes much worse for people who eat hydrogenated fats.
4. Trans fatty acids block the body's production of naturally occurring anti-inflammatories.
5. Trans fats are a source of immune system problems. They are incorporated into the cell membrane, where they increase cell membrane permeability making them more susceptible to infection.
6. Trans fats block the body's ability to metabolize and use the essential fatty acids, causing muscle fatigue and skin problems.

Most foods that are fried or deep-fried can be prepared in other ways e.g. broiling, baking or grilling. All sources of hydrogenated fats must be cut out of the diet. It is a type of food that is not compatible with health.

NOTES:

11. Luncheon meats

Luncheon meats, such as tined meats and hot dogs are packaged and processed foods that contain preservatives, coloring, additives, flavor enhancers and coloring that are not compatible with a healthy diet. The average person on a standard Western diet consumes over 10 pounds of chemical additives a year, which puts an untold amount of stress on the body. The liver has to detoxify and eliminate even the smallest amount of an additive. Over time this can place an enormous strain on the body's eliminative capacities.

One of the main problems is the sodium nitrite found in about 99% of all processed tinned meats and hot dogs. Nitrites are added to make the meat bright red and also to kill spores of Clostridium botulinum. What is less well known is the link between sodium nitrite and cancer. Nitrites become nitrosamines in the stomach, when then combine with stomach acid. Nitrosamines are a known carcinogen.

By staying away from processed and packaged meats, you will be much healthier.

NOTES:

12. Margarine

Margarine is a man-made, chemically altered fat. Margarine was developed as the great healthy, easy-to-spread, cholesterol free alternative to butter, because it was made out of vegetable oil. Unfortunately margarine is none of these. It is not even a food.

Margarine is 100% hydrogenated oil and is full of Trans fatty acids. A type of unnatural, man-made fat that has been linked with the following health problems:

1. Cancer: high levels of trans fats have been associated with an increased risk of breast cancer
2. Trans fats have been linked with increased platelet stickiness, which is associated with coronary heart disease
3. Pain and inflammation becomes much worse for people who eat hydrogenated fats.
4. Trans fatty acids block the body's production of naturally occurring anti-inflammatories.
5. Trans fats are a source of immune system problems. They are incorporated into the cell membrane, where they increase cell membrane permeability making them more susceptible to infection.
6. Trans fats block the body's ability to metabolize and use the essential fatty acids, causing muscle fatigue and skin problems.

The body does not know how to deal with trans fatty acids, as they are a new introduction into the food chain. We do not have the mechanisms to digest them and they tend to hang around the body for very long periods of time. The half-life for a trans fatty acid is 3-4 months i.e. it takes 3-4 months for the body to decrease in half the level of a recently ingested trans fatty acid.

People are under the impression that eating margarine will cause them to be healthier. Nothing could be further from the truth. Butter, used in moderation, is by far the most acceptable and healthy choice. Margarine will cause an essential fatty acid deficiency. Please consult your clinician about ways to increase the amounts of these essential fatty acids in your diet.

NOTES:

13. Milk products

Modern dairy and milk products are a far cry from the dairy used by our ancestors. Modern dairy products are a highly processed food. Pasteurization and homogenization, not to mention the hormones and antibiotics pumped into the cows, chemically alter the milk, making it an unsafe product to consume.

Most commercial milk products are pasteurized and homogenized. Pasteurization is a process whereby milk is partially heated (to 145 to 161 degrees F), but not boiled. The intent of this process is to kill microorganisms, which could be living in the milk. During this process, casein, the protein in the milk is altered or denatured and rendered more difficult to digest. In addition, naturally occurring enzymes, which would help in the digestion of the milk, are damaged or destroyed.

Homogenization is a process whereby the cream (fat) portion of milk, which normally floats on top, is emulsified with the non-fat portion. This process makes the fat in milk nearly indigestible, and allows the enzyme Xanthine oxidase in the cream to enter the bloodstream instead of being excreted, as would normally occur. When this enzyme enters the heart and arteries, it damages cell membranes, creating scar tissue. Cholesterol deposits accumulate on the scarred areas and can clog the arteries. This is what is commonly known as atherosclerosis.

Another problem with modern dairy is the increasing number of sensitivities or allergies to milk. One such condition is lactose intolerance, which is a deficiency of the enzyme lactase. This enzyme breaks down lactose, contained in the whey portion of milk, into smaller units for proper metabolism. There can also be difficulties with casein (milk protein) digestion. The symptoms of dairy sensitivity or allergy commonly include stomach pain, heartburn, and abdominal discomfort such as gas, bloating, or cramping, and other complaints such as runny or stuffy nose, sinus headache, sore throat, earaches and infections. If you think you may have an allergy or food sensitivity, ask your clinician for information on testing.

Raw Dairy

The best sources of dairy are goat's dairy and raw dairy products. Raw dairy is a controversial subject. From a nutritional perspective, raw cow's milk is superior to pasteurized milk in terms of its beneficial enzymes and natural protein structure. Make sure it is certified free of harmful microorganisms. Some counties may have provisions for certifying dairy herds to produce raw milk for human consumption, and such certified raw milk may be available in your area.

14. Radiation Exposure

Radiation is one of the ways to treat cancer by aiming a beam of high-energy radiation at the cancer in the hopes of killing the cancer cells. This treatment obviously has many side effects and takes its toll out on the body. A good diet is essential for someone undergoing radiation treatment. Please talk to your physician about ways to further assess the impact that radiation is having on your body, and ways to strengthen the body through diet, lifestyle and nutrition.

NOTES:

15. Refined flour/ Baked goods

Refined flour is any type of flour that has had the germ or bran removed. This yields white flour that is devoid of all naturally present nutrients. The list of nutrients lost in the processing of grains is enormous and includes B vitamins, many minerals, fiber, essential fatty acids and other vitamins. The body must rely on nutrients present in other foods or rob its own stores of nutrients to be able to digest, assimilate and utilize refined flour.

There are two main problems with the regular consumption of refined flour and baked goods:

1. The high sugar content of such foods
2. The presence of hydrogenated fats in almost every commercially prepared baked food.

Regular consumption of products containing refined flour will play havoc on blood sugar regulation. The refined flour is quickly broken down into sugar, which causes a rapid increase in blood sugar. The body responds to high blood sugar by secreting insulin, a hormone that lowers blood sugar levels. Often the large amount of insulin released causes the blood sugar to fall too low. A reaction called reactive hypoglycemia. If this happens on a regular basis a ricochet effect of high blood sugar and low blood sugar begins to occur, leading to insulin resistance and a pre-diabetic state.

The presence of hydrogenated fats in almost every commercially prepared baked food is a major health concern. Hydrogenated fats are full of trans fats. A type of unnatural, man-made fat that has been linked with an increased risk of cancer, coronary heart disease, increased pain and inflammation and an inability to properly metabolize essential fatty acids.

The regular use of refined flour or baked goods can have a strong impact on your brain chemistry. Refined sugars, flours, and baked goods, and other substances such as candy and other sweets, alcohol and certain drugs, will interfere with the receptors in the brain for neurotransmitters. The brain identifies that the receptor for a certain neurotransmitter is already filled, so it reduces the amount of neurotransmitters it produces. As the levels of neurotransmitters drop you begin to crave alcohol or refined sugars to fill newly emptied receptors in the brain. At some point you will no longer be able to fill the receptors with these "empty" foods and substances. At this point you will begin to experience mood swings and an even more intense craving for alcohol or refined sugars. To correct these imbalances you may require amino acid therapy. Ask your doctor about using L-Tyrosine, GABA, L-Taurine, L-Glutamine, and DL-Phenylalanine to help correct the imbalance in brain chemistry caused by regular refined flour and baked goods consumption.

Craving of refined flours is often a sign of wheat sensitivity and allergy. Please consult with your clinician on ways to detect and safely treat allergies.

16. Vitamins and minerals

An enormous amount of research has come out about the benefits of the regular and routine use of vitamins and minerals. They should be viewed as essential, based on their enormous health impact. It is estimated that over 100 million Americans take some form of nutritional supplementation on a regular basis. Supplementation is useful because of nutrient deficient diets and nutrient deficient soils, which leaves foods lacking in even the basic levels of key, essential nutrients.

It is important to remember that not all supplements are created equal. Many brands in the health food stores contain synthetic nutrients that are foreign to the body at best and potentially contaminated at worst. There is also the problem of inaccurate labeling i.e. a product having less of an ingredient than appears on the label. Knowing the source of your supplements is essential for both good quality and value. Buying supplements from your physician assures that the quality and value are maintained.

One company that is dedicated to excellence and value is Biotics Research. They specialize in the whole foods approach to supplementation. Their supplements are food form and they use vegetable cultures, which are rich in antioxidants, as their tableting base. This ensures proper tablet breakdown and absorption of nutrients.

NOTES:

17. Water, distilled

The quality of municipal tap water is questionable. Recent reports have indicated that many municipal water authorities are in violation of clean water standards. Significant levels of organic and inorganic chemicals such as pesticides, insecticides, fertilizers and lead, have been found in municipal water supplies. Unfortunately many of these pollutants are difficult to get rid of using the common purification methods that are in place in many areas of the country today. Studies have linked these pollutants with an increased risk of birth defects, mental disorders, cancer and many other health problems. Other pollutants such as fecal coliform bacteria, parasites and other water born pathogens have been reported in municipal water supplies.

Given the above information, a good, high quality water filtration system is a sound and healthy investment. Unfortunately, distilled water is not. Distilled water may not remove all of the organic chemicals from the water, and it also removes all of the minerals. Some practitioners believe that we should not consume distilled water, because it acts as a vacuum and requires the body to use its own stores of minerals to balance it out. There are better methods of water filtration, which include reverse osmosis, charcoal filtering and deionization. These are all acceptable methods of water treatment.

NOTES:

18. Water, tap

The quality of municipal tap water is questionable. Recent reports have indicated that many municipal water authorities are in violation of clean water standards. Significant levels of organic and inorganic chemicals such as pesticides, insecticides, fertilizers and lead, have been found in municipal water supplies. Unfortunately many of these pollutants are difficult to get rid of using the common purification methods that are in place in many areas of the country today. Studies have linked these pollutants with an increased risk of birth defects, mental disorders, cancer and many other health problems. Other pollutants such as fecal coliform bacteria, parasites and other water born pathogens have been reported in municipal water supplies.

Tap water also contains chlorine and in some cases fluoride, both of which are toxic to the body. It is best to filter your tap water before consuming it. A good, high quality water filtration system is a sound and healthy investment. Methods such as reverse osmosis, distillation, charcoal filtering and deionization are acceptable methods of water treatment.

NOTES:

19. Water, well

The quality of much of the ground water in this country is questionable. Runoff pollution from fields and roads can cause significant levels of organic and inorganic chemicals such as pesticides, insecticides, fertilizers, arsenic and other heavy metals in well water.

Unfortunately many people with well water do not routinely test their water quality and fail to use adequate filtration methods. Studies have linked these pollutants with an increased risk of birth defects, mental disorders, cancer and many other health problems. Bacterial contamination can occur if the well has not been properly sealed.

It is my recommendation to test your well water for organic and inorganic contaminants at least once a year. Depending on the results it is best to filter your well water before consuming it. A good, high quality water filtration system is a sound and healthy investment. Methods such as reverse osmosis, distillation, charcoal filtering and deionization are acceptable methods of water treatment.

NOTES:

20. Diet often for weight control

Frequent dieting for weight control will cause the metabolism of the body to slow down. The body moves into a starvation mode when the caloric intake falls below a certain level. One of the organs that gets most affected by frequent dieting is the thyroid. The thyroid is like the accelerator in your car. It helps accelerate the body's metabolism. Frequent dieting can cause a low-functioning thyroid and a sluggish metabolism geared more to weight gain than weight loss.

One of the other problems with frequent dieting is the intake of complete and whole foods diminish. Most people in this country are on the verge of nutritional deficiencies. Frequent dieting can push you into an overt nutrient deficiency due to an incomplete consumption of all the required nutrients. If you diet regularly you need to be careful to maintain a high nutritional content of the diet.

You can only lose weight by eating less than your body burns up as energy in a day. Your body consumes a certain number of calories just to maintain basic body functions; this is called your metabolic rate. An increase in physical activity will obviously greatly increase the number of calories burned as energy.

It is essential to exercise to lose weight. Frequent dieting without exercise will cause the "set-point" phenomenon. After a few days of restricted caloric intake, the body adjusts by lowering the base metabolic rate, thus permitting a more efficient use of calories. This biological defense mechanism makes losing weight while dieting progressively more difficult.

Frequent dieting also puts your body into the yo-yo syndrome; the continual cycle of losing and gaining weight. This syndrome makes it much harder for your body to lose weight each time. The metabolism will slow down, the body will go into conservation or starvation mode and the body gets used to operating at a slower metabolism.

It is important to not only shed the extra pounds, but also look at the habits, which cause you to gain weight in the first place. Regular exercise, healthy dietary choices and habits, proper food preparation and certain behavioral changes will go a long way to keeping the pounds off. Please consult with your clinician for safe and effective methods to lose weight before you begin your next diet.

NOTES:

LIFESTYLE

21. Times you exercise per week (1 = 1X/ week, 2 = 2 – 4 X/week, 3 = 5 X/week)
22. Changed jobs (3= within last 2 months, 2= within last 6 months, 1= within last 12 months.)
23. Divorced (3= within last 6 months, 2= within last year, 1= within last 2 years)
24. Work over 60 hours/week (3= always, 2= usually, 1= occasionally, 0= never)

21. Times you exercise per week (1 = once a week, 2 = 2-4 times/week, 3 = 5 times a week)

Exercise is an essential part of life. The type of exercise you do is not important. It is the fact that you do it that matters. A brief walk is better than nothing. Exercise can take what ever form you like: jogging, bicycling, tennis, swimming, dancing, skiing, badminton-anything.

The benefits of regular aerobic exercise are enormous.

1. Your lungs operate more efficiently
2. Your blood vessels become enlarged, making them more flexible thus reducing the resistance to blood flow
3. You significantly increase the oxygen supply, causing optimum oxygenation of your red blood cells
4. The tissues of your body get supplied with more oxygen
5. It does wonders for the heart
6. It helps you eat, digest and eliminate waste better by increasing the flow of lymphatic fluid around the body
7. When you exercise your body produces naturally occurring substances called endorphins. Endorphins help improve mood, relieves depression and helps you deal with stress better and helps you sleep better.
8. It will help change your resting basal metabolic rate, so that when you are not exercising you burn up more calories

It is beyond the scope of this narrative to give you exact, personalized information on the type, duration, frequency and intensity of a prescribed exercise program.

Please consult with your clinician for ways to introduce exercise into your routine.

NOTES:

22. Changed jobs (3= within last 2 months, 2= within last 6 months, 1= within last 12 months.)

A recent change in your working environment is a source of significant stress on your body.
When a person is under a lot of stress, normal organ functions become compromised. The adrenal glands, which produce hormones that provide the stress response, are especially vulnerable. If a stress continues over a long time, the adrenals eventually begin to weaken in their ability to keep up, and symptoms of adrenal hypo-function appear. The classic response to a stressful situation is the "fight or flight response". The blood supply to skeletal and heart muscles, brain, skin, and lungs increases. The body evolved to use the "flight or fight response" very infrequently. Unfortunately in our modern lifestyle our body has to deal with Fight or Flight type responses to stressful situations on a regular, if not daily basis. During this response the blood supply to the kidneys, liver, stomach and intestines diminishes. As a result, digestion, detoxification, and elimination are reduced.

Stress also increases your nutritional requirements. Increased stress leads to an increased demand for B vitamins, zinc and vitamin C. It is important to replace these either via the diet or through nutritional supplementation. Some people handle stress by over-eating, with cravings for ice cream, sweets, candy, and other foods with low nutritional value. Unfortunately the intake of these high sugar, high calorie and low nutrient foods will only exacerbate the problem, and may lead to other health problems.

Please consult with your clinician for ways to cope with stress.

NOTES:

23. Divorced (3= within last 6 months, 2= within last year, 1= within last 2 years)

A recent change in your marital status is a source of significant stress on your body. When a person is under a lot of stress, normal organ functions become compromised. The adrenal glands, which produce hormones that provide the stress response, are especially vulnerable. If a stress continues over a long time, the adrenals eventually begin to weaken in their ability to keep up, and symptoms of adrenal hypo-function appear. The classic response to a stressful situation is the "fight or flight response". The blood supply to skeletal and heart muscles, brain, skin, and lungs increases. The body evolved to use the "flight or fight response" very infrequently. Unfortunately in our modern lifestyle our body has to deal with Fight or Flight type responses to stressful situations on a regular, if not daily basis. During this response the blood supply to the kidneys, liver, stomach and intestines diminishes. As a result, digestion, detoxification, and elimination are reduced.

Stress also increases your nutritional requirements. Increased stress leads to an increased demand for B vitamins, zinc and vitamin C. It is important to replace these either via the diet or through nutritional supplementation. Some people handle stress by over-eating, with cravings for ice cream, sweets, candy and other foods with low nutritional value. Unfortunately the intake of these high sugar, high calorie and low nutrient foods will only exacerbate the problem, and may lead to other health problems.

Please consult with your clinician for ways to cope with stress.

NOTES:

24. Work over 60 hours/week (3= always, 2= usually, 1= occasionally, 0= never)

Working a lot of hours per week on a regular basis can be a source of significant stress on your body.

When a person is under a lot of stress, normal organ functions become compromised. The adrenal glands, which produce hormones that provide the stress response, are especially vulnerable. If a stress continues over a long time, the adrenals eventually begin to weaken in their ability to keep up, and symptoms of adrenal hypo-function appear. The classic response to a stressful situation is the "fight or flight response". The blood supply to skeletal and heart muscles, brain, skin, and lungs increases. The body evolved to use the "flight or fight response" very infrequently. Unfortunately in our modern lifestyle our body has to deal with Fight or Flight type responses to stressful situations on a regular, if not daily basis. During this response the blood supply to the kidneys, liver, stomach and intestines diminishes. As a result, digestion, detoxification, and elimination are reduced.

Stress also increases your nutritional requirements. Increased stress leads to an increased demand for B vitamins, zinc and vitamin C. It is important to replace these either via the diet or through nutritional supplementation. Some people handle stress by over-eating, with cravings for ice cream, sweets, candy, and other foods with low nutritional value. Unfortunately the intake of these high sugar, high calorie and low nutrient foods will only exacerbate the problem, and may lead to other health problems.

Please consult with your clinician for ways to cope with stress.

NOTES:

MEDICATIONS

25. Antacids
26. Anti-anxiety medications
27. Antibiotics
28. Anticonvulsants
29. Antidepressants
30. Antifungals
31. Aspirin/Ibuprofen
32. Asthma inhalers
33. Beta blockers
34. Birth control pills/Implant contraceptives
35. Chemotherapy
36. Cholesterol lowering medications
37. Cortisone and other steroids
38. Diabetic medications, insulin
39. Diuretics
40. Estrogen/Progesterone (pharmaceutical, prescription)
41. Estrogen/Progesterone (natural, non proscription)
42. Heart medications
43. High blood pressure medications
44. Laxatives
45. Recreational drugs
46. Relaxants/Sleeping pills
47. Testosterone (natural or prescription)
48. Thyroid medication
49. Tylenol/Acetaminophen
50. Ulcer medications
51. Sildenafal citrate (Viagra)

25. Antacids

Antacids come in many different forms, from the simple acid buffering medication found in Mylanta or Tums, to the acid blocking drugs Tagamet, Pepcid-AC, Prilosec, or Nexium. Some antacids are prescribed by a physician and are used to treat ulcers. Most of the time antacids are taken over the counter to relieve the discomfort of indigestion, usually following a heavy meal. The conventional wisdom is that the bloating and fullness is due to excess stomach acid. The truth is that most of the people needing to use antacids are actually suffering from hypochlorhydria, a condition marked by insufficient levels of stomach acid.

Sufficient stomach acid is essential for adequate digestion. It is important to improve digestion rather than reduce the body's ability to adequately digest our food. Improving the digestion, by treating the hypochlorhydria, will help to prevent the fullness and reduce the feeling that food is just sitting in the stomach.

Some people genuinely do produce excess stomach acid, and are at an increased risk for developing an ulcer. However, in my clinical experience, using in-office laboratory techniques to measure stomach acid levels, I have found excess stomach acid secretion to be very rare. If you are taking antacids to treat an ulcer you probably experience some relief with the medication. It is important to realize that the antacids are not helping to treat the ulcer, but merely reducing the irritation and pain.

Recent information has come out about a possible infectious link between ulcers and the bacteria Helicobacter pylori. It is my opinion that this link has more to do with the environment of the stomach being the ideal breeding ground for the H. pylori, rather than the pathogenic nature of the bacteria itself.

Treating the ulcer by focusing on the things that cause them is essential:

- Address the balance of the environment in the stomach by treating the hypochlorhydria
- Cut out the stomach irritants coffee and alcohol
- Reduce stress
- Quit smoking
- Take supplements to actually heal the damaged tissue and if necessary treat the H. pylori infection with natural medicine.

Please consult your physician for more information on treating ulcers naturally.

The use of acid blocking medications such as Tagamet, Pepcid-AC, Prilosec, and Nexium can lead to serious long term health problems. It is important to remember that stomach acid plays an essential role in not only digestion but vitamin and mineral absorption and protecting the digestive tract from infectious agents such as parasites and bacteria. You are putting your health at risk by taking a medication that totally blocks the production and release of stomach acid: nutritional deficiencies, B12 deficient anemia, calcium deficiency, osteoporosis and other serious health problems.

Please consult with your physician to explore ways to reduce your need for such drugs and begin the journey to renewed health.

26. Antianxiety Medications

Anxiety may have either a physiological or a psychological cause. Physiological causes include an increased autonomic response to fearful situations or impulses. These would result in the physiological manifestations often seen in panic attacks. Psychological causes of anxiety may have some emotional stress that precedes the bout of anxiety. The emotional stress may be easily identifiable, as in a loss of a job or a relationship, or it may be subconscious. Either way an environmental or social occurrence can trigger an anxiety episode.

There are many classes of drug that are designed to treat anxiety. These include Azaspirones (Buspar) that are used to treat Genralized Anxiety Disorder, Benzodiazepines (Ativan, Centrax, Dalmane, Klonopin, Librium, Paxipam, Restoril, Serax, Tranxene, and Xanax) that are used to panic disorders and social phobias, Beta Blockers (inderal and tenormin) that are used to calm certain anxiety symptoms, such as shaking, palpitations, and sweating, Tricyclic antidepressants (Adapin, Anafranil and Elavil) that are used to treat mood and anxiety-related disorders, and Selective Serotonin Re-uptake Inhibitors (SSRIs) (Prozac, Zoloft, Effexor, paxil, and Serxone) that are used to treat depression and panic disorders.

As with any drug you should be aware of the possible damage it can have on the liver and the rest of the body. Persons taking anti-anxiety drugs should avoid alcohol as there is a significant drug interaction that takes place with alcohol.

Some of the side-effects of anti-anxiety drugs include:

1. Weight gain- Keeping the weight at an optimal level is one of the main battles facing a person on anti-anxiety medication
2. Sexual dysfunction- a lack of sexual desire is another problem that affects people on anti-anxiety medication.
3. Lethargy

Natural alternatives to anti-anxiety medication include the following:

1. Kava kava extract
2. 5-hydroxy tryptophan
3. St. John's wort

27. Antibiotics

Antibiotics, when used sensibly, can be life saving. Unfortunately they have been misused and over prescribed to the point where more powerful drugs are needed to cope with antibiotic resistant strains of bacteria.

Antibiotics work by killing bacteria. They are not effective against viruses, parasites or yeast. They are very useful for dealing with an overwhelming infection that the body is having a hard time dealing with, but their use does not come without side effects. Not all bacteria in the body cause disease. There are different strains of bacteria in our body that help to keep us healthy. These bacteria are found in the digestive tract and include Lactobacillus acidophilus and bifidobacteria. Unfortunately antibiotics kill all bacteria, including the friendly kind in the intestines. If the friendly bacteria is not replaced you can become susceptible to additional infections of yeast, fungus and bacteria, which lead to digestive and other health problems. Care should be taken to re-introduce the friendly bacteria as soon as possible when taking antibiotics.

Another thing to remember is that the environment in the body and the strength of the immune system play an important role in preventing infections from taking hold. Antibiotics actually weaken the immune system by impairing the efficacy of white blood cells. They also put additional stress on the liver by reducing various nutrients needed by the liver for detoxification.

More and more people are experiencing antibiotic resistant infections. In most of these cases there are no other medical options other than using more and more powerful drugs. I recommend that you look at the cause of the infection and at the reason why your body has become a perfect place for these infections to thrive. In most cases it is case of weakened immunity and a damaged internal environment of the body. Use the following to increase your immunity and reduce the susceptibility that your body will become infected:

- Cut out or reduce the amount of refined sugar in the diet
- Exercise regularly
- Drink adequate amounts of water to stay hydrated
- Work on improving your digestion
- Regularly use hydrotherapy techniques to stimulate lymph flow
- Eat a well balanced diet
- Take regular supplements that stimulate the immune system e.g. Calcium-D-Glucarate

These will ensure that your body is not a good environment for bacteria growth and your immune system is strong enough to deal with any infections before they overwhelm the body.

28. Anticonvulsants

Anticonvulsant medications are used to treat seizures and epilepsy. Some of the common anticonvulsant medications that you may be taking include Phenobarbital, Dilantin or Tegretol. Seizures occur as a result of hyperactivity in the brain, and for many people anticonvulsant medication makes the difference between having a "normal life" and being a prisoner of their disease. There are different types of seizures: partial seizures, absence seizures (also called petit mal) and generalized seizures (also called Grand mal). Partial seizures are either simple or complex. Partial simple seizures consist of a single detectable dysfunction, which does not change during the episode and consciousness is maintained throughout. Partial complex seizures begin in a focal area and spread causing dulled or lost consciousness. Absence seizures are more common in children and teens and present as brief episodes of blank staring without convulsions. Generalized seizures begin with prolonged contraction and then whole body jerking.

Whatever the type of seizure you have, you are probably on some form of medication. It is important to remember that drugs are toxins to the body, and put extra stress on the liver and kidneys, the two organs that get rid of the drugs from the body. Many people on anticonvulsant medication are on Dilantin, a drug that is used to treat most forms of epilepsy. Do not stop taking this drug suddenly, as this may cause severe convulsions. Always talk with the prescribing physician before stopping Dilantin or any other drugs. There are a long list of known drugs that interact with Dilantin. Always tell a physician who is prescribing another drug that you are on Dilantin.

Functional medicine may help explain why you may be prone to epilepsy. Many disorders and diseases have origins in a disturbed function within the body. Some of the predisposing factors for epilepsy and seizures include:

- A heavy metal body burden
- Intestinal parasites
- Food sensitivities
- Reactive hypoglycemia
- And certain nutrient deficiencies such as magnesium, vitamin B6 and manganese.

Please consult with your practitioner about the functional changes that you can make to strengthen your body's foundation.

NOTES:

29. Antidepressants

Depression is a multi-factorial problem with many different contributing factors. Nutritional deficiencies, blood sugar dysregulation, stress, biochemical imbalances, smoking, drinking, prescription medications and even caffeine can contribute to depression. Some of the common causes of depression include:

- An overgrowth of yeast in the digestive system, which can rob the body of essential nutrients leading to nutrient deficiency
- Hypothyroidism
- Low blood sugar
- Allergies
- Poor adrenal function
- Essential fatty acid deficiencies
- Protein deficiency
- Poor digestion and absorption

Most physicians use antidepressants to treat depression. Many of the modern antidepressants work by increasing the activity of certain chemicals in the brain called neurotransmitters. They act to keep the neurotransmitters around longer by preventing their destruction or recycling. Most of the neurotransmitters in the brain are formed from amino acids, which are found in protein. Serotonin, for instance, is formed from the amino acid Tryptophan. Nutritional approaches to treating depression are as effective as using anti-depressants for many people, without the many side effects of drug treatment.

The regular use of candy and other sweets can have a strong impact on your brain chemistry causing an increase in mood disorders. Candy, and other substances such as refined sugars, flours, alcohol and certain drugs, will interfere with the receptors in the brain for key neurotransmitters. The brain identifies that the receptor for a certain neurotransmitter is already filled, so it reduces the amount of neurotransmitters it produces. As the levels of neurotransmitters drop you begin to crave alcohol or refined sugars to fill newly emptied receptors in the brain. At some point you will no longer be able to fill the receptors with these “empty” foods and substances. At this point you will begin to experience mood swings, depression, and an even more intense craving for alcohol or refined sugars. To correct these imbalances you may require amino acid therapy. Ask your doctor about using L-Tyrosine, GABA, L-Taurine, L-Glutamine, and DL-Phenylalanine to help correct the imbalance in brain chemistry caused by regular candy bar or refined sugar consumption

You can start by taking some positive steps to re-address the balance in your life: Eat a good, healthy diet low in refined sugar, high in fiber and essential fatty acids. It is important to include plenty of good quality protein, as the amino acids in protein form the building blocks for all of the neurotransmitters in the brain.

Please discuss the various nutritional methods of treating depression with your physician.

30. Antifungals

Antifungal drugs work by killing yeast and fungus. They are not effective against viruses, parasites or bacteria. They can be useful for dealing with an overwhelming yeast infection that the body is having a hard time dealing with, but their use does not come without side effects. They put a considerable stress on the liver and kidneys, which have the task of detoxifying and eliminating the drugs. Many times a yeast infection occurs after taking antibiotics due to the destruction of friendly bacteria in the digestive system that leaves the body open for colonization by unfriendly yeast. Taking appropriate levels of Lactobacillus acidophilus and bifidus soon after using antibiotics will prevent this from happening.

Another thing to remember is that the environment in the body and the strength of the immune system play an important role in preventing yeast from taking hold in the body. Use the following to increase your immunity and reduce the susceptibility that your body will become infected:

- Cut out or reduce the amount of refined sugar in the diet
- Exercise regularly
- Drink adequate amounts of water to stay hydrated
- Work on improving your digestion
- Regularly use hydrotherapy techniques to stimulate lymph flow
- Eat a well balanced diet
- Take regular supplements that stimulate the immune system e.g. Calcium-D-Glucarate

These will ensure that your body is not a good environment for yeast growth and your immune system is strong enough to deal with any infections before they overwhelm the body.

Please consult your physician for ways to naturally treat yeast infections using diet and nutrition.

NOTES:

31. Aspirin/Ibuprofen

Aspirin and ibuprofen are painkillers that provide temporary relief for minor problems. If you take painkillers on a regular basis for headaches and aches and pains it is important to remember that they are not getting at the primary cause for the pain, and are just masking the symptoms. For instance if you take pain killers regularly for headaches would it not be more effective to find out the cause of the headaches rather than relying on a band aid to cover the symptom? The results of this questionnaire and further testing may uncover the real cause of the aches and pains in the body, thus providing a real solution.

Unfortunately the use of aspirin or Ibuprofen use does not come without potential side effects: stomach irritation, stomach bleeding and ulcers and increased intestinal hyperpermeability that can lead to allergies. These drugs also have effects outside of their role in relieving pain. Aspirin will knock out the clotting ability of your platelets, and will depress your body temperature thus preventing the body from mounting a fever if needed to deal with infections. Additionally all drugs are essentially toxins to the body, and need to be detoxified and eliminated by the liver and kidneys, causing increased stress on these already overworked organs.

In many cases increasing the levels of Essential fatty acids in the diet can go a long way to helping with pain and inflammation, the reasons why many people resort to painkillers such as aspirin or ibuprofen in the first place.

Please consult with your physician for ways to reduce the amount of pain killers you have to take. Many times identifying key imbalances in the body can make a huge difference in the amount of painkillers you may need for your condition.

NOTES:

32. Asthma inhalers

Asthma has been on the increase over the last 20 years due primarily to increased stress on the immune system, increased pollution of air, water and food, earlier weaning of infants and an earlier introduction of solid foods, resulting in an increase in foods that a person is allergic or sensitive too. It is currently estimated that over 4 million people in the United States suffers from asthma or allergies.

Asthma inhalers come in two different forms: bronchodilators and steroids.

Bronchodilators such as Ventolin, Proventil, Alupen and Metaprel act on the smooth muscle in the bronchi if the lungs open up the airways rapidly during a mild or moderate asthma attack. Bronchodilators are available in inhaler and pill form. The inhaler is preferred because the chances of side effects are minimized. These medications are extremely effective for "asthma attacks" but their effectiveness begins to wear off after a few hours, requiring larger and larger doses. Inhalers are not without side effects. They can cause the following side effects:

- Dry mouth and throat
- Increased heart rate and blood pressure
- Insomnia
- Anxiety.

The use of steroid containing inhalers such as Beclovent, Beconase and Azmacort, has increased over the last few years. They work by reducing the production of pro inflammatory and pro allergic compounds in the body. They are only effective in preventing asthma attacks and are pretty much useless in an acute attack. The use of steroid inhalers does not come without side effects. They include:

- An increased risk of yeast overgrowth in the mouth and throat
- Allergic reactions
- Dryness of the mouth and sore throat

Long-term use may increase the risk of developing a respiratory tract infection. This is due to the immune suppressing effects of corticosteroids.

Asthma is a condition that responds well to alternative medicine. Please consult with your physician about ways to treat asthma naturally and begin to reduce your dependence on asthma inhalers.

NOTES:

33. Beta blockers

Beta-blockers are drugs for high blood pressure that block the binding of a substance called epinephrine to a particular cellular receptor known as a beta-receptor. The effect is to reduce heart rate and decrease the force of contraction in the heart. Some common beta-blockers include Secratal, Tenormin, Lopressor, Levatol and Inderal. Beta blockers are also used to treat angina and certain arrhythmias in the heart. In these cases Beta blockers are not only ineffective but may actually contribute the condition they are trying to prevent.

The common side effects of beta blockers include:

- Cold hands and feet
- Impaired mental function
- Fatigue
- Dizziness
- Depression
- Lethargy
- Reduced libido and impotence.

Beta blockers reduce the amount of blood being pumped by the heart, which reduces the amount of blood and oxygen to the extremities, hence cold hands and feet and impotence. Beta blockers will also increase cholesterol and serum triglyceride levels.

It is important to remember that drugs are toxins to the body, and put extra stress on the liver and kidneys, the two organs that get rid of the drugs from the body. **Do not stop taking this drug suddenly**, as this may cause severe withdrawal symptoms including headache, increased heart rate and dramatic increase in blood pressure. Always talk with the prescribing physician before stopping your beta blocker or any other drugs.

High blood pressure is a condition that responds well to diet, lifestyle and supplemental treatment. Talk to your physician about natural ways to treat high blood pressure

NOTES:

34. Birth Control Pills / Implant Contraceptives

Birth control pills and implants are powerful hormones that prevent pregnancy. One of the questions you may want to ask yourself is “are birth control pills or implant contraceptives the safest contraceptive option for me”? The list of adverse effects, which are both psychological and physiological, seems to grow each year. The convenience of the pill or implant is obvious, but many women suffer from headaches, bloating, nausea, irregular bleeding, breast tenderness, weight gain, an increased risk of heart attack and stroke, and other unpleasant side effects. The long-term effects include high blood pressure, liver tumor, gallbladder disease and depression. Temporary infertility has been associated with using the pill, and especially implant contraceptives.

Oral and implant contraceptives also have nutritional effects on the body, causing a number of vitamin and mineral deficiencies in the body, including folic acid and vitamin B6, which can lead to other symptoms.

If you decide that you still want to take the pill, it is essential that you eat a good diet, exercise and take a good nutritional supplement to replace those that your body is losing. Please talk to your physician for ways to help your body while you are on the pill. Also it may be wise to look at other alternatives that are less damaging to the body.

NOTES:

35. Chemotherapy

Chemotherapy is a strong chemical treatment for many forms of cancer. It puts an enormous burden and stress on your body, in addition to the stress your body is already under dealing with cancer. It is therefore very important to maintain good dietary and lifestyle habits whilst undergoing chemotherapy.

One of the common side effects of most chemotherapy drugs is nutritional deficiency, especially the vitamin folic acid, which is an essential nutrient for cell repair and immune function. It is important to discuss your increased nutritional needs with your physician, who can help put you on a nutritional program that will provide your body with good quality and highly absorbable nutrients.

As with all drugs, chemotherapy is a toxin to the body. It puts additional demands on the liver and kidneys, which have to detoxify and eliminate the drugs from the body. It is important to avoid the many things that can increase the burden on these overworked organs: sugar and refined sugars, hydrogenated oils, smoking, chemical additives and processed foods.

NOTES:

36. Cholesterol lowering medications

The most common cholesterol lowering medications are a family of drugs called Statins. They include Atorvastatin (Lipitor), fluvastatin (Lescol), lovastatin (Mevacor, Altocor), pravastatin (Pravachol), simvastatin (Zocor), and rosuvastatin (Crestor). These drugs work to lower cholesterol by inhibiting the enzyme called HMG CoA reductase that makes cholesterol in the liver.

Another family of cholesterol lowering drugs are the bile acid sequestrants. Cholestyramine (Questran, Questran Light, Prevalite, LoCholest), colestipol (Colestid), and colesevelam (WelChol) are commonly prescribed bile acid sequestrants. They work by binding with cholesterol-containing bile acids in the intestine, which are subsequently excreted in the stool.

Some of the many problems of cholesterol lowering medications include:

1. Interferance with Coenzyme Q10 metabolism. HMG CoA reductase, the enzyme that produces cholesterol, is also the enzyme that produces CoQ10, which is an essential nutrient for the production of energy and is found in highest levels in the mitochondria of heart muscle cells. Decreasing levels of CoQ10 are associated with cardiovascular disease.
2. Stomach and/or intestinal dysfunction (nausea, vomiting, gas, indigestion, diarrhea, cramps, and bloating)
3. increasing liver and kidney dysfunction
4. Muscle soreness, pain, weakness, and even increased muscle breakdown

It is essential that you have a conversation with your clients about the side effects and potential dangers of long-term use of cholesterol lowering medications. A conversation about the role of cholesterol in the body and ways to naturally lower cholesterol is a must. Remember, only the prescribing physician can change a client's prescription medication. Educate your client about the changes you want them to make and have a conversation with the prescribing physician and let them know that you are working with their client to lower their cholesterol naturally and you expect their cholesterol levels to be lowered using these methods. It is always worth asking the prescribing physician when they were planning on reducing or stopping the use of these medications.

37. Cortisone and other steroids

Cortisol is a hormone produced by the adrenal glands, which are two organs located above the kidneys. Cortisone is a synthetic form of cortisol and is prescribed as an anti-inflammatory drug under the common names Prednisone or Prednisolone. It is also used topically as hydrocortisone cream for the control of itching and other skin ailments.

Cortisone is a powerful drug with wide reaching action in the body, and is associated with many unpleasant side effects. Cortisone has many undesirable metabolic effects in the body when used as a drug. It will cause the following:

- Increase in blood sugar
- Muscle wasting with protein loss
- Deposition of excess fat around the face and other parts of the body, giving the characteristic puffy features.
- It will cause the adrenal glands to stop functioning properly, leading to physiological adrenal hypofunction.

Some other side effects include:

- Osteoporosis from calcium loss
- Water retention
- Poor wound healing
- Muscle weakness or atrophy
- Ulcers and weakening of the connective tissue leading to thinning of the skin and stretch marks.

It is very difficult to get off cortisone once you have been on it for a while. If you are worried about these possible side effects it is best to talk to your prescribing physician. It is not my place to tell you to not take this or any other drug. It is my aim to provide you with up to date education as to the effects of drugs, lifestyle, diet and exercise.

NOTES:

38. Diabetic medications, Insulin

Diabetic medication includes insulin and various oral hypoglycemic drugs. Diabetes can be split into two categories: Insulin-dependent diabetes and non-insulin dependent diabetes. For the former group taking insulin is a necessity. There is overwhelming evidence that adult onset diabetes is responsive to dietary changes and nutritional supplementation. Dietary regulation and awareness are important in all cases of diabetes, and in some cases diet alone may control the disease. A whole food diet that has no refined and concentrated sugar, is high in protein and essential fatty acids and low in slow-acting or low glycemic carbohydrates is recommended. If one is overweight, a diet low in calories is also suggested. The avoidance of processed, commercial, empty-calorie foods, which are deficient in essential vitamins and minerals, will help the body regenerate those organs that may be damaged. Studies show that treating food sensitivities reduces dependence on insulin and helps regulate blood glucose levels.

Studies have shown that a diet high in fiber helps reduce insulin or oral hypoglycemic drugs used to maintain blood glucose levels. Up to 100 grams of fiber are recommended per day. Please consult your physician to discuss ways to implement a diet and nutritional program to help with your diabetes.

Oral hypoglycemic drugs, like all drugs, are toxins to the body. They put additional demands on the liver and kidneys, which have to detoxify and eliminate the drugs from the body. It is important to avoid the many things that can increase the burden on these overworked organs: sugar and refined sugars, hydrogenated oils, smoking, chemical additives and processed foods.

Insulin is a life-saving drug for people suffering from insulin-dependent diabetes, a condition marked by the destruction of the cells in the pancreas that produce insulin. Unfortunately insulin is often used in adult-onset or non-insulin dependent diabetes, a condition that is very responsive to dietary changes and nutritional supplementation, and if managed properly can be treated without the need for drug intervention.

For insulin dependent diabetics there is strong evidence that diet and nutritional supplementation can help with not only blood sugar control but also many of the conditions associated with long term diabetes: retinopathies, chronic infections, leg ulcers, and nerve and kidney damage. Dr. Richard Bernstein's book "Dr. Bernstein's diabetes solution" is a good resource for the natural treatment and management of diabetes. Dr. Bernstein is a long-term survivor of insulin dependent diabetes, and shares his first hand knowledge of how he controlled his type 1 diabetes.

Please see the handout in the appendix on Recommendations for controlling blood sugar for more information.

NOTES:

39. Diuretics

Diuretics are drugs used to treat high blood pressure. They work by accelerating the elimination of water from the body, and thus reduce the volume of fluid in the blood. The reduction of the fluid in the blood reduces the blood pressure. One of the problems with the diuretic drugs is the loss of electrolytes in the urine, especially potassium. Some of the common diuretics include Lasix, Corzide, Aldoclor and Midamor. There are different categories of diuretic drugs: Thiazides, loop diuretics and potassium-sparing diuretics. Thiazide diuretics are some of the most commonly prescribed diuretics because they work at lower dosages and are often used in combination with other heart medications.

Unfortunately they cause the loss of potassium and magnesium in the urine. Interestingly enough these are two nutrients that have well documented use in treating high blood pressure. Thiazide diuretics also increase cholesterol and serum triglycerides, and worsen blood sugar control. Typical side effects include increased blood sugar, increased uric acid levels, muscle weakness and cramps caused by potassium loss and decreased libido and impotence.

It is important to remember that drugs are toxins to the body, and put extra stress on the liver and kidneys, the two organs that get rid of the drugs from the body. There may be problems if you suddenly stop taking this medication. Always talk with the prescribing physician before stopping any drugs.
High blood pressure is a condition that responds well to diet, lifestyle and supplemental treatment. Talk to your physician about natural ways to treat high blood pressure.

NOTES:

40. Estrogen/Progesterone (Pharmaceutical prescription)

Estrogen and progesterone are commonly prescribed to treat the side effects of menopause, such as hot flashes, vaginal dryness, and to prevent osteoporosis. The most common prescription for estrogen is a drug hormone called Premarin. What many people do not realize is that Premarin is not a naturally occurring hormone in the human body. It is an equine estrogen obtained from pregnant mares urine, hence the name Premarin. It is about 20 times more active than the equivalent estrogen in the body and has a long list of side effects including an increased risk for breast cancer, endometrial cancer, high blood pressure, abnormal vaginal bleeding and weight gain. So we have a drug that hopes to reduce the risk of osteoporosis while being a potential promoter of breast and endometrial cancer.

Synthetic progesterone in the form of Provera is often used in combination with Premarin to decrease the cancer side effects. They have their own list of side effects including increased risk of blood clots, stroke and blindness. It caused breast and uterine cancers when administered to laboratory mammals.

In the last few years a number of natural hormones have emerged. They are synthesized from wild yam and are identical to the estrogens and progesterone in your body. Progesterone cream can be bought in the health food store. It is important to remember that the quality of such products varies from company to company, and the amount of progesterone in each product varies enormously. Natural estrogens can usually be obtained from your alternative physician.

It is important to have your hormone levels checked every six months with salivary hormone testing to make sure you are not taking too much.

Menopause is a condition that responds very well to dietary, lifestyle and nutritional medicine. Please consult with your physician about ways to reduce your need for such mediations.

NOTES:

41. Estrogen / Progesterone (natural, non-prescription)

In the last few years a number of natural hormones have emerged. They are synthesized from wild yam and are identical to the estrogens and progesterone in your body. Progesterone cream can be bought in the health food store. It is important to remember that the quality of such products varies from company to company, and the amount of progesterone in each product varies enormously. Natural estrogens can usually be obtained from your alternative physician. It is important to have your hormone levels checked every six months with salivary hormone testing to make sure you are not taking too much.
Menopause is a condition that responds very well to dietary, lifestyle and nutritional medicine. Please consult with your physician about ways to reduce your need for such mediations.

Hormones are chemicals that your body produces in very small amounts and get delivered to the rest of the body by the blood stream. Hormones are used for treating various disorders including the side effects of menopause and hypothyroidism. The liver is partly responsible for keeping hormone levels in balance by breaking down hormones and prepares them for excretion. If the liver is compromised in any way, the hormones remain unchanged in circulation and can continue to stimulate the body. This puts stress on the body. If you continue to take hormones it is important to keep the liver healthy.

For some people hormone therapy can be very helpful. For example taking natural estrogen and progesterone after a hysterectomy can help maintain function and taking thyroid hormone can make all the difference.

If taking hormones please talk to your physician about ways to keep the liver healthy, and to discuss alternatives to the hormones themselves that may have considerable less side effects.

NOTES:

42. Heart medications

Heart medication falls into a number of different categories: blood pressure control, arrhythmia control and anti-angina medication to name but a few. The heart is a system that responds well to diet, lifestyle and nutrition. Many times the heart is just a mirror for deeper problems within the body. Changing the diet, reducing the amount of processed and refined foods and exercising can make a profound difference. Please talk to your physician about ways to start working on the foundational issues that affect your body, and begin to treat the heart naturally.

NOTES:

43. High blood pressure medications

High blood pressure is a condition that responds well to diet, lifestyle and nutrition. The mainstream approach is to treat hypertension with beta-blockers, diuretic, calcium channel blockers etc. This may be helpful in acute cases or situations when the blood pressure is very high. For most people a natural approach can reduce their dependence on such medication, which is not without significant side effects.

Many times the heart is just a mirror for deeper problems within the body. Changing the diet, reducing the amount of processed and refined foods and exercising can make a profound difference. Please talk to your physician about ways to start working on the foundational issues that affect your body, and ways to treat blood pressure naturally.

NOTES:

44. Laxatives

Laxatives are a very commonly used over the counter medication for constipation. Constipation is almost endemic in this country, judging from the size of the laxative section in the local drug store. Constipation is a subjective symptom where stools are too hard, too small, too infrequent, difficult to expel, or when a person has a feeling of incomplete evacuation after the bowel movement is over. Other objective signs are fewer than *3-5* stools per week, or more than 3 days without a stool. The average time it takes for food to make it through the gastrointestinal tract is 50-100 hours. The optimum time is 17-30 hours. From a functional perspective you could be considered constipated if a day passes without a bowel movement.

The most common cause of constipation is a lack of dietary fiber and adequate hydration. Many people do not take their supplementary fiber with adequate amounts of water. This can make the constipation much worse, and cause the stool to be harder and more difficult to pass. Treating constipation is a process of trying one approach, seeing if it works and if it doesn't moving to the next step. The most likely causes of constipation in a functional list are: lack of fiber, lack of adequate hydration, a deficiency in pancreatic enzymes and hydrochloric acid, biliary congestion with a need for bile salts, dysbiosis, food allergies and a low functioning thyroid. Constipation is also a sign of magnesium deficiency.
Please see your physician to discuss ways to treat your constipation naturally and get you off the laxatives.

NOTES:

45. Recreational drugs

Recreational drugs have significant health risks attached to their use. They place considerable strain on the body from the adrenal glands that are too often over stimulated by recreational drugs, to the liver and kidneys, which have to detoxify and eliminate the drug from the body. If the drug use is combined with smoking, alcohol and a poor diet, you are placing your body at more risk for developing serious problems later on. Some drugs act as immune suppressants, leaving the body wide open for opportunistic infections. The overall impact on the body is a profound alteration in the internal environment or terrain. Increased exposure to free radicals, pH changes and a systemic loss of minerals and vitamins provide even more stress on the body.

If you are using recreational drugs please talk to your physician about ways to improve the diet, and begin a nutritional supplement program that will help lessen the impact of recreational drugs on the body.

NOTES:

46. Relaxants/Sleeping pills

Relaxants and sleeping pills refer to a class of drugs called sedatives. They either help the muscles relax or act on the nervous system to help with sleep. Next to antibiotics, sleeping pills are the most prescribed class of medication. Many people use these drugs to combat insomnia. It is important to take a step back and look at why you need to take this drug. Insomnia can have many causes, including depression, stress, anxiety and tension. Various foods, drinks and medications also have an impact on your ability to sleep.
There are two categories of sedatives: antihistamines and benzodiazepines. Antihistamines prevent the release of histamine, which causes you to feel drowsy and sleepy. Benzodiazepines such as Halcion, Valium and Librium are some of the primary drugs prescribed for insomnia and anxiety. Other drugs include Ativan, Clonipin, Resotril and Xanax. They act to block the arousal centers of the brain, are not to be used long term due to their addictive qualities and can cause abnormal sleep patterns. They can produce many side effects including dizziness, drowsiness, and impaired coordination. They should not be used with alcohol.

There are a number of dietary and lifestyle factors that you can try to deal with the insomnia. Eliminate caffeine and all stimulants from the diet; avoid nocturnal hypoglycemia by eating a good-quality snack 20-30 minutes before going to bed, learn to relax more by doing some kind of relaxation techniques, and exercise.
Please discuss stress with your physician who will be able to help you with diet, lifestyle and other natural ways to treat stress and insomnia.

NOTES:

47. Testosterone (natural or prescription)

Testosterone is a steroid hormone that is produced by both men and women. Primarily a male sex hormone produced in the testes, testosterone is also produced in the ovaries and adrenal glands of women. Testosterone is responsible for sex drive in both men and women.

Levels of testosterone begin to decline with age in a process called andropause. Some of the symptoms of declining testosterone levels include:

1. Decreased energy and stamina
2. Decreased mental clarity
3. Decreased sex drive
4. decreased musle and increased fat
5. Depression
6. irritability
7. Increased risk of cancer and cardiovascular disease

Clients may have been prescribed testosterone by another prescribing physician as a means to counter these unfortunate effects of aging. Many people report positive effects from taking supplemental testosterone including feeling stronger, having a better sex drive, increased muscle tone, and more stamina in general. Testosterone has also been shown to have a beneficial effect on cardiovascular health, and also bone development.

Supplemental testosterone is not without its side effects and you should be aware of these and discuss them with your clients that are taking supplemental testosterone.

Side effects:

1. Unopposed testosterone in men can be problematic if the levels are not checked regularly. Some men have reported that they have increased irritability, are quick to anger, and feel more aggressive.
2. Another problem is the effect of unopposed testosterone on the prostate. Benign Prostatic Hypertrophy (BPH) may be caused by increased levels of a hormone called di-hydrotestosterone (DHT), which stimulates prostate growth. Testosterone can easily be turned into DHT in men supplementing testosterone. High levels of DHT have also been implicated in male pattern baldness.
3. Testosterone cannot be used in men with a risk of prosatate cancer or with active prostate cancer as it can accelerate the growth of tumors. Regular checks of the PSA are essential for men taking testosterone.
4. Women who are taking testosterone shold get their levels checked regularly as increased levels of testosterone can lead to the development of masculine features such as increased body hair on the face.

48. Thyroid medication

Thyroid medication is designed to replace or augment the amount of thyroid hormone your body is producing. It is usually prescribed after a physician discovers from a blood test that your body is not producing enough hormone on its own. The thyroid gland is a small organ located at the base of the neck. It produces thyroid hormone, which acts as a sort of accelerator to your body's metabolism. Without adequate thyroid hormone, the metabolism slows down; you feel tired, have slower reflexes and feel cold. Thyroid hormone is designed to ameliorate that imbalance.

There maybe underlying nutritional deficiencies that make it more difficult for the body to produce enough of its own thyroid hormone, or a situation in which the cells of the body become more resistant to thyroid hormone. In each of these cases a thorough nutritional evaluation of the thyroid and other organ systems will allow this to be corrected, so that you may be able to discontinue or at least reduce your current dose. Please talk to your physician about ways to treat the thyroid naturally.

NOTES:

49. Tylenol/Acetaminophen

Tylenol or acetaminophen is a painkiller that provides temporary relief for minor problems. If you take painkillers on a regular basis for headaches and aches and pains it is important to remember that they are not getting at the primary cause for the pain, and are just masking the symptoms. For instance if you take pain killers regularly for headaches would it not be more effective to find out the cause of the headaches rather than relying on a band aid to cover the symptom? The results of this questionnaire and further testing may uncover the real cause of the aches and pains in the body, thus providing a real solution.
Unfortunately the use of Tylenol or acetaminophen does not come without potential side effects: stomach irritation, stomach bleeding and ulcers, increased intestinal hyperpermeability that can lead to allergies. Tylenol, more than the other non-steroidal anti-inflammatory painkillers, puts tremendous stress on the liver. In order for it to be detoxified effectively, the liver will produce a very toxic intermediary substance. If the liver is dealing with alcohol at the same time as trying to detoxify the Tylenol or is trying to detoxify too much Tylenol, high levels of this toxic intermediary may be formed. Hundreds of people die each year from the liver damage caused by using alcohol or taking more than the recommended amount of Tylenol. Remember, all drugs are essentially toxins to the body, and need to be detoxified and eliminated by the liver and kidneys, causing increased stress on these already overworked organs. Please consult with your physician to discuss ways to reduce your dependence on this medication.

NOTES:

50. Ulcer medications

Some people genuinely do produce excess stomach acid, and are at an increased risk for developing an ulcer. If you are taking antacids to treat an ulcer you probably experience some relief with the medication. It is important to realize that the antacids are not helping to treat the ulcer, but merely reducing the irritation and pain. Recent information has come out about a possible infectious link between ulcers and the bacteria Helicobacter pylori. It is my opinion that this link has more to do with the environment of the stomach being the ideal breeding ground for the H. pylori, rather than the pathogenic nature of the bacteria itself. Treating the ulcer by focusing on the things that cause them is essential. Re-addressing the balance of the environment in the stomach by treating the hypochlorhydria, cutting out the stomach irritants coffee and alcohol, reducing stress and quitting smoking, taking supplements to actually heal the damaged tissue and if necessary treating the H. pylori infection with natural medicine. Please consult your physician for more information on treating ulcers naturally.

NOTES:

51. Sildenafil citrate (Viagra)

Sildenafil citrate is the chemical name for the prescription drug Viagra, which is the drug used to treat erection difficulties, such as erectile dysfunction. Another drug called Levitra has just reached the market and is an alternative to Viagra.

Many people think of Viagra and Levitra as drugs to treat impotence. However, impotence is a fairly general term that includes erectile difficulties, lack of sexual desire, and a failure to ejaculate. Viagra was developed to treat erectile dysfunction and works by increasing blood flow to the penis. It is not a hormone or an aphrodisiac, and has been used by many men who complain of impotence. Once taken Viagra and Levitra begin to work as quickly as 30 minutes and the effect lasts for up to 4 hours.

Erectile dysfunction is a problem that has been getting a lot of press since Viagra came on the market. It is estimated that between 15 and 30 million men complain of erectile dysfunction. Taking a pill to increase the blood flow to the penis is a classic case of treating the symptom ond not the cause. Viagra does nothing to help resolve the underlying problem of why there is a decrease in blood flow to the penis in the first place. There are of course men for whom Viagra is the only solution to their erectile dysfunction. These would include elderly men that have a physical cause of their erectile dysfunction, including disease, injury, and side effects to medication. But for many men focusing on the organic cause of low blood flow to the periphweral tissues in the first place would be a good thing to focus on.

Some of the many causes of erectile dysfunction include:

1. Damage to the nerves- this may be caused by an undetected B12 deficiency and diabetes
2. Damage to the arteries- atherosclerotic changes in the arteries can lead to arterial damage as can an increase in levels of homocysteine.
3. Diseases such as diabetes, atherosclerosis, kidney disease, alcoholism, peripheral vascular disease, multiple sclerosis, and neurological diseases are the cause of an estimated 70% of erectile dysfunction.
4. Roughly 40% of men with Diabetes have erectile dysfunction. Assessing blood sugar regulation can be very helpful in addressing this issue.
5. Medications such as blood pressure drugs, antihistamines, antidepressants, tranquilizers, appetite suppressants, and cimetidine (an acid-blocking drug) can cause erectile dysfunction.
6. Psychological anxiety, stress, guilt, low self-esteem, and fear of sexual failure.
7. Smoking, which damages the microvasculature
8. Homronal irregularities such as low levels of testosterone.

The take-home message is this: a client reporting that they take Viagra on their NAQ should be evaluated for many of the above potential causes of their erectile dysfunction.

UPPER GASTROINTESTINAL SYSTEM

52. Belching or gas one hour after eating
53. Heartburn or acid reflux
54. Bloating shortly after eating (within 1 hour)
55. Vegan (no dairy, meat, fish or eggs)
56. Bad breath (halitosis)
57. Loss of taste for meat
58. Sweat has a strong odor
59. Stomach upset by taking vitamins
60. Sense of excess fullness after meals
61. Do you feel like skipping breakfast?
62. Do you feel better if you don't eat?
63. Sleepy after meals
64. Fingernails chip, peel or break easily
65. Anemia unresponsive to iron
66. Stomach pains or cramps
67. Diarrhea, chronic
68. Diarrhea shortly after meals
69. Black or tarry colored stools
70. Undigested food in stool

52. Belching or gas one hour after a meal

Belching or gas one hour after a meal is a strong indication of digestive dysfunction with either hypochlorhydria or pancreatic insufficiency. The delayed nature of the belching or gas may point to a pancreatic insufficiency over hypochlorhydria. Lack of pancreatic secretions in the small intestine can lead to putrification of proteins or fermentation of carbohydrates, giving off gas as a by-product. Clients may also complain of bloating in the mid to lower abdomen. Further testing will allow you to determine whether or not this problem is due to hypochlorhydria in the stomach or pancreatic insufficiency in the small intestine.

Clinical experience has shown that these two conditions are often linked and share a common etiology:

- Sympathetic dominance
- Antacid drug use
- Excess sugar and refined foods
- Chronic overeating
- Constant snacking between meals
- Excess carbohydrate and alcohol consumption
- Nutrient deficiencies, especially zinc and thiamin
- H-Pylori infection

As mentioned in the list above, zinc deficiency is closely associated with hypochlorhydria and should therefore be assessed as well.

1° Indication

Pancreatic insufficiency with pancreatic enzyme need

Further assessment	1. Check Ridler enzyme point for tenderness 1 inch below xyphoid and over to the right edge of the rib cage 2. Check for tenderness in the Chapman reflex for the pancreas located in the 7th intercostal space 3. Increased urinary sediment levels

2° Indication

Digestive dysfunction with hydrochloric acid need

Further assessment	1. Check Ridler HCL reflex for tenderness 1 inch below xyphoid and over to the left edge of the rib cage 2. Check for tenderness in the Chapman reflex for the stomach and upper digestion located in 6th intercostal space on the left 3. Gastric acid assessment using Gastrotest 4. Increased urinary indican levels

3° Indication

Zinc insufficiency

Further assessment	1. Check for a positive zinc tally: A client holds a solution of aqueous zinc sulfate in their mouth and tells you if and when they can taste it. An almost immediate very bitter taste indicates the client does not need zinc. Clients who are zinc deficient will report no taste from the solution.

Other indications

Biliary stasis
Toxic bowel

Supplemental Support

1. Betaine HCL, Pepsin, and pancreatin
2. Pancreatic Enzymes
3. Nutritional zinc
4. Bromelain, cellulase, lipase, and amylase
5. Beet juice, taurine, vitamin C and pancreolipase
6. Lactobacillus acidophilus and Bifidobacterium bifidus

Lifestyle changes

Please see handout in the appendix on Diet to aid digestion

NOTES:

53. Heartburn or acid reflux

Most of your clients assume that heartburn or acid reflux is due to a hyperacidity in their stomachs. Their first course of action before consulting with you is to use an over-the-counter antacid or acid blocker. They may have already consulted their MD and gotten a prescription for an acid blocking drug. Whatever the case, symptoms of heartburn or acid reflux are a perfect excuse for you to educate your clients on the importance of stomach acid and the rarity in clinical practice of hyperacidity. Clinical experience testing the pH of client's stomachs has shown that very few people who complain of acid reflux or heartburn are hyperacid. Most of the time, it has to do with an inappropriate timing of stomach acid secretion leading to increased acid secretion when there is no food in the stomach, leading to irritated and inflamed mucosa.

For many people the problem is most likely due to low stomach acid secretion or hypochlorhydria, which can also lead to irritated and inflamed mucosa. Hypochlorhydria sets up the ideal environment for an infection by Helicobacter pylori, an opportunistic bacterium that seems to prefer the chronically irritated environment of the gastric mucosa. H. pylori is associated with gastric ulcers. It is important to rule out H. pylori with clients that have a history of heartburn or acid reflux.

Frequent or chronic heartburn may have a structural component to it too. Hiatal hernia, an outpouching of the stomach lining through the diaphragm, is associated with frequent or chronic heartburn.

Another cause of heartburn or acid reflux is a weak or sensitive esophageal sphincter. The main culprit in this case is overeating, which causes gastric juices to enter through a stretched esophageal sphincter into the esophagus.

Other causes of acid reflux include:

- Obesity
- Cigarette smoking
- Chocolate
- Fried foods
- Carbonated beverages
- Alcohol
- Coffee

Many of the above foods or conditions cause acid reflux by increasing intra-abdominal pressure, a condition which forces gastric contents up into the esophagus, or irritate the esophageal sphincter decreasing the muscular tone of the sphincter.

<u>1° Indication</u>
Gastric irritation with possible ulcer and/or H. pylori infection. May be an indication of gastric hyperacidity.

Further assessment	1. Test for H. pylori 2. Gastric assessment with Gastrotest to determine ambient stomach pH

Other indications

1. Hypochlorhydria
2. Pancreatic insufficiency
3. Biliary stasis
4. Hiatal hernia
5. Helicobacter pylori infection

Supplemental Support

1. Gut healing nutrients and demulscents
2. Chlorophyllins
3. Nutrients that protect the gut from infection
4. Nutrients that heal the intestines
5. Beet juice, taurine, vitamin C and pancreolipase
6. Pancreatic Enzymes

Note: Betaine HCL, Pepsin, and pancreatin may be indicated if client is hypochlorhydric, but make sure to heal mucosa before introducing supplemental HCL.

NOTES:

54. Bloating shortly after eating (within 1 hour)

Bloating shortly after eating (within 1 hour) is an indication of digestive dysfunction with either hypochlorhydria or pancreatic insufficiency. The quick onset of bloating shortly after eating strongly suggests hypochlorhydria as the cause. Low stomach acid can cause gas to build up in the stomach. This is caused by the putrification and fermentation of the stomach content.

Hypochlorhydria has a number of possible etiologies:

- Sympathetic dominance
- Antacid drug use
- Excess sugar and refined foods
- Chronic overeating
- Constant snacking between meals
- Excess carbohydrate and alcohol consumption
- Nutrient deficiencies, especially zinc and thiamin
- H-Pylori infection

Many of the above can lead to irritation of the gastric mucosa causing a decreased output of acid from the parietal cells.

Zinc deficiency is closely associated with hypochlorhydria and should therefore be assessed.

1° Indication

Digestive dysfunction with hydrochloric acid need

Further assessment	1. Check Ridler HCL reflex for tenderness 1 inch below xyphoid and over to the left edge of the rib cage 2. Check for tenderness in the Chapman reflex for the stomach and upper digestion located in 6th intercostal space on the left 3. Gastric acid assessment using Gastrotest 4. Check for a positive zinc tally: A client holds a solution of aqueous zinc sulfate in their mouth and tells you if and when they can taste it. An almost immediate very bitter taste indicates the client does not need zinc. Clients who are zinc deficient will report no taste from the solution. 5. Increased urinary indican levels

2° Indication

Pancreatic insufficiency with pancreatic enzyme need

Further assessment	1. Check Ridler enzyme point for tenderness 1 inch below xyphoid and over to the right edge of the rib cage 2. Check for tenderness in the Chapman reflex for the pancreas located in the 7th intercostal space 3. Increased urinary sediment levels

Other indications

Toxic bowel

Supplemental Support

1. Betaine HCL, Pepsin, and pancreatin
2. Pancreatic Enzymes
3. Bromelain, cellulase, lipase, and amylase
4. Beet juice, taurine, vitamin C and pancreolipase
5. Water soluble fiber and nutrients to support colon health
6. Lactobacillus acidophilus and Bifidobacterium bifidus

Lifestyle changes

1. Chew food thoroughly and eating slowly. Most people eat too fast and swallow air with their food; these can be a major cause of bloating.
2. Please see handout in the appendix on the Diet to aid digestion

NOTES:

55. Are you a vegan (no dairy, meat, fish or eggs)?

Vegans tend to be deficient in B12, an essential nutrient that is difficult to obtain with a vegan diet. Many vegans consume a large portion of their calories from carbohydrates. A high intake of carbohydrates has been linked with an increased risk of developing hypochlorhydria. Adequate stomach acid is essential for the proper absorption of vitamin B12. Vegans are therefore compromised on the supply end and the digestion end of the B12 issue.

A thorough assessment of the upper digestive tract is essential in vegan clients to ensure that the correct mechanism for adequate B12 digestion and absorption is in place. Zinc deficiency has been associated with hypochlorhydria and should therefore be assessed.

1° Indication

Assess for digestive dysfunction for possible hydrochloric acid need

Further assessment	1. Check Ridler HCL reflex for tenderness 1 inch below xyphoid and over to the left edge of the rib cage 2. Check for tenderness in the Chapman reflex for the stomach and upper digestion located in 6th intercostal space on the left 3. Gastric acid assessment using Gastrotest 4. Check for a positive zinc tally: A client holds a solution of aqueous zinc sulfate in their mouth and tells you if and when they can taste it. An almost immediate very bitter taste indicates the client does not need zinc. Clients who are zinc deficient will report no taste from the solution. 5. Increased urinary indican levels

Supplement support

1. Betaine HCL, Pepsin, and pancreatin
2. Nutritional zinc
3. Pancreatic Enzymes
4. Bromelain, cellulase, lipase, and amylase

Lifestyle changes

Please see the handout in the appendix on the Diet to aid digestion

NOTES:

56. Bad breath (halitosis)

Bad breath or halitosis is an indication of a disturbed digestive system. It is indicative of a bowel toxemia in either the small or large intestine with an overgrowth of bacteria or yeast. Some of the causes of bowel toxemia include:

- Hypochlorhydria
- Slow peristalsis or slow bowel transit time and bowel sluggishness
- Constipation
- Exposure to excessive chemicals in the water, food, air, and drugs
- Abnormal bowel flora: yeast/Candida, parasites or bacteria

Bowel toxemia normally starts with a pre-existing hypochlorhydria. Proteins that are not digested and broken down adequately in the stomach form the substrate for bacteria and yeast to proliferate, which produce excess amounts of toxic metabolites. The liver detoxifies toxins produced from the gut. If the liver is not functioning optimally or if the amount of toxin production overwhelms its metabolic capacities, the toxins can enter systemic circulation. The halitosis is a result of these toxic metabolites forming on the breath.

If the digestive system is assessed and any dysfunction is corrected, the chances are that the halitosis will resolve. Halitosis can, of course, be from poor dental hygiene.

<u>1° Indication</u>

Dysbiosis caused by an overgrowth of bacteria or yeast

Further assessment	1. Increased urinary indican levels 2. Stool analysis- either comprehensive digestive analysis or a parasite profile 3. Check for tenderness in the Chapman reflex for the colon located bilaterally along the iliotibial band on the thighs. Palpate the colon for tenderness and tension. 4. Check for tenderness in the Chapman reflex for the small intestine located on the 8th, 9th and 10th intercostal spaces near the tip of the rib. Also palpate four quadrants in a 2" to 3" radius around the umbilicus for tenderness and tension

<u>2° Indication</u>

Pancreatic enzyme need or hydrochloric acid

Further assessment	**Pancreatic enzymes** 1. Check Ridler enzyme point for tenderness 1 inch below xyphoid and over to the right edge of the rib cage 2. Check for tenderness in the Chapman reflex for the pancreas located in the 7th intercostal space 3. Increased urinary sediment levels **Hydrochloric acid** 1. Check Ridler HCL reflex for tenderness 1 inch below xyphoid and over to the left edge of the rib cage 2. Check for tenderness in the Chapman reflex for the stomach

	and upper digestion located in 6th intercostal space on the left 3. Gastric acid assessment using Gastrotest 4. Check for a positive zinc tally: A client holds a solution of aqueous zinc sulfate in their mouth and tells you if and when they can taste it. An almost immediate very bitter taste indicates the client does not need zinc. Clients who are zinc deficient will report no taste from the solution. 5. Increased urinary indican levels

Supplemental Support

1. Micro Emulsified Oregano
2. Nutrients that heal the intestines
3. Betaine HCL, Pepsin, and pancreatin
4. Water soluble fiber and nutrients to support colon health
5. Multiple nutrients that support the immune system
6. Pancreatic Enzymes
7. Broad spectrum proteolytic enzymes
8. Lactobacillus acidophilus and Bifidobacterium bifidus

Lifestyle changes:

Please see the handouts in the appendix on the Dysbiosis diet and the Diet to aid digestion

NOTES:

57. Loss of taste for meat

This is a symptom strongly suggestive of digestive dysfunction with incomplete digestion of proteins. The most likely cause of this is hypochlorhydria. Hypochlorhydria is a very common problem and leads to a number of digestive complaints including H. pylori infection, bowel toxemia, dysbiosis, pancreatic insufficiency and leaky gut syndrome.

Hypochlorhydria has a number of possible etiologies that include:

- Sympathetic dominance
- Antacid drug use
- Excess sugar and refined foods
- Chronic overeating
- Constant snacking between meals
- Excess carbohydrate and alcohol consumption
- Nutrient deficiencies, especially zinc and thiamin
- H-Pylori infection

Many of the above can lead to irritation of the gastric mucosa causing a decreased output of acid from the parietal cells. One of the side effects of this process is a loss of taste for protein, and especially meat.

I have talked to a number of parents who have expressed exasperation that their young children eat all of the carbohydrate on their plates but will not touch the protein. In my experience giving the child a low dose of supplemental HCL prior to the meal usually results in the protein being eaten. The low dose form or HCL I recommend is Betaine HCL mixed with pepsin, and Pancreatin. Each tablet should ideally contain 150mg of betaine HCL, pepsin and pancreatin 4X.

Zinc deficiency is closely associated with hypochlorhydria and I recommend assessing zinc levels in all clients complaining of digestive complaints.

<u>1° Indication</u>

Digestive dysfunction with hydrochloric acid, pepsin and protease need

Further assessment	1. Check Ridler HCL reflex for tenderness 1 inch below xyphoid and over to the left edge of the rib cage 2. Check for tenderness in the Chapman reflex for the stomach and upper digestion located in 6th intercostal space on the left 3. Gastric acid assessment using Gastrotest 4. Check for a positive zinc tally: A client holds a solution of aqueous zinc sulfate in their mouth and tells you if and when they can taste it. An almost immediate very bitter taste indicates the client does not need zinc. Clients who are zinc deficient will report no taste from the solution. 5. Increased urinary indican levels

Supplement support

1. Betaine HCL, Pepsin, and pancreatin
2. Nutritional zinc
3. Pancreatic Enzymes
4. Bromelain, cellulase, lipase, and amylase

Lifestyle changes

Please see the handout in the appendix on the diet to aid digestion

58. Sweat has a strong odor

Sweat having a strong odor is a sign of need for liver or kidney support. It is also a sign of possible magnesium deficiency. The sweat glands are another excretory organ, and the more toxic the body, the more toxic the sweat is likely to be. With adequate liver detoxification and kidney excretion, it is less likely that the sweat glands and the skin in general will act as a primary excretory organ.

Another possible cause is bowel toxemia. Bowel toxemia normally starts with a pre-existing hypochlorhydria. Proteins that are not digested and broken down adequately in the stomach form the substrate for bacteria and yeast to proliferate, which produce excess amounts of toxic metabolites. The liver detoxifies toxins produced from the gut. If the liver is not functioning optimally or if the amount of toxin production overwhelms its metabolic capacities, the toxins can enter systemic circulation. The sweat serves a major excretory function and if the kidney or liver is dysfunctional the body will use the skin as a route of elimination. The toxic metabolites usually have a strong odor that can be smelt on the breath and in the urine as well as in the sweat.

1° Indication

Liver congestion with detoxification problems

Further assessment	1. Check for tenderness in the Chapman reflex for the liver-gallbladder located over the 6th intercostal space on the right side 2. Check for tenderness in the Liver point located on the 3rd rib, 3 " to the right of the sternum, at the costochondral junction. 3. Check for tenderness underneath the right rib cage 4. Increased SGOT, SGPT on a blood chemistry panel 5. Assess for Hepato-biliary congestion with the Acoustic Cardiogram (ACG), which will show post-systolic rounding due to increased backpressure on the pulmonic and aortic valve. It may also show through to the tricuspid valve if chronic. 6. Various labs do liver detoxification panels

2° Indication

Need to support kidney function to promote adequate elimination

Further assessment	1. Check for tenderness in the Chapman reflex for the kidneys located 1" lateral and 1" superior from the umbilicus on the medial margin of the Rectus abdominus muscle. Have clients tighten stomach muscles to palpate. 2. Check for an increase in blood pressure when the client goes from standing to supine 3. Routine and functional 24-hour urinalysis 4. Blood chemistry renal function panel

Other indications

Bowel toxemia

Supplemental Support

1. Nutrients to support Phase II liver detoxification
2. Herbs that cleanse the liver
3. Glutathione, cysteine, and glycine
4. Powdered detoxification support formula
5. Plant source molybdenum
6. Calcium d-glucarate
7. Multiple nutrients for supporting renal function
8. Kidney tissue (neonatal bovine)
9. Culture of Beet Juice containing Arginase
10. Magnesium
11. Pyridoxal-5-phosphate

Lifestyle changes

Please see the handouts in the appendix on "How to keep the liver healthy". You may also want to put your clients on a dysbiosis diet to deal with the toxic bowel.

NOTES:

59. Stomach upset by taking vitamins

This is a clear sign of hypochlorhydria and a need for supplemental HCL. Low stomach acid can cause discomfort when taking supplemental vitamins. Hypochlorhydria is a very common problem and leads to a number of digestive complaints including H. pylori infection, bowel toxemia, dysbiosis, pancreatic insufficiency and leaky gut syndrome.

Hypochlorhydria has a number of possible etiologies that include:

- Sympathetic dominance
- Antacid drug use
- Excess sugar and refined foods
- Chronic overeating
- Constant snacking between meals
- Excess carbohydrate and alcohol consumption
- Nutrient deficiencies, especially zinc and thiamin
- H-Pylori infection

Many of the above can lead to irritation of the gastric mucosa causing a decreased output of acid from the parietal cells. Sensitivity to supplements is one of the potential side effects of this process.

I have noticed clinically that many people with hypochlorhydria are sensitive to zinc and feel nauseated taking supplemental zinc. Zinc deficiency is strongly associated with hypochlorhydria because zinc is an essential nutrient in the production of HCL from the parietal cells. I recommend that you assess for zinc levels in all clients suffering from gastrointestinal complaints. It is also worth noting that people who have a difficulty swallowing their supplements may also by in need of supplemental HCL.

1° Indication

Hypochlorhydria with hydrochloric acid need

Further assessment	1. Check Ridler HCL reflex for tenderness 1 inch below xyphoid and over to the left edge of the rib cage 2. Check for tenderness in the Chapman reflex for the stomach and upper digestion located in 6th intercostal space on the left 3. Check for a positive zinc tally: A client holds a solution of aqueous zinc sulfate in their mouth and tells you if and when they can taste it. An almost immediate very bitter taste indicates the client does not need zinc. Clients who are zinc deficient will report no taste from the solution. 4. Gastric acid assessment using Gastrotest 5. Increased urinary indican levels

Supplemental support

1. Betaine HCL, Pepsin, and pancreatin

Lifestyle changes: Please see the handout on the diet to aid digestion

60. Sense of excess fullness after meals

A sense of fullness after meals is an indication of digestive dysfunction with either hypochlorhydria or pancreatic insufficiency. Hypochlorhydria leads to a decreased efficiency in protein digestion, so the body retains food in the stomach to prolong digestion. This leads to a feeling of excessive fullness. Another cause of excessive fullness may be the production of gas in the stomach or small intestine. This leads to a feeling of being bloated. .

Hypochlorhydria is a very common problem and leads to a number of digestive complaints including H. pylori infection, bowel toxemia, dysbiosis, pancreatic insufficiency and leaky gut syndrome. Hypochlorhydria has a number of possible etiologies that include:

- Sympathetic dominance
- Antacid drug use
- Excess sugar and refined foods
- Chronic overeating
- Constant snacking between meals
- Excess carbohydrate and alcohol consumption
- Nutrient deficiencies, especially zinc and thiamin
- H-Pylori infection

Zinc levels should be assessed because insufficient production of stomach HCL is strongly associated with Zinc deficiency.

<u>1° Indication</u>

Digestive dysfunction with hydrochloric acid need

Further assessment	1. Check Ridler HCL reflex for tenderness 1 inch below xyphoid and over to the left edge of the rib cage 2. Check for tenderness in the Chapman reflex for the stomach and upper digestion located in 6th intercostal space on the left 3. Gastric acid assessment using Gastrotest 4. Check for a positive zinc tally: A client holds a solution of aqueous zinc sulfate in their mouth and tells you if and when they can taste it. An almost immediate very bitter taste indicates the client does not need zinc. Clients who are zinc deficient will report no taste from the solution. 5. Increased urinary indican levels

<u>2° Indication</u>

Pancreatic insufficiency with pancreatic enzyme need

Further assessment	1. Check Ridler enzyme point for tenderness 1 inch below xyphoid and over to the right edge of the rib cage 2. Check for tenderness in the Chapman reflex for the pancreas located in the 7th intercostal space 3. Increased urinary sediment levels

Other indications

1. Biliary stasis
2. Toxic bowel

Supplemental Support

1. Betaine HCL, Pepsin, and pancreatin
2. Pancreatic Enzymes
3. Bromelain, cellulase, lipase, and amylase
4. Beet juice, taurine, vitamin C and pancreolipase
5. Water soluble fiber and nutrients to support colon health
6. Lactobacillus acidophilus and Bifidobacterium bifidus

Lifestyle changes

Please see the handout in the appendix on the Diet to aid digestion

NOTES:

61. Do you feel like skipping breakfast?

This is a sign of HCL or pancreatic enzyme need. This is a pattern seen in clients who eat a large dinner very fast without chewing it properly. Unfortunately this causes the food to stay in the digestive system for a longer period of time, and in the morning they are still digesting and do not feel hungry. Encourage the client to break this habit by eating a smallish breakfast, having regular meals throughout the day and encouraging an earlier, lighter dinner. Zinc deficiency has been associated with hypochlorhydria and should therefore be assessed.

1° Indication

Hydrochloric acid or Pancreatic enzyme need

Further assessment	**Hydrochloric acid** 1. Check Ridler HCL reflex for tenderness 1 inch below xyphoid and over to the left edge of the rib cage 2. Check for tenderness in the Chapman reflex for the stomach and upper digestion located in 6th intercostal space on the left 3. Gastric acid assessment using Gastrotest 4. Check for a positive zinc tally: A client holds a solution of aqueous zinc sulfate in their mouth and tells you if and when they can taste it. An almost immediate very bitter taste indicates the client does not need zinc. Clients who are zinc deficient will report no taste from the solution. 5. Increased urinary indican levels **Pancreatic enzymes** 1. Check Ridler enzyme point for tenderness 1 inch below xyphoid and over to the right edge of the rib cage 2. Check for tenderness in the Chapman reflex for the pancreas located in the 7th intercostal space 3. Increased urinary sediment levels

Other indications

Hypoglycemia with glycogen storage problem. Client can skip breakfast but needs 2-3 cups of coffee to get their blood sugar up.

Supplemental Support

1. Betaine HCL, Pepsin, and pancreatin
2. Pancreatic Enzymes
3. Bromelain, cellulase, lipase, and amylase
4. Beet juice, taurine, vitamin C and pancreolipase

Lifestyle changes

Please see the handout in the appendix on the Diet to aid digestion

62. Do you feel better if you don't eat?

For many people eating has become an uncomfortable process. This is mainly due to an inflamed gastric mucosa that is irritated by food and digestive juices. For others eating is synonymous with heartburn and acid reflux. Interestingly enough these two patterns share a common etiology: hypochlorhydria and low pancreatic enzyme output leading to a damaged, irritated and inflamed gastric lining.

Most of your clients assume that the pain they experience with eating is caused by hyperacidity in their stomachs. Their first course of action before consulting with you is usually to use an over-the-counter antacid or acid blocker. They may have already consulted their MD and gotten a prescription for an acid blocking drug. Whatever the case, the pain they experience is most likely due to low stomach acid secretion or hypochlorhydria, which can also lead to irritated and inflamed mucosa. Hypochlorhydria sets up the ideal environment for an infection by Helicobacter pylori, an opportunistic bacterium that seems to prefer the chronically irritated environment of the gastric mucosa. H. pylori is associated with gastric ulcers. It is important to rule out H. pylori with clients that have a history of heartburn or acid reflux.

Many clients will tell you that eating causes frequent or chronic heartburn. It is important that heartburn may have a structural component to it too. Hiatal hernia, an outpouching of the stomach lining through the diaphragm, is associated with frequent or chronic heartburn.

Another cause of heartburn or acid reflux is a weak or sensitive esophageal sphincter. The main culprit in this case is overeating, which causes gastric juices to enter through a stretched esophageal sphincter into the esophagus. Other causes include:

- Obesity
- Cigarette smoking
- Chocolate
- Fried foods
- Carbonated beverages
- Alcohol
- Coffee

Many of the above foods or conditions cause acid reflux by increasing intra-abdominal pressure, a condition which forces gastric contents up into the esophagus, or irritate the esophageal sphincter decreasing the muscular tone of the sphincter.

Acid reflux, hernia and reflux are all common reasons why clients may say they feel better if they do not eat. It is important to thoroughly assess the digestive system and to look at the types of food your clients are eating. Sometimes it is simply a case of changing the foods they eat.

<u>1° Indication</u>
Hydrochloric acid or Pancreatic enzyme need leading to an irritated gastric mucosa

Further assessment	**Hydrochloric acid** 1. Check Ridler HCL reflex for tenderness 1 inch below xyphoid and over to the left edge of the rib cage

	2. Check for tenderness in the Chapman reflex for the stomach and upper digestion located in 6th intercostal space on the left 3. Gastric acid assessment using Gastrotest 4. Check for a positive zinc tally: A client holds a solution of aqueous zinc sulfate in their mouth and tells you if and when they can taste it. An almost immediate very bitter taste indicates the client does not need zinc. Clients who are zinc deficient will report no taste from the solution. 5. Increased urinary indican levels **Pancreatic enzymes** 1. Check Ridler enzyme point for tenderness 1 inch below xyphoid and over to the right edge of the rib cage 2. Check for tenderness in the Chapman reflex for the pancreas located in the 7th intercostal space 3. Increased urinary sediment levels

Supplemental Support

1. Betaine HCL, Pepsin, and pancreatin 2. Pancreatic Enzymes 3. Bromelain, cellulase, lipase, and amylase 4. Beet juice, taurine, vitamin C and pancreolipase

<u>Lifestyle changes</u>

Please see the handout in the appendix on the Diet to aid digestion

NOTES:

63. Sleepy after meals

Being sleepy after meals is a sign of blood sugar dysregulation, or inadequate digestion, which leaves a heavy amount of food in the digestive system that needs to be digested. An increased carbohydrate load in a meal, without adequate protein and fat to provide a balance, will lead to an increase in insulin. Increased insulin will lower the blood sugar very rapidly, leading to a concomitant lowering of the blood glucose. This causes post-prandial sleepiness. This is a common complaint after lunch, which tends to be a meal heavily weighted towards carbohydrates. Having the correct protein carbohydrate ratio in each meal will increase energy after the meal and ensure that the energy is long lasting.

Clients with digestive dysfunction also complain of being sleepy after meals. This is due to a large amount of energy being used up by the body to digest food in an environment that is lacking the necessary gastric juices and enzymes. It is important to remember that the symptom of being sleepy after meals is not just a problem with blood sugar dysregulation. Consider that clients with this symptom may also be suffering from hypochlorhydria, which is a very common problem and leads to a number of digestive complaints including H. pylori infection, bowel toxemia, dysbiosis, pancreatic insufficiency and leaky gut syndrome.

Hypochlorhydria has a number of possible etiologies that include:

- Sympathetic dominance
- Antacid drug use
- Excess sugar and refined foods
- Chronic overeating
- Constant snacking between meals
- Excess carbohydrate and alcohol consumption
- Nutrient deficiencies, especially zinc and thiamin
- H-Pylori infection

Zinc deficiency has also been associated with hypochlorhydria and should therefore be assessed.

1° Indication

Blood sugar dysregulation

Further assessment	1. Check for tenderness in the Chapman reflex for the liver-gallbladder located over the 6th intercostal space on the right side 2. Check for tenderness in the Liver point located on the 3rd rib, 3 " to the right of the sternum, at the costochondral junction. 3. Check for tenderness underneath the right rib cage 4. Check for tenderness or nodularity in the right thenar pad, which is a pancreas indicator if tender 5. Check for tenderness in the Chapman reflex for the pancreas located in the 7th intercostal space on the left 6. Check for tenderness or guarding at the head of the pancreas located in the upper left quadrant of the abdominal region 1/2 to 2/3 of the way between the umbilicus and the angle of the ribs

Further Assessment	7. Check for tenderness in the inguinal ligament bilaterally, an adrenal indicator 8. Check for tenderness at the medial knee bilaterally, at the insertion of the sartorius muscle at the Pes Anserine. This is an adrenal indicator. 9. Check for a paradoxical pupillary reflex by shining a light into a client's eye and grading the reaction of the pupil. A pupil that fails to constrict indicates adrenal exhaustion 10. Check for the presence of postural hypotension. A drop of more than 10 points is an indication of adrenal insufficiency. 11. Check for a chronic short leg due to a posterior-inferior ilium. An adrenal indicator when confirmed with postural hypotension and a paradoxical pupillary response. 12. Check fasting blood glucose 13. Run a six-hour glucose-insulin tolerance test.

2° Indication

Digestive dysfunction with hydrochloric acid need

Further assessment	1. Check Ridler HCL reflex for tenderness 1 inch below xyphoid and over to the left edge of the rib cage 2. Check for tenderness in the Chapman reflex for the stomach and upper digestion located in 6th intercostal space on the left 3. Gastric acid assessment using Gastrotest 4. Check for a positive zinc tally: A client holds a solution of aqueous zinc sulfate in their mouth and tells you if and when they can taste it. An almost immediate very bitter taste indicates the client does not need zinc. Clients who are zinc deficient will report no taste from the solution. 5. Increased urinary indican levels

3° Indication

Pancreatic insufficiency with pancreatic enzyme need

Further assessment	1. Check Ridler enzyme point for tenderness 1 inch below xyphoid and over to the right edge of the rib cage 2. Check for tenderness in the Chapman reflex for the pancreas located in the 7th intercostal space 3. Increased urinary sediment levels

Supplemental Support

1. Multiple nutrients for blood sugar handling problems 2. Adrenal tissue (neonatal bovine) and adaptogenic herbs for adrenal function 3. High dose synthetic vitamin B complex 4. Nutritional zinc 5. Betaine HCL, Pepsin, and pancreatin 6. Pancreatic enzymes

Lifestyle changes

Please see the handout in the appendix on the Recommendations for controlling blood sugar and the Diet to aid digestion

64. Fingernails chip, peel or break easily

Fingernails that chip, break or peel easily are a sign of hypochlorhydria and a number of nutritional deficiencies: protein, trace minerals and essential fatty acids. The protein and trace mineral deficiencies are caused by low stomach acid and pancreatic insufficiency.

Hypochlorhydria is a very common problem and leads to a number of digestive complaints including H. pylori infection, bowel toxemia, dysbiosis, pancreatic insufficiency and leaky gut syndrome. Hypochlorhydria has a number of possible etiologies that include:

- Sympathetic dominance
- Antacid drug use
- Excess sugar and refined foods
- Chronic overeating
- Constant snacking between meals
- Excess carbohydrate and alcohol consumption
- Nutrient deficiencies, especially zinc and thiamin
- H-Pylori infection

Many of the above can lead to irritation of the gastric mucosa causing a decreased output of acid from the parietal cells. It is essential that we have enough stomach acid to adequately digest and break down our foods. Protein and trace minerals especially rely on this process to make the nutrients available for absorption and assimilation into the blood stream. The fingernails are composed of structural molecules that are assimilated from the food we eat. Without optimum digestion we cannot adequately absorb these structural molecules and the fingernails become weak and brittle. Assessing for digestive function and ensuring good quality nutrients in the diet will allow the fingernails to strengthen over time.

1° Indication

Protein and mineral deficiency secondary to maldigestion

Further assessment	**Hydrochloric acid** 1. Check Ridler HCL reflex for tenderness 1 inch below xyphoid and over to the left edge of the rib cage 2. Check for tenderness in the Chapman reflex for the stomach and upper digestion located in 6th intercostal space on the left 3. Gastric acid assessment using Gastrotest 4. Check for a positive zinc tally: A client holds a solution of aqueous zinc sulfate in their mouth and tells you if and when they can taste it. An almost immediate very bitter taste indicates the client does not need zinc. Clients who are zinc deficient will report no taste from the solution. 5. Increased urinary indican levels **Pancreatic enzymes** 1. Check Ridler enzyme point for tenderness 1 inch below xyphoid and over to the right edge of the rib cage 2. Check for tenderness in the Chapman reflex for the pancreas located in the 7th intercostal space 3. Increased urinary sediment levels

2° Indication
Essential fatty acid deficiency.

Further assessment	4. Oral pH less than 7.2 indicates essential fatty acid deficiency 5. Repeated muscle challenge. This challenge involves a simple, normal muscle test repeated once per second, 20 times with regular intensity. As in a standard muscle test, the joint is positioned in such a way that the muscle to be tested is shortened. The practitioner applies pressure to the joint to lengthen the muscle, until a "locking" is noted. A positive result occurs when "locking" of the muscle and joint does not occur, indicating deficient free fatty acids. 6. Fatty acid profile via laboratory testing of blood

Other indications
1. Biliary insufficiency- need for bile salts
2. B Complex deficiency
3. Magnesium and vitamin B6 are needed as co-factors in fat metabolism

Supplemental Support
1. Betaine HCL, Pepsin, and pancreatin
2. Pancreatic enzyme
3. Bromelain, cellulase, lipase, and amylase
4. Multiple mineral without iron or copper
5. Broad spectrum amino acids
6. Flax Seed Oil caps
7. Blackcurrant Seed oil
8. EPA and DHA from fish oil
9. Mixed fatty acids (walnut, hazelnut, sesame, and apricot)
10. Beet juice and bile salts
11. Phosphatidylcholine

Lifestyle changes
Please see handout in the appendix on the Diet to aid digestion

NOTES:

65. Anemia unresponsive to iron

An anemia that is not responsive to iron may be sign of digestion and/or absorption problems. The client may not be absorbing the supplemental iron due to a low amount of stomach acid. Also, many doctors give iron for an anemia before considering its true cause. An anemia that is unresponsive to iron may be due to some other nutritional deficiency, especially B12 and folic acid. Vitamin B12 requires adequate stomach acid for its absorption. Zinc deficiency has been associated with hypochlorhydria and should therefore be assessed.

1° Indication

Digestion and/or absorption problems due to low stomach acid

Further assessment	1. Check Ridler HCL reflex for tenderness 1 inch below xyphoid and over to the left edge of the rib cage 2. Check for tenderness in the Chapman reflex for the stomach and upper digestion located in 6th intercostal space on the left 3. Gastric acid assessment using Gastrotest 4. Check for a positive zinc tally: A client holds a solution of aqueous zinc sulfate in their mouth and tells you if and when they can taste it. An almost immediate very bitter taste indicates the client does not need zinc. Clients who are zinc deficient will report no taste from the solution. 5. Increased urinary indican levels

2° Indication

Anemia that is not due to iron deficiency

Further assessment	1. CBC and blood chemistry screen. If MCV is above 90, the client may be B12 and folic acid deficient

Supplemental Support

1. Betaine HCL, Pepsin, and Pancreatin 2. Pancreatic enzymes 3. Nutritional zinc 4. Vitamin B12 and folic acid 5. B vitamin complex

NOTES:

66. Stomach pains or cramps

Stomach pains or cramps can be an indication of an acute abdomen, which needs to be thoroughly assessed. If pathology is ruled out consider the following as causes of generalized inflammation: foods allergies, upper GI bleeding, gastritis and Irritable Bowel Syndrome (IBS).

Also consider that the client may be suffering from a dysbiotic bowel, a possible parasitic infection, or they are allergic to certain food. A client that is allergic to gluten will complain of stomach crams and pain, as will a client that is lactose intolerant. There are many good labs that allow you to make accurate assessments of your clients' gastrointestinal environment and possible food allergies.

Checking the Chapman reflex for the stomach is a good general indicator for dysfunction in the upper bowel and inflammation in the upper GI, especially in clients with a poor tolerance for supplemental HCL or digestive enzymes. The reflexes for the small and large intestine are good general indicators for dysfunction further down the digestive tract.

1° Indication

Assess upper gastrointestinal system

Further assessment	1. Check for tenderness in the Chapman reflex for the stomach and upper digestion located in 6th intercostal space on the left 2. Check Ridler HCL reflex for tenderness 1 inch below xyphoid and over to the left edge of the rib cage 3. Gastric acid assessment using Gastrotest 4. Check for a positive zinc tally: A client holds a solution of aqueous zinc sulfate in their mouth and tells you if and when they can taste it. An almost immediate very bitter taste indicates the client does not need zinc. Clients who are zinc deficient will report no taste from the solution. 5. Increased urinary indican levels 6. Increased urine sediment levels

2° Indication

Assess lower gastrointestinal system

Further assessment	1. Increased urinary indican and sediment levels 2. Stool analysis- either comprehensive digestive analysis or a parasite profile 3. Check for tenderness in the Chapman reflex for the colon located bilaterally along the iliotibial band on the thighs. Palpate the colon for tenderness and tension. 4. Check for tenderness in the Chapman reflex for the small intestine located on the 8th, 9th and 10th intercostal spaces near the tip of the rib. Also palpate four quadrants in a 2" to 3" radius around the umbilicus for tenderness and tension 5. Increased secretory IgA on stool analysis

Supplemental Support

1. Betaine HCL, Pepsin, and pancreatin
2. Pancreatic Enzymes
3. Nutritional zinc
4. Bromelain, cellulase, lipase, and amylase
5. Beet juice, taurine, vitamin C and pancreolipase
6. Lactobacillus acidophilus and Bifidobacterium bifidus

Lifestyle changes: Please see handout in the appendix on Diet to aid digestion

NOTES:

67. Diarrhea, chronic

Diarrhea refers to an increased frequency, volume, or fluidity of stool and is a common symptom of many conditions. Diarrhea is usually a mild episode lasting just a few days and is a way for the body to cleanse itself of irritants. However, it can also be an indication of a serious underlying condition. Diarrhea can be due to a variety of causes including infections or overgrowth of bacteria, viruses, or parasites (sometimes secondary to antibiotic use); the use of laxatives or medications causing increased motility; inflammatory bowel disease; malabsorption; emotional stress; and food allergies.

The main dangers of Diarrhea include dehydration and mineral or electrolyte imbalance, malabsorption, weight loss, or the presence of a more serious underlying condition. Below are some general recommendations to control Diarrhea. If Diarrhea lasts for more than a few days, is severe and acute, contains blood or pus, or is associated with a high fever, weight loss, listlessness, severe cramping, or vomiting, see your clinician. Its cause must be determined and treated.

Generally, if the cause is in the small intestine, the Diarrhea is characterized by large quantities of water and/or fatty stools; if the Diarrhea is due to disease in or of the colon, the stool are frequent and often accompanied by blood, mucus or pus; it the disease is rectal in origin, there are often frequent movements of a small amount of stool.

<u>1° Indication</u>
Intestinal parasites and/or dysbiosis

Further assessment	1. CBC to see if eosinophils or basophils are elevated 2. Stool test for ova and parasite can help detect which parasite, if any, is present. Start with one random stool. If no parasite is found and the index of suspicion is high repeat the stool test, but this time do a purged sample with either a large bolus of vitamin C or magnesium sulfate. Collect the next two stools for testing.

<u>2° Indication</u>
Malabsorption- assess small and large intestine

Further assessment	1. Check for tenderness in the Chapman reflex for the colon located bilaterally along the iliotibial band on the thighs. Palpate the colon for tenderness and tension. 2. Check for tenderness in the Chapman reflex for the small intestine located on the 8th, 9th and 10th intercostal spaces near the tip of the rib. Also palpate four quadrants in a 2" to 3" radius around the umbilicus for tenderness and tension 3. Increased urinary indican and sediment 4. Decreased bowel transit time. Have a client check their bowel transit time. Give 6 "00" caps of activated charcoal and ask them to record how long it takes for the black to appear and to go completely away.

Other indications

1. Too much vitamin C or magnesium can make stool loose
2. Lactose intolerance
3. Consumption of sorbitol, mannitol and other types of insoluble sugars

Supplemental Support

1. Bentonite Clay
2. Micro Emulsified Oregano
3. Water soluble fiber and nutrients to support colon health
4. Nutrients that heal the intestines
5. Gut healing nutrients and demulscents
6. Betaine HCL, Pepsin, and pancreatin
7. Pancreatic enzymes
8. Chlorophyllins

Lifestyle changes

Please see the handout in the appendix on recommendations for Diarrhea

NOTES:

68. Diarrhea shortly after meals

Diarrhea shortly after meals is most often an indication of food intolerance. The body will often attempt to remove an intolerant or irritating food by causing diarrhea. It is also a sign of biliary insufficiency, especially if there is fat in the stool, a condition called steatorrhea. Irritable bowel syndrome (IBS) is characterized by loose stools shortly after meals.

<u>1° Indication</u>

Assess upper gastrointestinal system

Further assessment	1. Check for tenderness in the Chapman reflex for the stomach and upper digestion located in 6th intercostal space on the left 2. Check Ridler HCL reflex for tenderness 1 inch below xyphoid and over to the left edge of the rib cage 3. Gastric acid assessment using Gastrotest 4. Check for a positive zinc tally: A client holds a solution of aqueous zinc sulfate in their mouth and tells you if and when they can taste it. An almost immediate very bitter taste indicates the client does not need zinc. Clients who are zinc deficient will report no taste from the solution. 5. Increased urinary indican levels 6. Increased urine sediment levels

<u>2° Indication</u>

Malabsorption- assess small and large intestine

Further assessment	1. Check for tenderness in the Chapman reflex for the colon located bilaterally along the iliotibial band on the thighs. Palpate the colon for tenderness and tension. 2. Check for tenderness in the Chapman reflex for the small intestine located on the 8th, 9th and 10th intercostal spaces near the tip of the rib. Also palpate four quadrants in a 2" to 3" radius around the umbilicus for tenderness and tension 3. Increased urinary indican and sediment 4. Decreased bowel transit time. Have a client check their bowel transit time. Give 6 "00" caps of activated charcoal and ask them to record how long it takes for the black to appear and to go completely away. Various dyes, including beets, and un-popped popcorn can also be used.

<u>3° Indication</u>

Biliary insufficiency with possible biliary stasis

Further assessment	1. Check for tenderness underneath the right rib cage 2. Check for tenderness and nodulation on the web between thumb and fore-finger of right hand 3. Check for tenderness in the Chapman reflex for the liver-gallbladder located over the 6th intercostal space on the right side

Other indications

1. Dysbiosis
2. Too much vitamin C or magnesium can make stool loose
3. Lactose intolerance
4. Consumption of sorbitol, mannitol and other types of insoluble sugars

Supplemental Support

1. Betaine HCL, Pepsin, and pancreatin
2. Pancreatic Enzymes
3. Nutritional zinc
4. Water soluble fiber and nutrients to support colon health
5. Beet juice, taurine, vitamin C and pancreolipase with or without bile salts
6. Gut healing nutrients and demulscents
7. Lactobacillus acidophilus and Bifidobacterium bifidus
8. Chlorophyllins

Lifestyle changes

Please see the handout in the appendix on recommendations for Diarrhea

NOTES:

69. Black or tarry stools

Black or tarry stools are usually a result of bleeding into upper GI tract. This is a serious sign and needs immediate investigation to rule out pathology (ulcer, Crohn's disease, colitis, cancer etc.). Also enquire whether your clients are consuming iron, charcoal or bismuth products. Bismuth is found in over the counter medication, such as Pepto-Bismol and other nutritional supplements. When bismuth oxidizes in the GI tract it turns black, and could therefore stain the stool. A heavy meat diet can also cause black stools.

1° Indication

Bleeding in the gastrointestinal tract

Further assessment	1. Test for occult blood 2. Refer to gastroenterologist for further evaluation and assessment

NOTES:

70. Undigested food in stool

Undigested food in the stool is usually suggestive of a client not chewing their food well. It is also associated with a pancreatic insufficiency with a need for digestive enzymes and/or hypochlorhydria with a need for supplemental stomach acid.

Hypochlorhydria is a very common problem and leads to a number of digestive complaints including H. pylori infection, bowel toxemia, dysbiosis, pancreatic insufficiency and leaky gut syndrome.

Hypochlorhydria has a number of possible etiologies that include:

- Sympathetic dominance
- Antacid drug use
- Excess sugar and refined foods
- Chronic overeating
- Constant snacking between meals
- Excess carbohydrate and alcohol consumption
- Nutrient deficiencies, especially zinc and thiamin
- H-Pylori infection

Many of the above can lead to irritation of the gastric mucosa causing a decreased output of acid from the parietal cells. Low stomach acid results in a decreased output of enzymes from the pancreas. The body requires a strongly acidic stimulus from food exiting the stomach to trigger a large output of digestive enzymes from the pancreas into the small intestine. Without this stimulus food entering the small intestine does not get digested adequately leaving undigested food to remain in the stool.

Hypochlorhydria has also been associated with Zinc deficiency, which should be assessed.

<u>1° Indication</u>

Pancreatic enzyme insufficiency with a need for pancreatic enzyme supplementation

Further assessment	1. Check Ridler enzyme point for tenderness 1 inch below xyphoid and over to the right edge of the rib cage 2. Check for tenderness in the Chapman reflex for the pancreas located in the 7th intercostal space 3. Increased urinary sediment levels 4. Chymotrypsin levels on a digestive stool analysis

<u>2° Indication</u>

Digestive dysfunction with hydrochloric acid need

Further assessment	1. Check Ridler HCL reflex for tenderness 1 inch below xyphoid and over to the left edge of the rib cage 2. Check for tenderness in the Chapman reflex for the stomach and upper digestion located in 6th intercostal space on the left 3. Gastric acid assessment using Gastrotest

	4. Check for a positive zinc tally: A client holds a solution of aqueous zinc sulfate in their mouth and tells you if and when they can taste it. An almost immediate very bitter taste indicates the client does not need zinc. Clients who are zinc deficient will report no taste from the solution. 5. Increased urinary indican levels

Supplemental Support

1. Pancreatic Enzymes
2. Bromelain, cellulase, lipase, and amylase
3. Betaine HCL, Pepsin, and pancreatin

Lifestyle changes

Please see the handout in the appendix on the Diet to aid digestion

NOTES:

LIVER AND GALLBLADDER

71. Pain between shoulder blades
72. Stomach upset by greasy foods
73. Greasy or shiny stools
74. Nausea
75. Sea, car or airplane sickness, motion sickness
76. History of morning sickness (1 = yes, 0 = no)
77. Light or clay collared stools
78. Dry skin, itchy feet and/or skin peels on feet
79. Headache over the eye
80. Gallbladder attacks (0 = never, 1 = years ago, 2 = within last year, 3 = within past 3 months)
81. Gallbladder removed (1 = yes, 0 = no)
82. Bitter taste in mouth, especially after meals
83. Become sick if you were to drink wine
84. Easily intoxicated if you were to drink wine
85. Easily hung over if you were to drink wine
86. Alcohol per week (0 = < 3/ week, 1 = < 7/ week, 2 = < 14/ week, 3 = > 14/week)
87. Recovering alcoholic (1 = yes, 0 = no)
88. History of drug or alcohol abuse (1 = yes, 0 = no)
89. History of hepatitis (1 = yes, 0 = no)
90. Long term use of prescription and/or recreational drugs (1 = yes, 0 =no)
91. Sensitive to chemicals (perfume, cleaning agents, etc.)
92. Sensitive to tobacco smoke
93. Exposure to diesel fumes
94. Pain under right side of rib cage
95. Hemorrhoids or varicose veins
96. NutraSweet (aspartame) consumption
97. Bothered by aspartame (NutraSweet)
98. Chronic fatigue or Fibromyalgia

71. Pain between shoulder blades

Pain between the shoulder blades is a sign of gallbladder stasis due to referred pain from the gallbladder radiating up into the shoulder area. This is not a very strong or specific sign, as many other things can cause pain between the shoulder blades including nerve irritation, nerve impingement, bursitis, frozen shoulder, weak pectoralis muscles etc.

1° Indication

Gallbladder dysfunction with biliary stasis and need for liver support

Further assessment	1. Check for tenderness underneath the right rib cage 2. Check for tenderness and nodulation on the web between thumb and fore-finger of right hand 3. Check for tenderness in the Chapman reflex for the liver-gallbladder located over the 6th intercostal space on the right side 4. Blood chemistry and CBC testing for SGOT, SGPT, GGT

Other indications
1. Nerve irritation
2. Weak pectoralis minor muscles

Supplemental Support

1. Beet juice, taurine, vitamin C and pancreolipase with or without bile salts
2. Inositol
3. Phosphatidylcholine
4. Herbs that cleanse the liver
5. Broad spectrum proteolytic enzymes

Lifestyle changes

Please see the handout in the appendix on Healthy lifestyle for a healthy gallbladder.

NOTES:

72. Stomach upset by greasy foods

Fats in the diet require adequate bile production from the liver and adequate bile release from the gallbladder to be properly emulsified and digested. A client who has a stomach upset by greasy foods is in need of gallbladder support. The bile is probably too thick and needs thinning. If the bile does not properly emulsify fats, they can lead to irritation of the small intestine, especially if the fats are from hydrogenated oils.

This client may need to take supplementary bile salts to help with the fat emulsification. Another possible cause is pancreatic insufficiency. The pancreas produces lipase, which aids in the digestion of the emulsified fat.

1° Indication

Biliary stasis due to gallbladder dysfunction

Further assessment	1. Check for tenderness underneath the right rib cage 2. Check for tenderness and nodulation on the web between thumb and fore-finger of right hand 3. Check for tenderness in the Chapman reflex for the liver-gallbladder located over the 6th intercostal space on the right side 4. Blood chemistry and CBC testing for SGOT, SGPT, GGT

2° Indication

Pancreatic insufficiency with pancreatic enzyme need, especially lipase

Further assessment	1. Check Ridler enzyme point for tenderness 1 inch below xyphoid and over to the right edge of the rib cage 2. Check for tenderness in the Chapman reflex for the pancreas located in the 7th intercostal space 3. Increased urinary sediment levels, especially calcium oxalate levels, which are typically elevated in these cases

Other indications

1. Excess fats, especially hydrogenated oils and saturated fats
2. Refined foods in the diet

Supplemental Support

1. Beet juice, taurine, vitamin C and pancreolipase with or without bile salts
2. Phosphatidylcholine
3. Pancreatic enzymes

Lifestyle changes

Please see the handout in the appendix on Healthy lifestyle for a healthy gallbladder

NOTES:

73. Greasy or shiny stools

Greasy or shiny stools are an indication of hepato-biliary dysfunction. Fats in the diet require adequate bile production from the liver and adequate bile release from the gallbladder to be properly emulsified and digested. Decreased output of bile from the gallbladder will cause fat to remain undigested in the small intestine, leading to steatthorea or greasy/shiny stools. There is a strong need for bile salts to help with the emulsification of fats.

Also consider that this client is consuming large amounts of hydrogenated/trans fatty acids or has an excess of difficult to digest fats such as those from deep fried foods. Large levels of these "fake" fats make it difficult for the body to digest and break down the fat in the digestive tract leading to fat being eliminated in the stool.

Another possible cause is pancreatic insufficiency. The pancreas produces lipase, which aids in the digestion of the emulsified fat.

1° Indication

Need for supplementary bile salts

Further assessment	1. Check for tenderness underneath the right rib cage 2. Check for tenderness and nodulation on the web between thumb and fore-finger of right hand 3. Check for tenderness in the Chapman reflex for the liver-gallbladder located over the 6th intercostal space on the right side 4. Blood chemistry and CBC testing for SGOT, SGPT, GGT 5. Increased urinary sediment levels, especially calcium oxalate levels, which are typically elevated in these cases

2° Indication

Pancreatic insufficiency with pancreatic enzyme need, especially lipase

Further assessment	1. Check Ridler enzyme point for tenderness 1 inch below xyphoid and over to the right edge of the rib cage 2. Check for tenderness in the Chapman reflex for the pancreas located in the 7th intercostal space 3. Increased urinary sediment levels, especially calcium oxalate levels, which are typically elevated in these cases

Supplemental Support

1. Beet juice, taurine, vitamin C and pancreolipase with or without bile salts

Lifestyle changes

Please see the handout on "Healthy lifestyle for a healthy gallbladder" for lifestyle and dietary recommendations on how to keep the gallbladder healthy.

74. Nausea

Nausea is often seen with digestive dysfunction. One of the most common causes of nausea is biliary insufficiency or stasis, a condition called cholestasis. The bile is an essential route of elimination of toxins from the liver. When the flow of bile is inhibited toxins can build up in the body leading to a feeling of nausea. Inhibition of bile flow can be caused by a number of different factors, including liver damage. Liver damage can be mild, in the form of an early onset of hepatitis, or severe as is the case in full blown hepatitis. Liver dysfunction that impairs bile flow can have a number of different symptoms including digestive disturbances and nausea. Other digestive causes include inadequate levels of stomach acid, pancreatic insufficiency and excess stomach acid. An irritated mucosal lining of the digestive tract can also cause nausea.

1° Indication

Biliary insufficiency with possible biliary stasis

Further assessment	1. Check for tenderness underneath the right rib cage 2. Check for tenderness and nodulation on the web between thumb and fore-finger of right hand 3. Check for tenderness in the Chapman reflex for the liver-gallbladder located over the 6th intercostal space on the right 4. Blood chemistry and CBC testing for SGOT, SGPT, GGT

2° Indication

Pancreatic insufficiency and stomach acid deficiency

Further assessment	**Pancreatic enzymes** 1. Check Ridler enzyme point for tenderness 1 inch below xyphoid and over to the right edge of the rib cage 2. Check for tenderness in the Chapman reflex for the pancreas located in the 7th intercostal space 3. Increased urinary sediment levels **Hydrochloric acid** 1. Check Ridler HCL reflex for tenderness 1 inch below xyphoid and over to the left edge of the rib cage 2. Check for tenderness in the Chapman reflex for the stomach and upper digestion located in 6th intercostal space on the left 3. Gastric acid assessment using Gastrotest 4. Check for a positive zinc tally: A client holds a solution of aqueous zinc sulfate in their mouth and tells you if and when they can taste it. An almost immediate very bitter taste indicates the client does not need zinc. Clients who are zinc deficient will report no taste from the solution. 5. Increased urinary indican levels

Other indications

1. Drugs/toxins
2. Pregnancy
3. Mechanical obstruction

Supplemental Support

1.	Beet juice, taurine, vitamin C and pancreolipase with or without bile salts
2.	Phosphatidylcholine
3.	Betaine HCL, Pepsin, and pancreatin
4.	Pancreatic enzymes
5.	Gut healing nutrients and demulscents (to soothe irritated mucosa)

Lifestyle changes

Please see the handout in the appendix on Healthy lifestyle for a healthy gallbladder

NOTES:

75. Sea, car or airplane sickness, motion sickness

The most common reason for motion sickness is a disturbance to equilibrium in the organs of balance in the inner ear. It is also a sign of a need for liver and gallbladder support.

1° Indication

Disturbance to inner ear

Further assessment	1. If severe refer to an Otolaryngologist for further assessment

2° Indication

Need for liver and gallbladder support

Further assessment	1. Check for tenderness in the Chapman reflex for the liver-gallbladder located over the 6th intercostal space on the right side 2. Check for tenderness in the Liver point located on the 3rd rib, 3 " to the right of the sternum, at the costochondral junction. 3. Check for tenderness underneath the right rib cage

Supplemental Support

1. Beet juice, taurine, vitamin C and pancreolipase with or without bile salts
2. Nutrients to support Phase II liver detoxification
3. Herbs that cleanse the liver
4. Glutathione, cysteine, and Glycine

Lifestyle changes

- Read or listen to music while traveling and try to keep eyes from outdoor scenery as it flashes past.
- Sip steamy, hot drinks or hold moist, hot towels against the nose when traveling - dry air in vehicle dries out nasal passages.
- Sipping ginger tea
- Please see the handout in the appendix on Recommendations for keeping your liver healthy

NOTES:

76. History of morning sickness (1 = yes, 0 = no)

A history of morning sickness is an indication of liver insufficiency. Morning sickness corresponds with the increase in Beta HCG hormone, which, like most hormones, relies on the liver for proper detoxification and elimination. If the liver, and to some extent the gallbladder, is not able to detoxify hormones, the HCG can linger and cause the symptoms associated with morning sickness. There is a need for liver and gallbladder support, which should also decrease the likelihood of severe morning sickness in subsequent pregnancies.

1° Indication

Need for liver and gallbladder support

Further assessment	1. Check for tenderness in the Chapman reflex for the liver-gallbladder located over the 6th intercostal space on the right side 2. Check for tenderness in the Liver point located on the 3rd rib, 3 " to the right of the sternum, at the costochondral junction. 3. Check for tenderness underneath the right rib cage

Supplemental Support

1. Beet juice, taurine, vitamin C and pancreolipase with or without bile salts
2. Nutrients to support Phase II liver detoxification
3. Herbs that cleanse the liver
4. Glutathione, cysteine, and Glycine
5. Powdered detoxification support formula

Lifestyle changes

- Please see the handout in the appendix on Recommendations for keeping your liver healthy
- Periodic detoxification using the Nutriclear system will help the liver process and handle hormones more effectively

NOTES:

77. Light or clay colored stools

Light or clay colored stools are an indication of biliary insufficiency, which is an inability of the liver cells to produce adequate amounts of bile due to:

- Changes in metabolism (excess hydrogenated oils, excess refined foods, oxidative stress, low fat diets)
- Diseases affecting function (steatosis causing damage to hepatocytes, hepatitis)
- Diseases that reduce levels of hepatocytes (advanced cirrhosis)

There is a strong need for bile salts to help with the emulsification of fats. Fats in the diet require adequate bile production from the liver and adequate bile release from the gallbladder to be properly emulsified and digested. Bile is responsible for providing the pigment to the stool. Without bile the stool takes on a light or clay colored appearance. A client with clay colored stools is in need of gallbladder support, and is likely to become deficient in essential fatty acids if this is not corrected. There is also a difficulty in digesting fats in general, especially those from deep fried foods and hydrogenated oil.

1° Indication
Need for supplementary bile salts

Further assessment	1. Check for tenderness underneath the right rib cage 2. Check for tenderness and nodulation on the web between thumb and fore-finger of right hand 3. Check for tenderness in the Chapman reflex for the liver-gallbladder located over the 6th intercostal space on the right side 4. Blood chemistry and CBC testing for SGOT, SGPT, GGT

Other indications
1. Excess fats in the diet, especially hydrogenated fats
2. Refined foods in the diet

Supplemental Support

1. Beet juice, taurine, vitamin C and pancreolipase with or without bile salts

Lifestyle changes
Please see the handout in the appendix on Healthy lifestyle for a healthy gallbladder

NOTES:

78. Dry skin, itchy feet and/or skin peels on feet

Dry skin, itchy feet with skin peeling off the feet and heels are an indication of essential fatty insufficiency with a concomitant gallbladder dysfunction. All fats in the diet require adequate bile production from the liver and adequate bile release from the gallbladder to be properly emulsified and digested. An inability to emulsify the fats can lead to an essential fatty acid deficiency.

Dry skin, itchy feet and/or skin peeling off the feet is also associated with liver congestion. The liver can easily become overworked from the environmental pollution to the polluted food we put in our bodies. Persistent cracking of the heels indicates a liver gallbladder system that is congested and sluggish, and may be a sign of thyroid abnormality. Clinical experience has shown that cracked heels, when treated as a liver gallbladder issue, resolve quite quickly.

1° Indication

Essential fatty acid insufficiency.

Further assessment	1. Oral pH less that 7.2 indicates essential fatty acid deficiency 2. Repeated muscle challenge. This challenge involves a simple, normal muscle test repeated once per second, 20 times with regular intensity. As in a standard muscle test, the joint is positioned in such a way that the muscle to be tested is shortened. The practitioner applies pressure to the joint to lengthen the muscle, until a "locking" is noted. A positive result occurs when "locking" of the muscle and joint does not occur, indicating deficient free fatty acids. 3. Fatty acid profile via laboratory testing of blood

2° Indication

Liver and gallbladder congestion

Further assessment	1. Check for tenderness in the Chapman reflex for the liver-gallbladder located over the 6th intercostal space on the right 2. Check for tenderness in the Liver point located on the 3rd rib, 3 " to the right of the sternum, at the costochondral junction. 3. Check for tenderness underneath the right rib cage 4. Check for tenderness and nodulation on the web between thumb and fore-finger of right hand 5. Assess for Hepato-biliary congestion with the Acoustic Cardiogram (ACG), which will show post-systolic rounding due to increased backpressure on the pulmonic and aortic valve. It may also show through to the tricuspid valve if chronic.

Other indications

1. Calcium need
2. Need for liver detoxification

Supplemental Support

1. Flax seed oil Caps
2. Blackcurrant Seed Oil
3. EPA and DHA from fish oil
4. Mixed fatty acids (walnut, hazelnut, sesame, and apricot)
5. Phosphatidylcholine
6. Beet juice, taurine, vitamin C and pancreolipase with or without bile salts
7. Herbs that cleanse the liver
8. Glutathione, cysteine, and Glycine
9. Powdered detoxification support formula

Lifestyle changes

- Please see the handouts in the appendix on Healthy lifestyle for a healthy gallbladder

NOTES:

79. Headache over the eye

The gallbladder and liver meridians in the Chinese medicine system pass over the head. Liver and gallbladder congestion often causes headaches over the eye. They may also be due to a pancreatic dysfunction causing either a deficiency in digestive enzymes, or blood sugar dysregulation. If the headaches come in the afternoon or first thing in the morning, then treating the blood sugar dysregulation will be very helpful to prevent these types of headaches.

<u>1° Indication</u>

Liver and gallbladder congestion

Further assessment	1. Check for tenderness in the Chapman reflex for the liver-gallbladder located over the 6th intercostal space on the right side 2. Check for tenderness in the Liver point located on the 3rd rib, 3 " to the right of the sternum, at the costochondral junction. 3. Check for tenderness underneath the right rib cage 4. Check for tenderness and nodulation on the web between thumb and fore-finger of right hand 5. Assess for Hepato-biliary congestion with the Acoustic Cardiogram (ACG), which will show post-systolic rounding due to increased backpressure on the pulmonic and aortic valve. It may also show through to the tricuspid valve if chronic.

<u>2° Indication</u>

Pancreatic dysfunction with pancreatic enzyme need or need for blood sugar control.

Further assessment	1. Check Ridler enzyme point for tenderness 1 inch below xyphoid and over to the right edge of the rib cage 2. Check for tenderness in the Chapman reflex for the pancreas located in the 7th intercostal space on the left 3. Check for tenderness or guarding at the head of the pancreas located in the upper left quadrant of the abdominal region 1/2 to 2/3 of the way between the umbilicus and the angel of the ribs 4. Increased urinary sediment levels 5. Abnormal glucose tolerance

<u>Other indications</u>

1. B vitamin deficiency, especially riboflavin
2. Hidden food allergies

Supplemental Support

1. Phosphatidylcholine
2. Beet juice, taurine, vitamin C and pancreolipase with or without bile salts
3. Herbs that cleanse the liver
4. Multiple nutrients for blood sugar handling problems
5. Pancreatic enzymes

80. Gallbladder attacks (past or present)

A gallbladder attack, or a history of gallbladder attacks, is an indication of the presence of gallstones. Cholestasis, cholecystolithiasis and cholelithiasis are potentially serious problems and should be thoroughly evaluated with ultrasound for acuteness. Once any acute conditions have been ruled out the following can be considered.

Gallbladder symptoms are suggestive of congested bile with the build up of concentrated bile that can cause the precipitation of stones. Therapy must focus on keeping the bile thin and fluid. Bile salts, Iodine and phosphorous are all nutritional therapies for keeping bile thin. Hidden food allergies are another cause.

A gallbladder attack a number of years ago should not be overlooked. Many gallstones are considered silent when there are no associated symptoms. An attack in the past is a sign that an attack in the present may be imminent. Practice preventative medicine and determine the state of health of the gallbladder following the guidelines below.

While there is much evidence to support that a silent gallstone will remain just that, there is also evidence to suggest that if the risk factors associated with gallstone formation are not closely watched a silent gallstone may become symptomatic. Some of the risk factors associated with gallstone and gallbladder attacks include:

- Being female- women are 2 to 4 times more likely to develop gallstones than men. This may be due to increased cholesterol synthesis or suppression of bile acid formation by estrogens.
- Age- gallstone formation is common in people in their 40s and 50s, though gallstones have been found in young children and in the elderly.
- Race- gallstones are most common in Native Americans. This may be due to the rate of cholesterol in the bile.
- Obesity- cholesterol in the bile increases with an increase in body weight.
- Digestive dysfunction
- Prescription medications- certain medications such as oral contraceptives, estrogens and cholesterol lowering drugs (gemfibrozil and clofibrate)

1° Indication

Biliary stasis with thick, congested bile and the threat of gallstones

Further assessment	1. Check for tenderness underneath the right rib cage 2. Check for tenderness and nodulation on the web between thumb and fore-finger of right hand 3. Check for tenderness in the Chapman reflex for the liver-gallbladder located over 6th intercostal space on right side 4. Assess for Hepato-biliary congestion with the Acoustic Cardiogram (ACG), which will show post-systolic rounding due to increased backpressure on the pulmonic and aortic valve. It may also show through to the tricuspid valve if chronic. 5. Iodine test: Use a tincture of 2% iodine solution, and pain a 3" by 3" square on the client's abdomen. The client is to

	leave the patch unwashed until it disappears. The square should still be there in 24 hours. If it has disappeared, there is an indication of iodine need 6. Blood chemistry and CBC testing for SGOT, SGPT, GGT 7. Gallbladder ultrasound

2° Indication

Hidden food allergies

Further assessment	1. Finding and eliminating the hidden food allergies by what ever method you find successful from ELISA/RAST testing through Applied Kinesiology

Supplemental support

1. Beet juice, taurine, vitamin C and pancreolipase (if gall stones)
2. Beet juice and bile salts (if gallbladder removed)
3. Potassium iodide
4. Phosphatidylcholine
5. Pancreatic enzymes
6. Nutritional phosphorous
7. Multiple herbal anti-histamines

Lifestyle changes

- Please see the handouts in the appendix on Healthy lifestyle for a healthy gallbladder
- Avoidance of all identified food allergies
- Castor oil packs applied topically to the right upper quadrant

NOTES:

81. Gallbladder removed (1 = yes, 0 = no)

Gallbladder removal is one of the most commonly performed surgeries in this country. It is estimated that half a million gallbladders are removed in the US each year. The majority of these are removed because of the presence of gallstones. The removal of the gallbladder is often done as an emergency procedure in response to a severe gallbladder attack.

It has often been thought that the gallbladder is a redundant organ that can be removed without too much harm to the client. This could not be further from the truth. The gallbladder is an essential organ and people who have had their gallbladders removed are unable to adequately emulsify and digest fat. They may complain of digestive discomfort that can be attributed to irritation from bile that is continually dripping into the small intestine. Clients with their gallbladders removed need gallbladder support and bile salt supplementation.

Clients' without gallbladders are also likely to be deficient in essential fatty acids. It is essential to check EFA levels in clients with no gallbladders and begin to work on getting their bodies replete in the essential fats.

1° Indication

Need for supplementary bile salts

Further assessment	1. Check for tenderness underneath the right rib cage 2. Check for tenderness and nodulation on the web between thumb and fore-finger of right hand 3. Check for tenderness in the Chapman reflex for the liver-gallbladder located over the 6th intercostal space on the right side 4. Blood chemistry and CBC testing for SGOT, SGPT, GGT

2° Indication

Essential fatty acid insufficiency.

Further assessment	1. Oral pH less that 7.2 indicates essential fatty acid deficiency 2. Repeated muscle challenge. This challenge involves a simple, normal muscle test repeated once per second, 20 times with regular intensity. As in a standard muscle test, the joint is positioned in such a way that the muscle to be tested is shortened. The practitioner applies pressure to the joint to lengthen the muscle, until a "locking" is noted. A positive result occurs when "locking" of the muscle and joint does not occur, indicating deficient free fatty acids. 3. Fatty acid profile via laboratory testing of blood

Supplemental Support

1. Beet juice and bile salts

Lifestyle changes

Please see the handout in the appendix on Healthy lifestyle for a healthy gallbladder

82. Bitter taste in mouth, especially after meals

A bitter taste in the mouth, especially after meals, may be due to bile. This is a symptom of gallbladder dysfunction. Bile should not be regurgitated and you should consider gross pathology first, such as biliary or abdominal congestion, or gallstones, before beginning supplement protocols. Identifying and removing hidden food allergies may help.

1° Indication

Gallbladder dysfunction

Further assessment	1. Check for tenderness underneath the right rib cage 2. Check for tenderness and nodulation on the web between thumb and fore-finger of right hand 3. Check for tenderness in the Chapman reflex for the liver-gallbladder located over the 6th intercostal space on the right side 4. Assess for Hepato-biliary congestion with the Acoustic Cardiogram (ACG), which will show post-systolic rounding due to increased backpressure on the pulmonic and aortic valve. It may also show through to the tricuspid valve if chronic. 5. Iodine test: Use a tincture of 2% iodine solution, and paint a 3" by 3" square on the client's abdomen. The client is to leave the patch unwashed until it disappears. The square should still be there in 24 hours. If it has disappeared, there is an indication of iodine need 6. Blood chemistry and CBC testing for SGOT, SGPT, GGT 7. Gallbladder ultrasound

2° Indication

Hidden food allergies

Further assessment	1. Finding and eliminating the hidden food allergies by what ever method you find successful from ELISA/RAST testing through Applied Kinesiology

Supplemental support

1. Beet juice, taurine, vitamin C and pancreolipase (if gall stones)
2. Beet juice and bile salts (if gallbladder removed)
3. Potassium iodide
4. Phosphatidylcholine
5. Pancreatic enzymes
6. Nutritional phosphorous
7. Multiple herbal anti-histamines

Lifestyle changes

- Please see the handouts in the appendix on Healthy lifestyle for a healthy gallbladder
- Avoidance of all identified food allergies
- Castor oil packs applied topically to the right upper quadrant

83. Become sick if you were to drink wine

Wine, as opposed to other alcoholic beverages, often makes people sick. Most wines contain sulfites as a preservative, and many people are sensitive to sulfites, which can be toxic to the body. Sulfites are detoxified via the sulphodixation pathway in phase II liver detoxification.

Sulphoxidation is closely linked to the sulfation detoxification, which requires sulfur as a cofactor. Sulfoxidation uses an enzyme called sulphite oxidase to detoxify sulfur-containing molecules (foods and drugs). Sulphite molecules, which are used as preservatives and food additives, are also removed using sulfoxidation. Abnormal sulfoxidation makes it hard for the body to detoxify sulfites, which can cause food and drug sensitivities, especially in asthmatics. Sulphoxidation problems can be helped with supplemental molybdenum, an essential trace mineral for the sulphite oxidase enzyme. There may also be a deficiency in zinc, as zinc is an essential nutrient for the effective detoxification of alcohol via the enzyme alcohol dehydrogenase.

1° Indication

Sulfite sensitivity due to a molybdenum deficiency

Further assessment	1. Test for increased urinary sulfites 2. A decreased uric acid on a blood chemistry panel indicates molybdenum deficiency

2° Indication

Liver detoxification problems, especially phase I detoxification

Further assessment	1. Check for tenderness in the Chapman reflex for the liver-gallbladder located over 6th intercostal space on right side 2. Check for tenderness in the Liver point located on the 3rd rib, 3 " to the right of the sternum, at the costochondral junction. 3. Check for tenderness underneath the right rib cage 4. Increased SGOT, SGPT on a blood chemistry panel 5. Various labs do liver detoxification panels

3° Indicator

Zinc deficiency

Further assessment	1. Positive zinc tally: A client holds a solution of aqueous zinc sulfate in their mouth and tells you if and when they can taste it. An almost immediate very bitter taste indicates the client does not need zinc. Clients who are zinc deficient will report no taste from the solution.

Supplemental Support

1. Plant source of molybdenum
2. Nutrients to support Phase II liver detoxification
3. Herbs that cleanse the liver
4. Glutathione, cysteine, and Glycine
5. Powdered detoxification support formula

84. Easily intoxicated if you were to drink wine

This is a symptom of a need for liver support. The liver is the main organ of detoxification and a dysfunction in either of the two phases of detoxification can cause a build-up of alcohol in the body. An enzyme called alcohol dehydrogenase, which is a zinc dependent enzyme, detoxifies alcohol. Alcohol dehydrogenase is a rate limited enzyme i.e. it can only deal with a certain amount of alcohol at any one time. Zinc deficiency can prevent this enzyme from working at its optimal.

Alcohol is known to induce phase 1 detoxification in the body i.e. it speeds it up. This presents a problem to the body when the phase 2 portion of detoxification cannot "keep up". Phase I detoxification involves the oxidation, reduction and/or hydrolysis of a molecule to make it less toxic. High exposure to alcohol in phase 1 detoxification may deplete critical nutrients in phase 2 detoxification.

Phase II detoxification is a process of conjugation, which makes the molecule water-soluble, so that it can be removed from the body. This phase requires adequate levels of glycine and glutathione, along with many other different nutrients for adequate conjugation.

1° Indication

Liver detoxification problems, especially phase I and II detoxification

Further assessment	1. Check for tenderness in the Chapman reflex for the liver-gallbladder located over the 6th intercostal space on the right side 2. Check for tenderness in the Liver point located on the 3rd rib, 3 " to the right of the sternum, at the costochondral junction. 3. Check for tenderness underneath the right rib cage 4. Increased SGOT, SGPT on a blood chemistry panel 5. Various labs do liver detoxification panels

2° Indication

Zinc deficiency

Further assessment	1. Positive zinc tally: A client holds a solution of aqueous zinc sulfate in their mouth and tells you if and when they can taste it. An almost immediate very bitter taste indicates the client does not need zinc. Clients who are zinc deficient will report no taste from the solution.

Other indications

Molybdenum deficiency

Supplemental Support

1. Nutrients to support Phase II liver detoxification
2. Herbs that cleanse the liver
3. Glutathione, cysteine, and Glycine
4. Powdered detoxification support formula
5. Plant source of molybdenum

85. Easily get hung over if your were to drink wine

This is a clear sign of liver detoxification problems with an increased need for liver support. Alcohol is primarily detoxified by Phase I of the detoxification pathway, the phase that changes the molecular structure of a toxic molecule by oxidation, reduction or hydrolysis. Alcohol is known to induce phase 1 detoxification in the body i.e. it speeds it up. This presents a problem to the body when the phase 2 portion of detoxification cannot "keep up". Phase I detoxification involves the oxidation, reduction and/or hydrolysis of a molecule to make it less toxic. High exposure to alcohol in phase 1 detoxification may deplete critical nutrients in phase 2 detoxification.

Alcohol dehydrogenase is a zinc dependent enzyme, therefore zinc deficient people are less likely to be able to adequately detoxify alcohol. Acetaldehyde, the molecule that actually causes the effects of a hangover, needs to be detoxified by aldehyde oxidase, a molybdenum dependent molecule. Essential fatty acids, which have anti-inflammatory properties, may also be needed.

1° Indication

Liver detoxification problems, especially phase I detoxification

Further assessment	1. Check for tenderness in the Chapman reflex for the liver-gallbladder located over 6th intercostal space on right side 2. Check for tenderness in the Liver point located on the 3rd rib, 3 " to the right of the sternum, at the costochondral junction. 3. Check for tenderness underneath the right rib cage 4. Increased SGOT, SGPT on a blood chemistry panel 5. Various labs do liver detoxification panels

2° Indication

Zinc and molybdenum deficiency

Further assessment	1. Positive zinc tally: A client holds a solution of aqueous zinc sulfate in their mouth and tells you if and when they can taste it. An almost immediate very bitter taste indicates the client does not need zinc. Clients who are zinc deficient will report no taste from the solution. 2. Test for increased urinary sulfites may indicate a molybdenum deficiency 3. A decreased uric acid on a blood chemistry panel indicates molybdenum deficiency

Other indications

Essential fatty acid deficiency

Supplemental Support

1.	Nutrients to support Phase II liver detoxification and herbs that cleanse the liver
2.	Glutathione, cysteine, and Glycine and powdered detoxification support formula
3.	Plant source of molybdenum and Nutritional zinc
4.	Mixed fatty acids (walnut, hazelnut, sesame, and apricot)

86. Alcohol per week (0 = < 3/ week, 1 = < 7/ week, 2 = < 14/ week, 3 = > 14/week

Alcohol is a metabolic toxin that carries with it some health risks. Its impact on the body is far reaching causing irritation to the lining of the gastrointestinal tract, leading to increased intestinal permeability (Leaky gut syndrome), a condition that allows unwanted substances to move from the digestive tract into the bloodstream. A leaky gut can cause allergies because the unwanted material that is absorbed through the hyper-permeable digestive tract stimulates the immune system.

The regular use of alcohol can have a strong impact on your brain chemistry. Alcohol, and other substances such as refined sugars and flours and certain drugs, will interfere with the receptors in the brain for neurotransmitters. The brain identifies that the receptor for a certain neurotransmitter is already filled, so it reduces the amount of neurotransmitters it produces. As the levels of neurotransmitters drop you begin to crave alcohol or refined sugars to fill newly emptied receptors in the brain. At some point you will no longer be able to fill the receptors with these "empty" foods and substances. At this point you will begin to experience mood swings and an even more intense craving for alcohol or refined sugars. To correct these imbalances you may require amino acid therapy. Ask your doctor about using L-Tyrosine, GABA, L-Taurine, L-Glutamine, and DL-Phenylalanine to help correct the imbalance in brain chemistry caused by constant alcohol use.

The liver is also affected by alcohol. It takes the liver eight hours to detoxify one "measure of alcohol" i.e. one drink. During this time the other items that need detoxification are put on hold. Drinking daily may have long-term health repercussions. Excessive drinking varies from person to person, but it has long been recognized that the consumption of more than two drinks/day (two glasses of wine, two 12-ounces of beer, or two shots of spirits) can contribute to significant health problems: Intestinal Dysbiosis, leaky gut, blood sugar abnormalities, reactive hypoglycemia, multiple mineral-vitamin deficiency, sub clinical liver dysfunction, obesity, heart disease, liver disease and damage, and fetal alcohol syndrome if consumed even in low amounts during pregnancy. Alcohol is very high in calories and has virtually no nutritional value. The exact amount that will cause problems will vary from person to person. The occasional glass of wine or beer is unlikely to be a problem, it has been noted in some research that the occasional alcoholic beverage may actually have some benefits to human physiology. It is clear that the overuse or alcohol abuse does not.

Additionally frequent alcohol consumption can cause nutritional deficiencies. A daily multiple vitamin and mineral supplement, along with a broad spectrum antioxidant foormula will be a preventative step.

87. Recovering alcoholic (1 = yes, 0 = no)

Long-term alcohol use can have a wide spread effect on the body: nutritional deficiencies, liver damage, and damage to the gastrointestinal tract, increased susceptibility to oxidative stress, blood sugar dysregulation, and hypoglycemia and B vitamin deficiency. A recovering alcoholic should be applauded and encouraged for taking the right step for their long-term health and well-being. It is the clinician's responsibility to act as an ally.

For many alcoholics, their body responds to alcohol as if it were sugar. A recovering alcoholic, therefore, may be more likely to turn to sugar as a substitute for alcohol. If they are suffering from depression, dizziness, fatigue, feeling weak and shaky or have frequent headaches, especially first thing in the morning or in the afternoon, assess for blood sugar dysfunction. Unfortunately an addiction to sugar makes it more difficult to stop wanting alcohol.

1° Indication

Blood sugar dysregulation and hypoglycemia.

Further assessment	1. Check for tenderness in the Chapman reflex for the liver-gallbladder located over the 6th intercostal space on the right 2. Check for tenderness in the Liver point located on the 3rd rib, 3 " to the right of the sternum, at the costochondral junction. 3. Check for tenderness underneath the right rib cage Check for tenderness in the Chapman reflex for the pancreas located in the 7th intercostal space on the left 4. Check for tenderness or guarding at the head of the pancreas located in the upper left quadrant of the abdominal region 1/2 to 2/3 of the way between the umbilicus and the angel of the ribs 5. Check for tenderness or nodularity in the right thenar pad, which is a pancreas indicator if tender 6. Check for tenderness in the inguinal ligament bilaterally, an adrenal indicator 7. Check for tenderness at the medial knee bilaterally, at the insertion of the sartorius muscle at the Pes Anserine. This is an adrenal indicator.

Other indications

1. B vitamin deficiency
2. Increased oxidative stress on the body
3. Increased intestinal hyperpermeability
4. An increased need for liver support

Supplemental Support

1. Multiple nutrients to support sugar handling problems
2. Adrenal tissue (neonatal bovine) and adaptogenic herbs to support adrenal function
3. Beet juice, taurine, vitamin C and pancreolipase
4. Herbs that cleanse the liver
5. Broad spectrum antioxidants and bioflavanoids
6. Nutrients that heal the intestines
7. Vitamin B complex

88. History of drug or alcohol abuse (1 = yes, 0 = no)

A history of drug or alcohol abuse can be an indication for an increased need for liver support. The liver is the main organ of detoxification and a dysfunction in either of the two phases of detoxification can caused by long term drug and alcohol use.
Phase I detoxification involves the oxidation, reduction and/or hydrolysis of a molecule to make it less toxic. Many of the enzymes in this phase require molybdenum.

Phase II detoxification is a process of conjugation, which makes the molecule water-soluble, so that it can be removed from the body. This phase requires adequate levels of glycine and glutathione, along with many other different nutrients for adequate conjugation.

Long-tem dysfunction in the phase I and II pathways of detoxification can contribute to a problem called toxic loading, a build up of toxicity in the body. This can lead to various problems such as kidney damage and blood sugar dysregulation caused by an increased oxidative stress.

1° Indication

Increased need for liver support with possible long term liver detoxification problems, especially phase I and II detoxification

Further assessment	1. Check for tenderness in the Chapman reflex for the liver-gallbladder located over the 6th intercostal space on the right side 2. Check for tenderness in the Liver point located on the 3rd rib, 3 " to the right of the sternum, at the costochondral junction. 3. Check for tenderness underneath the right rib cage 4. Increased SGOT, SGPT on a blood chemistry panel 5. Various labs do liver detoxification panels

2° Indication

Assess for oxidative stress

Further assessment	1. Check for free radical activity in the body with the urine Oxidata test 2. Check for tissue levels of vitamin C with the lingual ascorbic acid test. Dry client's tongue and put one drop of blue reagent on centre of tongue and time the seconds it takes for the color to completely disappear. 20 seconds or less is an indication of sufficient vitamin C levels in the body. 3. Check for tissue ascorbic acid levels.

Other indications

1. Molybdenum and zinc deficiency
2. Blood sugar dysregulation with possible B vitamin deficiency
3. Increased intestinal hyperpermeability

Supplemental Support

1.	Nutrients to support Phase II liver detoxification
2.	Herbs that cleanse the liver
3.	Glutathione, cysteine, and Glycine
4.	Powdered detoxification support formula
5.	Beet juice, taurine, vitamin C and pancreolipase
6.	Plant source of molybdenum
7.	Nutritional zinc
8.	Broad spectrum antioxidants
9.	Nutrients that heal the intestines
10.	Vitamin B complex
11.	Multiple nutrients to support sugar handling problems
12.	Adaptogenic herbs to support adrenal function
13.	Adrenal tissue (neonatal bovine)

Lifestyle changes

Please see the handout in the appendix on Recommendations for keeping your liver healthy

NOTES:

89. History of hepatitis (1 = yes, 0 = no)

A history of hepatitis can be an indicator for an increased need for liver support. Hepatitis is an inflammatory and destructive process that destroys the hepatic cells and causes liver damage. The liver has the ability to regenerate itself given the correct environment. However, long-term damage to the hepatocytes from hepatitis is not reversible.

Supporting the many functions of the liver from protein synthesis, blood sugar regulation, detoxification, blood filtration etc. can be very helpful for people recovering from hepatitis.

1° Indication
Increased need for liver support with possible long term liver detoxification problems, especially phase I and II detoxification

Further assessment	1. Check for tenderness in the Chapman reflex for the liver-gallbladder located over the 6th intercostal space on the right side 2. Check for tenderness in the Liver point located on the 3rd rib, 3 " to the right of the sternum, at the costochondral junction. 3. Check for tenderness underneath the right rib cage 4. Increased SGOT, SGPT on a blood chemistry panel 5. Various labs do liver detoxification panels

Supplemental support

1. Nutrients to support Phase II liver detoxification
2. Herbs that cleanse the liver
3. Glutathione, cysteine, and Glycine
4. Powdered detoxification support formula
5. Plant source molybdenum

Lifestyle changes
Please see the handout in the appendix on Recommendations for keeping your liver healthy

NOTES:

90. Long term use of prescription medications (1 = yes, 0 =no)

Long-term use of prescription and over the counter medication will put increased stress on the liver's detoxification system. The liver is the main organ of detoxification and the constant need to detoxify prescription drugs can lead to a dysfunction in either of the two phases of detoxification. This can make the drugs less effective, or can cause the drug to stay in the body longer than it should be, leading to drug related side effects. Clients on long-term prescription drugs need extra liver support

Phase I detoxification involves the oxidation, reduction and/or hydrolysis of a molecule to make it less toxic. Phase 1 detoxification can actually produce an intermediate metabolite from a drug that is more dangerous and toxin than the drug being detoxified. A case in point it acetaminophen, which is converted in phase 1 into a substance called NAPQI, a liver specific toxin. Hopefully NAPQI is quickly detoxified in phase II before it can cause long term damage to the liver. Phase 1 detoxification can be slowed down or accelerated by various drugs, which can cause a drug to linger in the body. Medications such as cimetidine, benzodiazepines, anti-histamines, anti-fungal agents and oral contraceptives can inhibit phase 1 detoxification. This might become problematic if a client is on multiple drugs. Certain drugs, such as nicotine, steroids and phenobarbitol can cause the phase 1 process to speed up

Phase II detoxification is a process of conjugation, which makes the molecule water-soluble, so that it can be removed from the body. This phase requires adequate levels of glycine and glutathione, along with many other different nutrients for adequate conjugation. Long term use of prescription medications can lead to long-term nutrient deficiencies, because the 6 enzyme systems of phase 2 detoxification systems require large amounts of specific nutrients to work properly.

1° Indication

Increased need for liver support to help with possible long term liver detoxification problems, especially phase I and II detoxification

Further assessment	1. Check for tenderness in the Chapman reflex for the liver-gallbladder located over 6th intercostal space on right side 2. Check for tenderness in the Liver point located on the 3rd rib, 3 " to the right of the sternum, at the costochondral junction. 3. Check for tenderness underneath the right rib cage 4. Increased SGOT, SGPT on a blood chemistry panel 5. Various labs do liver detoxification panels

Supplemental Support

1. Nutrients to support Phase II liver detoxification
2. Herbs that cleanse the liver
3. Powdered detoxification support formula
4. Glutathione, Cysteine and Glycine

Lifestyle changes

Please see the handout in the appendix on Recommendations for keeping your liver healthy

91. Sensitive to chemicals (perfume, solvents, etc.)

Sensitivity to chemicals such as perfume is a very strong indicator for an increased need for liver support. The detoxification pathways in the liver require many nutritional co-factors. Phase I detoxification involves the oxidation, reduction and/or hydrolysis of a molecule to make it less toxic.

Sensitivity to perfumes etc. is a strong indicator of a need for sulfoxidation support in phase 2. Sulfoxidation uses an enzyme called sulphite oxidase to detoxify sulfur, aldehydes and ketone-containing molecules. Sulphite, aldehyde and ketone molecules, which are found in many perfumes, solvents and exhaust fumes, are removed using sulfoxidation. Abnormal sulfoxidation makes it hard for the body to detoxify these chemicals, which can cause sensitivities, especially in asthmatics. Sulphoxidation problems can be helped with supplemental molybdenum, an essential trace mineral for the sulphite oxidase enzyme.

This symptom may also be an indication of dysbiosis in the large intestine. A build-up of yeast such as Candida will increase the toxic load that the liver has to deal with. This is more likely in a person who eats a lot of refined sugar and has a history of antibiotic use.

1° Indication

Increased need for liver support and supplementary Molybdenum

Further assessment	1. Check for tenderness in the Chapman reflex for the liver-gallbladder located over the 6th intercostal space on the right 2. Check for tenderness in the Liver point located on the 3rd rib, 3 " to the right of the sternum, at the costochondral junction. 3. Check for tenderness underneath the right rib cage 4. Increased SGOT, SGPT on a blood chemistry panel 5. Various labs do liver detoxification panels 6. Decreased uric acid on a blood chemistry panel is an indication for molybdenum deficiency

2° Indication

Dysbiosis caused by an overgrowth of bacteria or yeast

Further assessment	1. Increased urinary indican levels 2. Stool analysis- either comprehensive digestive analysis or a parasite profile 3. Check for tenderness in the Chapman reflex for the colon located bilaterally along the iliotibial band on the thighs. Palpate the colon for tenderness and tension. 4. Check for tenderness in the Chapman reflex for the small intestine located on the 8th, 9th and 10th intercostal spaces near the tip of the rib. Also palpate four quadrants in a 2" to 3" radius around the umbilicus for tenderness and tension

Supplemental support

1. Nutrients to support Phase II liver detoxification
2. Herbs that cleanse the liver
3. Glutathione, Cysteine, and Glycine
4. Powdered detoxification support formula
5. Plant source molybdenum
6. Micro Emulsified Oregano
7. Nutrients that heal the intestines
8. Betaine HCL, Pepsin, and pancreatin
9. Water soluble fiber and colon health nutrients
10. Multiple nutrients that support the immune system

Lifestyle changes

Please see the handouts in the appendix on Recommendations for keeping your liver healthy and the Dysbiosis diet

NOTES:

92. Sensitive to tobacco smoke

Sensitivity to smoke is an indication of dysbiosis in the large intestine. A build-up of yeast such as Candida will increase the toxic load that the liver has to deal with. This is more likely in a person who eats a lot of refined sugar and has a history of antibiotic use.

It has also been associated with a need for increased liver support, as the liver is not doing an adequate job removing toxins. The detoxification pathways in the liver require many nutritional co-factors. Phase I detoxification involves the oxidation, reduction and/or hydrolysis of a molecule to make it less toxic. Sensitivity to smoke may indicate a need for molybdenum, a nutrient that is often deficient and is required for effective phase 2 detoxification. Either of these problems may be present simultaneously, as the liver is under the added stress of detoxifying the build-up of toxic metabolites produced by the Candida.

1° Indication

Increased need for liver support

Further assessment	1. Check for tenderness in the Chapman reflex for the liver-gallbladder located over the 6th intercostal space on the right side 2. Check for tenderness in the Liver point located on the 3rd rib, 3 " to the right of the sternum, at the costochondral junction. 3. Check for tenderness underneath the right rib cage

2° Indication

Dysbiosis caused by an overgrowth of yeast

Further assessment	1. Increased urinary indican levels 2. Stool analysis- either comprehensive digestive analysis or a parasite profile 3. Check for tenderness in the Chapman reflex for the colon located bilaterally along the iliotibial band on the thighs. Palpate the colon for tenderness and tension. 4. Check for tenderness in the Chapman reflex for the small intestine located on the 8th, 9th and 10th intercostal spaces near the tip of the rib. Also palpate four quadrants in a 2" to 3" radius around the umbilicus for tenderness and tension

Supplemental support

Liver support:
1. Nutrients to support Phase II liver detoxification
2. Herbs that cleanse the liver
3. Glutathione, cysteine, and Glycine
4. Powdered detoxification support formula

Dysbiosis:
1. Micro Emulsified Oregano
2. Nutrients that heal the intestines

3.	Betaine HCL, Pepsin, and pancreatin
4.	Water soluble fiber and colon health nutrients
5.	Multiple nutrients that support the immune system

Lifestyle changes

Please see the handouts in the appendix on Recommendations for keeping your liver healthy and the Dysbiosis diet

NOTES:

93. Exposure to diesel fumes

The body's detoxification system can be overwhelmed with exposure to diesel fumes, which is a strong indicator of a need for sulfoxidation support in phase 2 detoxification in the liver.

Sulfoxidation uses an enzyme called sulphite oxidase to detoxify sulfur, aldehydes and ketone-containing molecules. Sulphite, aldehyde and ketone molecules, which are found in many solvents and exhaust fumes, are removed using sulfoxidation. Abnormal sulfoxidation makes it hard for the body to detoxify these chemicals, which can cause sensitivities, especially in asthmatics. Sulphoxidation problems can be helped with supplemental molybdenum, an essential trace mineral for the sulphite oxidase enzyme.

Additionally, if the body is under a heavy toxic load to begin with, the exposure to diesel fumes can cause lingering problems of chemical toxicity. Diesel, unlike regular gasoline, has not had the lead removed. Exposure to diesel fumes can therefore contribute to a heavy metal burden in the body.

1° Indication

Increased need for liver support and supplementary Molybdenum

Further assessment	1. Check for tenderness in the Chapman reflex for the liver-gallbladder located over the 6th intercostal space on the right 2. Check for tenderness in the Liver point located on the 3rd rib, 3 " to the right of the sternum, at the costochondral junction. 3. Check for tenderness underneath the right rib cage 4. Increased SGOT, SGPT on a blood chemistry panel 5. Various labs do liver detoxification panels 6. Decreased uric acid on a blood chemistry panel is an indication for molybdenum deficiency

Other indications

Increased heavy metal body burden

Supplemental support

1. Nutrients to support Phase II liver detoxification
2. Herbs that cleanse the liver
3. Plant source molybdenum
4. Glutathione, Cysteine, and Glycine
5. Powdered detoxification support formula

Lifestyle changes

Please see the handout in the appendix on Recommendations for keeping your liver healthy

NOTES:

94. Pain under right side of rib cage

The gallbladder and liver are both located underneath the right rib cage. Pain in this area can be serious, so further investigation of possible pathology should be done before beginning supplemental protocols. If serious pathology is ruled out, then the most likely cause is biliary congestion with thick and congested bile, which can lead to bile stone precipitation.

A common condition of the biliary tract is called Biliary Stasis. This condition, marked by a thickening of the bile or in more advanced cases an actual obstruction of bile excretion into the bowel, can lead to an increase in size of the gallbladder, which must now store significantly greater amounts of bile. The gallbladder can become severely distended in biliary stasis, and in some cases be felt through the abdominal wall under the lower margin of the liver. The distension of the gallbladder can cause a dull aching pain under the right rib cage.

Therapy must focus on keeping the bile thin and fluid. Bile salts, Iodine and phosphorous are all nutritional therapies for keeping bile thin. Hidden food allergies are another cause.

1° Indication

Biliary stasis with thick, congested bile and the threat of gallstones

Further assessment	1. Check for tenderness underneath the right rib cage 2. Check for tenderness and nodulation on the web between thumb and fore-finger of right hand 3. Check for tenderness in the Chapman reflex for the liver-gallbladder located over 6th intercostal space on right side 4. Assess for Hepato-biliary congestion with the Acoustic Cardiogram (ACG), which will show post-systolic rounding due to increased backpressure on the pulmonic and aortic valve. It may also show through to the tricuspid valve if chronic. 5. Iodine test: Use a tincture of 2% iodine solution, and pain a 3" by 3" square on the client's abdomen. The client is to leave the patch unwashed until it disappears. The square should still be there in 24 hours. If it has disappeared, there is an indication of iodine need 6. Blood chemistry and CBC testing for SGOT, SGPT, GGT 7. Gallbladder ultrasound

Supplemental support

1. Beet juice, taurine, vitamin C and pancreolipase (if gall stones) 2. Beet juice and bile salts (if gallbladder removed) 3. Potassium iodide 4. Phosphatidylcholine 5. Pancreatic enzymes

Lifestyle changes

Please see the handout in the appendix on Healthy lifestyle for a healthy gallbladder

95. Hemorrhoids or varicose veins

Hemorrhoids are an indication of liver congestion. If the liver, which acts as a blood filter, becomes congested, the blood that flows into the liver from the digestive tract becomes backed up. Unfortunately the hemorrhoidal plexus is weak, and susceptible to forming varicosities and Hemorrhoids. Weakness in the blood vessels, due to bioflavonoid deficiency, can also contribute to the weakening of the plexus.

Always explore the possibility of liver congestion as a cause of hemorrhoids before resorting to more radical forms of therapy and surgery. Hemorrhoids often resolve themselves if the cause of liver congestion is dealt with. Some of the main causes of liver congestion include:

- Fiber poor diet
- Excessive calories
- Bowel toxicity and toxemia
- Leaky gut syndrome
- Dietary sources of free radicals: rancid oils and fats from fried foods, heated polyunsaturated fats, charred meats etc.)
- Trans-fatty acids (margarine, refined oils) and partially-hydrogenated oils.
- Blood sugar dysregulation: insulin resistance and fatty liver formation

1° Indication

Liver congestion

Further assessment	1. Check for tenderness in the Chapman reflex for the liver-gallbladder located over the 6th intercostal space on the right s 2. Check for tenderness in the Liver point located on the 3rd rib, 3 " to the right of the sternum, at the costochondral junction. 3. Check for tenderness underneath the right rib cage 4. Assess for Hepato-biliary congestion with the Acoustic Cardiogram (ACG), which will show post-systolic rounding due to increased backpressure on the pulmonic and aortic valve.

Other indications

Weakness in the blood vessels

Supplemental Support

1. Herbs that cleanse the liver
2. Beet juice, taurine, vitamin C and pancreolipase
3. Water soluble fiber and colon health nutrients
4. Emulsified vitamin A drops
5. Broad spectrum bioflavanoids and antioxidants
6. Nutrients that heal the intestines
7. EPA and DHA from fish oil

Lifestyle changes

- Please see the handout on keeping your liver healthy
- Avoid sitting for long periods of time and try aernating hot and cold sitz baths

96. NutraSweet (Aspartame) consumption
97. Bothered by Aspartame

Aspartame is a low-calorie sweetener used in foods and beverages and as a tabletop sweetener. It is sold under the name NutraSweet and is about 200 times sweeter than sugar. It is made by joining two amino acids, aspartic acid and phenylalanine and a small amount of methanol. Phenylalanine, as an amino acid, is quite stimulating to the body, especially when combined with caffeine. The ingredients of aspartame also interfere and compete with the essential amino acid L-tryptophan, which is essential for the synthesis of the neurotransmitter serotonin. Aspartame is used in many products including major brands of beverages, foods and other products such as cold cereals; drink mixes, gelatin, puddings, dairy products, and toppings. It loses its sweetness during long periods of storage and is not suitable for baking since heat causes the loss of sweetness. While there have been numerous studies, which argue its safety, many people have some very uncomfortable reactions from its use. Clients with phenylketonuria must not use it because of the release of phenylalanine during its metabolism.

H. J. Roberts, M. D., in his book *Aspartame (NutraSweet): Is It Safe?*, alerts us to the potential hazard of this sweetener. The book reports that aspartame may produce a wide variety of physical and mental symptoms. These may include convulsions, headaches, behavioral disorders and gastrointestinal problems.

In the United States the Aspartame Consumer Safety Network (ACSN) serves as a support group and clearinghouse for information. can write to them at PO Box 780634, Dallas, TX 75378. They produce a booklet called "The Deadly Deception," which reports such things as "85% of all complaints registered with the Food and Drug Administration (FDA), the US government agency that overseas food and drug safety, concerns aspartame's adverse reactions." Five deaths and at least seventy different symptoms have resulted from its use. Julia Ross, in her book "Diet Cure" reports that "so far, more than 10 thousand aspartame users have reported over 100 adverse symptoms, compiled by the Food and Drug Administration (FDA). They include everything from menstrual changes, weight gain, and headaches to severe depression, insomnia, and anxiety attacks."[4]

Everyone should avoid aspartame. Many people complain of headaches or dizziness after consuming aspartame. Aspartame releases methanol, a toxic chemical, when it is broken down in the digestive system. Methanol is converted into the toxic chemical acetaldehyde, which is further broken down by the enzyme aldehyde oxidase, a molybdenum dependent enzyme. If a client is bothered by aspartame they need additional liver support and molybdenum supplementation.

[4] Julia Ross, MA *The Diet Cure* (New York, NY: Penguin books , 1999), p.36-37

1° Indication

Increased need for liver support and supplementary Molybdenum

Further assessment	1. Check for tenderness in the Chapman reflex for the liver-gallbladder located over the 6th intercostal space on the right side 2. Check for tenderness in the Liver point located on the 3rd rib, 3 " to the right of the sternum, at the costochondral junction. 3. Check for tenderness underneath the right rib cage 4. Decreased uric acid on a blood chemistry panel is an indication for molybdenum deficiency

Supplemental support

1. Nutrients to support Phase II liver detoxification
2. Herbs that cleanse the liver
3. Glutathione, cysteine, and Glycine
4. Powdered detoxification support formula
5. Plant source of molybdenum

Lifestyle changes

Please see the handout in the appendix on Recommendations for keeping your liver healthy

NOTES:

98. Chronic Fatigue or Fibromyalgia

Chronic Fatigue Syndrome (CFS) describes a collection of the following symptoms:

- Recurrent fatigue
- Sore throat
- Low-grade fever
- Lymph node swelling
- Headache
- Muscle and joint pain
- Intestinal discomfort
- Emotional distress, and/or depression
- Loss of concentration

Much of the research has focused on identifying an infectious cause to CFS. The main culprit is Epstein Barr virus, along with a number of other viral agents (cytomegalovirus, varicella, various herpes viruses).

Fibromyalgia, like DFS has been getting a lot of attention over the past few years. The only difference in the diagnostic criteria for fibromyalgia and CFS is the requirement of musculoskeletal pain in fibromyalgia and fatigue in CFS.[5]

In my opinion the state of the terrain of the body is one of the most important places to focus attention in dealing with clients with chronic fatigue and fibromyalgia. Impaired immune function, liver dysfunction, stress, depression, hypothyroidism, hypoglycemia, adrenal exhaustion etc. all play a part in chronic fatigue and fibromyalgia.

It is also important to assess whether or not the client is getting enough sleep. There are a number of dietary causes of fatigue including a diet that is too high in refined sugars, multiple mineral and vitamin deficiencies and a person who is consuming the standard Western diet with too much coffee, alcohol and processed foods.

For clients with CFS and fibromyalgia focus on looking at the following causes: poor immune function, poor liver function, low adrenal function, low thyroid function, food allergies and/or digestive dysfunction.

<u>1° Indication</u>

Need for immune support

Further assessment	1. Check for tenderness in the Chapman reflex for the thymus located in the 5th intercostal space on the right near the sternum 2. Check for tenderness in the Chapman reflex for the lungs located bilaterally in the 3rd and 4th intercostal space near the sternum 3. Check for tenderness in the histamine point located at five o'clock on the pectoralis muscle in the intercostal space between the 5th and 6th rib on the right side only

[5] M.Murray and J. Pizzorno, *"Encyclopedia of natural medicine"* (California: Prima Publishing, 1998) p.363

	4. Assess the client for allergic tension. Take a full one-minute pulse sitting, then stand, wait 15 seconds and take another full minute pulse. If the standing pulse goes up by more than six beats, this is an indication of "allergic tension" 5. Assess the client's vitamin C status with the lingual and urinary ascorbic acid tests

2° Indication

Poor liver function

Further assessment	1. Check for tenderness in the Chapman reflex for the liver-gallbladder located over the 6th intercostal space on the right 2. Check for tenderness in the Liver point located on the 3rd rib, 3 " to the right of the sternum, at the costochondral junction. 3. Check for tenderness underneath the right rib cage 4. Increased SGOT, SGPT on a blood chemistry panel 5. Various labs do liver detoxification panels 6. Assess for Hepato-biliary congestion with the Acoustic Cardiogram (ACG), which will show post-systolic rounding due to increased backpressure on the pulmonic and aortic valve. It may also show through to the tricuspid valve if chronic. 7. Decreased uric acid on a blood chemistry panel is an indication for molybdenum deficiency

3° indication

Low adrenal function

Further assessment	1. Check for tenderness in the inguinal ligament bilaterally, an adrenal indicator 2. Check for tenderness at the medial knee bilaterally, at the insertion of the sartorius muscle at the Pes Anserine. This is an adrenal indicator. 3. Check for a paradoxical pupillary reflex by shining a light into a client's eye and grading the reaction of the pupil. A pupil that fails to constrict indicates adrenal exhaustion 4. Check for the presence of postural hypotension. A drop of more than 10 points is an indication of adrenal insufficiency. 5. Check for a chronic short leg due to a posterior-inferior ilium. An adrenal indicator when confirmed with postural hypotension and a paradoxical pupillary response. 6. Check the cortisol/DHEA rhythm with a salivary adrenal stress profile 7. Increased chloride in the urine is a sign of hypoadrenal function 8. Assess for adrenal insufficiency with the Acoustic Cardiogram (ACG), which will show static in both the systolic and diastolic rest phases. You will also see an elevated S2 sound.

4° Indication

Low thyroid function

Further assessment	1. Check for tenderness in the Chapman reflex for the thyroid located in the second intercostal space near the sternum on the right 2. Check for a delayed Achilles return reflex, which is a strong sign of a hypo-functioning thyroid 3. Check for general costochondral tenderness, which is a thyroid indicator 4. Check for pre-tibial edema, which is a sign of a hypo-functioning thyroid 5. Iodine test: Use a tincture of 2% iodine solution, and paint a 3" by 3" square on the client's abdomen. The client is to leave the patch unwashed until it disappears. The square should still be there in 24 hours. If it has disappeared, there is an indication of iodine need 6. Have client assess their basal metabolic temperature by taking their axillary temperature first thing in the morning for 5 straight days. An average temperature below 36.5°C is an indication of hypo-thyroidism

Other indications

1. Food allergies
2. Digestive dysfunction
3. Virus: Epstein-Barr

Supplemental Support

1. Nutrients to support phase II liver detoxification
2. Beet juice, taurine, vitamin C and pancreolipase
3. Herbs that cleanse the liver
4. Glutathione, cysteine, and Glycine
5. Adrenal tissue (neonatal bovine)
6. Adaptogenic herbs to support adrenal function
7. Multiple nutrients for blood sugar handling problems
8. Pyridoxal-5-phosphate
9. Multiple nutrients to support thyroid function with pituitary glandular
10. Potassium iodide
11. Multi-nutrients supporting fibromyalgia

Lifestyle changes

Please see the handout in the appendix on Recommendations for keeping your liver healthy and the Adrenal restoration measures

NOTES:

SMALL INTESTINE

99. Food allergies, sensitivities and intolerances
100. Abdominal bloating 1 to 2 hours after eating
101. Specific foods make you tired or bloated (1= yes, 0= no)
102. Pulse speeds after eating
103. Airborne allergies
104. Experience hives
105. Sinus congestion, "stuffy head"
106. Crave bread or noodles
107. Alternating constipation and Diarrhea
108. Crohn's disease
109. Wheat or grain sensitivity
110. Dairy sensitivity
111. Are there foods you could not give up (1 = yes, 0 = no)
112. Asthma, sinus infections, stuffy nose
113. Bizarre vivid or nightmarish dreams
114. Use over-the-counter pain medications
115. Feel spacey or unreal

99. Food allergies, sensitivities and intolerances

Allergies are overreactions of the immune system. The immune system is a very complex interconnected network, comprising the various different white blood cells (lymphocytes, granulocytes, macrophages, mast cells), as well as the entire system of mucous membranes throughout the body, but especially in the digestive system, where specialized lymphatic tissue, called Peyer's patches, plays an essential role in the Gut Associated Lymphoid Tissue or GALT. Another essential component of the immune system is the normally present bacterial colonies in the mucous membranes of the gut.

An allergy begins long before the manifestation of allergic like symptoms. The body has to be set up to respond to an allergen. This usually begins in early childhood. It takes a severely disturbed intestinal environment, the internal terrain of the body, to react allergenically. Unfortunately this disturbance to the intestinal environment often goes unnoticed, since it is chronic, and tends to build up over many years.

The disturbance to the intestinal environment is called dysbiosis. Dysbiosis can be described as an abnormal intestinal flora and an abnormally permeable intestinal mucous membrane. The intestinal flora, comprising of billions of bacteria, forms a fine film on the inside of the intestines. Everything you eat passes through this bacterial layer, which alters and filters the foodstuffs. When the intestinal flora is not intact, the absorptive ability of the intestinal mucous membranes becomes impaired.

Functional hypochlorhydria and pancreatic insufficiency causes the maldigestion of carbohydrates, fats and proteins. Large macromolecules are left undigested and form the substrate for dysbiosis formation. Over time the villi, the large absorptive surface of the intestines, becomes irritated and inflamed, which causes it to become less dense. The large, incompletely digested macromolecules, especially proteins, start to be able to penetrate the intestinal mucous membrane. With the destruction of the villi comes the reduction of the GALT and the secretory IgA, the body's first line defense against "foreign" invaders. Once in the bloodstream, the body's immune system recognizes the small protein or part of a protein as foreign, and produces antibodies against it. It is the reaction of the antibody/antigen complex that produces the classic allergy symptoms.

The body's second layer of defense lies in the liver. The liver normally screens the blood for antigens. On each pass through the body, the blood must pass through the liver for cleaning and detoxification. The liver normally takes these foreign substances and destroys them or gets them out of the body. Unfortunately liver dysfunction is a very common occurrence in our society. The destruction of foreign substances will not occur if the liver is not functioning as it should, if there is too much of the substance to get rid of easily or the liver's phase I and II detoxification pathways cannot destroy it.

Over 80% of the human immune system is situated alongside the intestines. It is therefore understandable that disturbances of the intestines and the intestinal flora place a tremendous overload on the immune system, which then often reacts "allergically" to otherwise quite innocuous proteins. Allergies are thus usually indirect ailments of the intestinal mucous membrane. Thus, in treating allergy clients, the greatest attention needs to be given to restoring the intestinal flora and the intestinal mucous membrane.

1° Indication

Dysbiosis- abnormal intestinal flora and increased intestinal hyperpermeability

Further assessment	1. Increased urinary indican and sediment levels 2. Stool analysis- either comprehensive digestive analysis or a parasite profile 3. Check for tenderness in the Chapman reflex for the colon located bilaterally along the iliotibial band on the thighs. Palpate the colon for tenderness and tension. 4. Check for tenderness in the Chapman reflex for the small intestine located on the 8th, 9th and 10th intercostal spaces near the tip of the rib. Also palpate four quadrants in a 2" to 3" radius around the umbilicus for tenderness and tension 5. Decreased secretory IgA on stool analysis

2° Indication

Liver congestion with detoxification problems, especially phase I and II detoxification

Further assessment	1. Check for tenderness in the Chapman reflex for the liver-gallbladder located over the 6th intercostal space on the right side 2. Check for tenderness in the Liver point located on the 3rd rib, 3 " to the right of the sternum, at the costochondral junction. 3. Check for tenderness underneath the right rib cage 4. Increased SGOT, SGPT on a blood chemistry panel 5. Various labs do liver detoxification panels

Other indications

1. Hypochlorhydria
2. Pancreatic insufficiency
3. Adrenal hypofunction
4. Mineral deficiency

Supplemental Support

Multiple herbal anti-histamines **Liver support:** 1. Nutrients to support Phase II liver detoxification 2. Herbs that cleanse the liver 3. Glutathione, cysteine, and Glycine 4. Powdered detoxification support formula 5. Plant source molybdenum	**Dysbiosis:** 1. Micro Emulsified Oregano 2. Nutrients that heal the intestines 3. L-Glutamine 4. Betaine HCL, Pepsin, and pancreatin 5. Water soluble fiber and colon health nutrients 6. Multiple nutrients that support the immune system 7. Lactobacillus acidophilus and Bifidobacterium bifidus

Lifestyle Changes

Please refer to the handouts in the appendix on the Dysbiosis diet and Recommendations for keeping the liver healthy

100. Abdominal bloating 1 to 2 hours after eating

Abdominal bloating one to two hours after eating is an indication of digestive dysfunction with pancreatic insufficiency and/or hypochlorhydria with a need for stomach acid supplementation. The delayed nature of the bloating suggests that the cause lies in the small intestine, and to some extent the colon.

Common causes of abdominal bloating 1 to 2 hours after eating include:

- Hypochlorhydria
- Pancreatic insufficiency
- Bowel toxemia
- Dysbiosis

1° Indication

Pancreatic insufficiency with pancreatic enzyme need

Further assessment	1. Check Ridler enzyme point for tenderness 1 inch below xyphoid and over to the right edge of the rib cage 2. Check for tenderness in the Chapman reflex for the pancreas located in the 7th intercostal space 3. Increased urinary sediment levels

2° Indication

Digestive dysfunction with hydrochloric acid need

Further assessment	1. Check Ridler HCL reflex for tenderness 1 inch below xyphoid and over to the left edge of the rib cage 2. Check for tenderness in the Chapman reflex for the stomach and upper digestion located in 6th intercostal space on the left 3. Gastric acid assessment using Gastrotest 4. Check for a positive zinc tally: A client holds a solution of aqueous zinc sulfate in their mouth and tells you if and when they can taste it. An almost immediate very bitter taste indicates the client does not need zinc. Clients who are zinc deficient will report no taste from the solution. 5. Increased urinary indican levels

Other indications

Toxic bowel

Supplemental Support

1. Pancreatic Enzymes 2. Bromelain, cellulase, lipase, and amylase 3. Beet juice, taurine, vitamin C and pancreolipase 4. Water soluble fiber 5. Lactobacillus acidophilus and Bifidobacterium bifidus

Lifestyle Changes

Please see handout in the appendix on the Diet to aid digestion

101. Specific foods make you tired or bloated (1= yes, 0= no)

Any kind of bloating after a meal is a sign of digestive dysfunction with HCL deficiency and/or pancreatic insufficiency. It is important to isolate the offending foods that cause the bloating. This can be done with an in-depth diet diary, a process where the client writes down everything they put in their mouths with a list of symptoms. Well-known offenders are diets high in refined foods, and low in vegetables and fiber.

It is essential that people slow down their eating and chew each mouthful thoroughly. This will prevent swallowing air, which is a well-known cause of bloating.

1° Indication

Digestive dysfunction with hydrochloric acid need

Further assessment	1. Check Ridler HCL reflex for tenderness 1 inch below xyphoid and over to the left edge of the rib cage 2. Check for tenderness in the Chapman reflex for the stomach and upper digestion located in 6th intercostal space on the left 3. Check for a positive zinc tally: A client holds a solution of aqueous zinc sulfate in their mouth and tells you if and when they can taste it. An almost immediate very bitter taste indicates the client does not need zinc. Clients who are zinc deficient will report no taste from the solution. 4. Gastric acid assessment using Gastrotest 5. Increased urinary indican levels

2° Indication

Pancreatic insufficiency with pancreatic enzyme need

Further assessment	1. Check Ridler enzyme point for tenderness 1 inch below xyphoid and over to the right edge of the rib cage 2. Check for tenderness in the Chapman reflex for the pancreas located in the 7th intercostal space 3. Increased urinary sediment levels

Other indications

Toxic bowel

Supplemental Support

1. Betaine HCL, Pepsin, and pancreatin
2. Pancreatic Enzymes
3. Bromelain, cellulase, lipase, and amylase
4. Beet juice, taurine, vitamin C and pancreolipase
5. Water soluble fiber and colon health nutrients capsules
6. Lactobacillus acidophilus and Bifidobacterium bifidus

Lifestyle changes

- Chew food thoroughly and eating slowly. Most people eat too fast and swallow air with their food; these can be a major cause of bloating. See handout on Diet to aid digestion.

102. Pulse speeds after eating
103. Airborne allergies
104. Experience hives

The above three questions have one thing in common- Allergies. Dr. Arthur Coca discovered that the speeding up of the pulse after consuming a food is a strong indication of allergies. Hives are often due to allergies too. They can manifest as both an immediate or delayed reaction.

Allergies are overreactions of the immune system. The immune system is a very complex interconnected network, comprising the various different white blood cells (lymphocytes, granulocytes, macrophages, mast cells), as well as the entire system of mucous membranes throughout the body, but especially in the digestive system, where specialized lymphatic tissue, called Peyer's patches, plays an essential role in the Gut Associated Lymphoid Tissue or GALT. Another essential component of the immune system is the normally present bacterial colonies in the mucous membranes of the digestive system.

An allergy begins long before the manifestation of allergic like symptoms. The body has to be set up to respond to an allergen. This usually begins in early childhood. It takes a severely disturbed intestinal environment, the internal terrain of the body, to react allergenically. Unfortunately this disturbance to the intestinal environment goes unnoticed, since it is chronic, and tends to build up over many years.

The disturbance to the intestinal environment is called dysbiosis. Dysbiosis can be described as an abnormal intestinal flora and an abnormally permeable intestinal mucous membrane. The intestinal flora, comprising of billions of bacteria, forms a fine film on the inside of the intestines. Everything you eat passes through this bacterial layer, which alters and filters the foodstuffs. When the intestinal flora is not intact, the absorptive ability of the intestinal mucous membranes becomes impaired.

Functional hypochlorhydria and pancreatic insufficiency causes the maldigestion of carbohydrates, fats and proteins. Large macromolecules are left undigested and form the substrate for dysbiosis formation. Over time the villi, the large absorptive surface of the intestines, becomes irritated and inflamed, which causes it to become less dense. The large, incompletely digested macromolecules, especially proteins, start to be able to penetrate the intestinal mucous membrane. With the destruction of the villi comes the reduction of the GALT and the secretory IgA, the body's first line defense against "foreign" invaders. Once in the bloodstream, the body's immune system recognizes the small protein or part of a protein as foreign, and produces antibodies against it. It is the reaction of the antibody/antigen complex that produces the classic allergy symptoms.

The body's second layer of defense lies in the liver. The liver normally screens the blood for antigens. On each pass through the body, the blood must pass through the liver for cleaning and detoxification. The liver will normally take these foreign substances and destroy them or get them out of the body. Unfortunately liver dysfunction is a very common occurrence in our society. The destruction of foreign substances will not occur if the liver is not functioning as it should, if there is too much of the substance to get rid of easily or the liver's phase I and II detoxification pathways cannot destroy it.

Over 80% of the human immune system is situated alongside the intestines. It is therefore understandable that disturbances of the intestines and the intestinal flora place a tremendous overload on the immune system, which then often reacts "allergically" to otherwise quite innocuous proteins. Allergies are thus usually indirect ailments of the intestinal mucous membrane. Thus, in treating allergy clients, the greatest attention needs to be given to restoring the intestinal flora and the intestinal mucous membrane.

1° Indication

Dysbiosis- abnormal intestinal flora and increased intestinal hyperpermeability

Further assessment	1. Increased urinary indican and sediment levels 2. Stool analysis- either comprehensive digestive analysis or a parasite profile 3. Check for tenderness in the Chapman reflex for the colon located bilaterally along the iliotibial band on the thighs. 4. Palpate the colon for tenderness and tension. 5. Check for tenderness in the Chapman reflex for the small intestine located on the 8th, 9th and 10th intercostal spaces near the tip of the rib. Also palpate four quadrants in a 2" to 3" radius around the umbilicus for tenderness and tension 6. Increased secretory IgA on stool analysis

2° Indication

Liver congestion with detoxification problems, especially phase I and II detoxification

Further assessment	1. Check for tenderness in the Chapman reflex for the liver-gallbladder located over the 6th intercostal space on the right 2. Check for tenderness in the Liver point located on the 3rd rib, 3 " to the right of the sternum, at the costochondral junction. 3. Assess for Hepato-biliary congestion with the Acoustic Cardiogram (ACG), which will show post-systolic rounding due to increased backpressure on the pulmonic and aortic valve. 4. Increased SGOT, SGPT on a blood chemistry panel 5. Various labs do liver detoxification panels

Other indications

1. Hypochlorhydria and pancreatic insufficiency
2. Adrenal hypofunction

Supplemental Support

Multiple herbal anti-histamines **Liver support:** 1. Nutrients to support Phase II detox 2. Herbs that cleanse the liver 3. Glutathione, cysteine, and Glycine 4. Powdered detoxification support formula 5. Plant source molybdenum	**Dysbiosis:** 1. Micro Emulsified Oregano 2. Nutrients that heal the intestines 3. L-Glutamine 4. Betaine HCL, Pepsin, and pancreatin 5. Lactobacillus acidophilus and Bifidobacterium bifidus

105. Sinus congestion, "stuffy head"

Chronic sinus congestion can be an indication of chronic dysbiosis in both the small intestine and more importantly in the sinuses themselves. New research has linked a chronic fungal infection with chronic sinus infections. Many people with chronic sinus congestion have had numerous courses of antibiotics to treat the infection, with no success. This can also contribute the dysbiosis in the small intestine. Another possible cause of sinus congestion is a need for HCL.

1° Indication

Dysbiosis

Further assessment	1. Increased urinary indican and sediment levels 2. Stool analysis- either comprehensive digestive analysis or a parasite profile 3. Check for tenderness in the Chapman reflex for the colon located bilaterally along the iliotibial band on the thighs. Palpate the colon for tenderness and tension. 4. Check for tenderness in the Chapman reflex for the small intestine located on the 8th, 9th and 10th intercostal spaces near the tip of the rib. Also palpate four quadrants in a 2" to 3" radius around the umbilicus for tenderness and tension

2° Indication

Digestive dysfunction with hydrochloric acid need

Further assessment	1. Check Ridler HCL reflex for tenderness 1 inch below xyphoid and over to the left edge of the rib cage 2. Check for tenderness in the Chapman reflex for the stomach and upper digestion located in 6th intercostal space on the left 3. Check for a positive zinc tally: A client holds a solution of aqueous zinc sulfate in their mouth and tells you if and when they can taste it. An almost immediate very bitter taste indicates the client does not need zinc. Clients who are zinc deficient will report no taste from the solution. 4. Gastric acid assessment using Gastrotest 5. Increased urinary indican levels

Supplemental Support

1. Micro Emulsified Oregano
2. Nutrients that heal the intestines
3. Betaine HCL, Pepsin, and pancreatin
4. Water soluble fiber and nutrients to support healthy colon
5. L-Glutamine
6. Multiple nutrients that support the immune system
7. Lactobacillus acidophilus and Bifidobacterium bifidus

Lifestyle changes

Please see the handout in the appendix on the Dysbiosis diet

106. Crave bread or noodles

Many people crave the foods they are allergic to. Unfortunately a wheat sensitivity or allergy is a common, unrecognized allergen. Therefore the craving of bread and noodles may be a sign of an unrecognized allergy. Most people associate an allergy with the full-blown immediate reaction, e.g. breaking out in hives after eating peanuts. Hidden allergies usually take longer to manifest with a reaction taking place anywhere from 24 to 72 hours later. This makes it very difficult to identify the offending food.

People with hidden allergies have many chronic health problems that they probably do not associate with any particular food. But one of the things we have to look at is the reason or cause of the sensitivity or allergy in the first place. The answer lies in the digestive tract.
Functional hypochlorhydria and pancreatic insufficiency causes the maldigestion of carbohydrates, fats and proteins. Large macromolecules are left undigested and form the substrate for bacterial growth leading to a dysbiosis. Over time the villi, the large absorptive surface of the intestines, becomes irritated and inflamed, which causes it to become less dense. The large macromolecules, especially proteins, can then penetrate the intestinal mucous membrane. Once in the bloodstream, the body's immune system will recognize the small protein or part of a protein as foreign, and produces antibodies against it. It is the reaction of the antibody/antigen complex that produces the classic allergy symptoms. A congested liver allows these allergens to circulate freely in the bloodstream, without being identified and destroyed.

Therefore, the underlying cause of the allergy needs to be addressed by thoroughly assessing the digestive and liver system and beginning therapy to restore the gut, and promote healthy liver function. Treatment calls for the identification and avoidance of the offending foods. Occasionally when the offending food is avoided, the symptoms can flare-up for 4-5 days. This can last for a short while, but the end result is the client feels better. We can also provide adjunctive nutritional therapy to help the client.

<u>1° Indication</u>
Dysbiosis- abnormal intestinal flora and increased intestinal hyperpermeability

Further assessment	1. Increased urinary indican and sediment levels 2. Stool analysis- either comprehensive digestive analysis or a parasite profile 3. Check for tenderness in the Chapman reflex for the colon located bilaterally along the iliotibial band on the thighs. Palpate the colon for tenderness and tension. 4. Check for tenderness in the Chapman reflex for the small intestine located on the 8th, 9th and 10th intercostal spaces near the tip of the rib. Also palpate four quadrants in a 2" to 3" radius around the umbilicus for tenderness and tension 5. Decreased secretory IgA on stool analysis

2° Indication

Liver congestion with detoxification problems, especially phase I and II detoxification

Further assessment	1. Check for tenderness in the Chapman reflex for the liver-gallbladder located over the 6th intercostal space on the right side 2. Check for tenderness in the Liver point located on the 3rd rib, 3 " to the right of the sternum, at the costochondral junction. 3. Check for tenderness underneath the right rib cage 4. Assess for Hepato-biliary congestion with the Acoustic Cardiogram (ACG), which will show post-systolic rounding due to increased backpressure on the pulmonic and aortic valve. It may also show through to the tricuspid valve if chronic. 5. Increased SGOT, SGPT on a blood chemistry panel

Other indications

1. Hypochlorhydria
2. Pancreatic insufficiency
3. Adrenal hypofunction
4. Mineral deficiency

Supplemental Support

Multiple herbal anti-histamines

Liver support:

1. Nutrients to support Phase II liver detoxification
2. Herbs that cleanse the liver
3. Glutathione, cysteine, and Glycine
4. Powdered detoxification support formula
5. Plant source molybdenum

Dysbiosis:

1. Micro Emulsified Oregano
2. Nutrients that heal the intestines
3. L-Glutamine
4. Betaine HCL, Pepsin, and pancreatin
5. Water soluble fiber and colon health nutrients
6. Multiple nutrients that support the immune system
7. Lactobacillus acidophilus and Bifidobacterium bifidus

Lifestyle changes

Please refer to the handouts in the appendix on the Dysbiosis diet and Recommendations for keeping the liver healthy

NOTES:

107. Alternating constipation and diarrhea

Alternating constipation and diarrhea is a symptom of irritable bowel syndrome (IBS). IBS is one of the most common gastrointestinal disorders that affect mostly women. Some of the other symptoms of IBS include:

- Abdominal pain and distension
- Hypersecretion of colonic mucous
- Flatulence
- Nausea
- Anxiety or depression
- Relief of pain with bowel movements

The irritation can come from food allergies, dysbiosis with an overgrowth of Candida, increased intestinal hyperpermeability or parasites. Another cause is increased stress and adrenal overload.

1° Indication

Irritated bowel due to Candida and leaky gut syndrome

Further assessment	1. Increased urinary indican and sediment levels 2. Stool analysis- either comprehensive digestive analysis or a parasite profile 3. Check for tenderness in the Chapman reflex for the colon located bilaterally along the iliotibial band on the thighs. Palpate the colon for tenderness and tension. 4. Check for tenderness in the Chapman reflex for the small intestine located on the 8th, 9th and 10th intercostal spaces near the tip of the rib. Also palpate four quadrants in a 2" to 3" radius around the umbilicus for tenderness and tension 5. Decreased secretory IgA on stool analysis

2° Indication

Stress and adrenal overload

Further assessment	1. Check for unilateral tenderness in the inguinal ligament 2. Check for a paradoxical pupillary reflex by shining a light into a client's eye and grading the reaction of the pupil. A pupil that fails to constrict indicates adrenal exhaustion 3. Check for the presence of postural hypotension. A drop of more than 10 points is an indication of adrenal insufficiency 4. Check for tenderness in the medial knee at the insertion of the sartorius muscle at the Pes Anserine. 5. Assess for adrenal insufficiency with the Acoustic Cardiogram (ACG), which will show static in both the systolic and diastolic rest phases. You will also see an elevated S2 sound. 6. Check for a chronic short leg due to posterior-inferior ilium 7. Lab test: An adrenal stress index measurement of the

	cortisol/DHEA ratio can indicate the severity of adrenal stress

Other indications

Food allergies

Supplemental Support

1. Micro Emulsified Oregano
2. Nutrients that heal the intestines
3. Betaine HCL, Pepsin, and pancreatin
4. Water soluble fiber and nutrients to support healthy colon
5. L-Glutamine
6. Multiple nutrients that support the immune system
7. Lactobacillus acidophilus and Bifidobacterium bifidus
8. Adrenal tissue (neonatal bovine)
9. Adaptogenic herbs to support adrenal function
10. Multiple nutrients to support sugar handling problems

Lifestyle changes

Please see handout in the appendix on the Dysbiosis diet

NOTES:

108. Crohn's disease

Crohn's disease is a non-specific inflammatory disease that usually affects the terminal ileum of the small intestine. It is characterized by inflammatory lesions called granulomas, though about 40% of sufferers do not appear to have well developed lesions.[6] The lesions may not be localized to just the small intestine. Lesions have been known to appear in the mouth, esophagus, stomach, duodenum, jejunum, and colon.

Crohn's disease presents with chronic diarrhea and abdominal pain. The lesion itself is ulcerative in nature and causes chronic damage to the lining of the intestines causing malabsorption, nutritional deficiencies and weight loss.

1° Indication

Assess small intestine

Further assessment	1. Check for tenderness in the Chapman reflex for the colon located bilaterally along the iliotibial band on the thighs. Palpate the colon for tenderness and tension. 2. Check for tenderness in the Chapman reflex for the small intestine located on the 8th, 9th and 10th intercostal spaces near the tip of the rib. Also palpate four quadrants in a 2" to 3" radius around the umbilicus for tenderness and tension 3. Increased urinary indican levels 4. Decreased secretory IgA on stool analysis

2° Indication

Assess the colon.

Further assessment	1. Check for tenderness in the Chapman reflex for the colon located bilaterally along the iliotibial band on the thighs. 2. Palpate the colon for tenderness and tension.

Supplemental support

1. Gut healing nutrients and vitamin U
2. Nutrients that heal the intestines
3. L-Glutamine
4. Betaine HCL, Pepsin, and pancreatin
5. Consider using a powdered detoxification formula as a meal replacement

NOTES:

[6] M.Murray and J. Pizzorno, *"Encyclopedia of natural medicine"* (California: Prima Publishing, 1998) p.587

109. Wheat or grain sensitivity

Wheat or grain sensitivity is suggestive of a gluten allergy or sensitivity. Even a mild sensitivity to wheat can cause the characteristic lesion of celiac disease: the shortening and flattening of the villi in the small intestine. This can lead to malabsorption, increased intestinal hyperpermeability and increased congestion with allergy like symptoms. If left untreated or unidentified a chronic alternating diarrhea and constipation can occur. Treatment involves following a gluten free diet and avoiding all sources of gluten.

1° Indication

Assess small intestine

Further assessment	1. Check for tenderness in the Chapman reflex for the colon located bilaterally along the iliotibial band on the thighs. Palpate the colon for tenderness and tension. 2. Check for tenderness in the Chapman reflex for the small intestine located on the 8th, 9th and 10th intercostal spaces near the tip of the rib. Also palpate four quadrants in a 2" to 3" radius around the umbilicus for tenderness and tension 3. Increased urinary indican levels 4. Decreased secretory IgA on stool analysis

2° Indication

Assess the colon.

Further assessment	1. Check for tenderness in the Chapman reflex for the colon located bilaterally along the iliotibial band on the thighs. 2. Palpate the colon for tenderness and tension.

Supplemental support

1. Gut healing nutrients and vitamin U
2. Nutrients that heal the intestines
3. L-Glutamine
4. Betaine HCL, Pepsin, and pancreatin

Lifestyle Changes

Please see the handout in the appendix on Foods to be avoided on a gluten free diet

NOTES:

110. Dairy sensitivity

A dairy sensitivity is an indication of lactose intolerance. The cells of the small intestine produce lactase, the enzyme that breaks lactose down. Dairy sensitivity is a strong indicator for small intestine support and/or the nutrients to help the lining of the small intestine heal.
The incomplete digestion of food due to a chronic pancreatic insufficiency can lead to increased irritation of the small intestine. Irritation can also be caused by dysbiosis. An overgrowth of unfriendly bacteria and yeast causes inflammation to the cells of the small intestine, which start to produce less lactase due to cell death. If the client continues to consume dairy, the irritation and cell death continues leading to chronic increased intestinal hyperpermeability and malabsorption

1° Indication

Need for small intestine support and/or increased intestinal hyperpermeability

Further assessment	1. Check for tenderness in the Chapman reflex for the colon located bilaterally along the iliotibial band on the thighs. Palpate the colon for tenderness and tension. 2. Check for tenderness in the Chapman reflex for the small intestine located on the 8th, 9th and 10th intercostal spaces near the tip of the rib. Also palpate four quadrants in a 2" to 3" radius around the umbilicus for tenderness and tension 3. Increased urinary indican levels 4. Decreased secretory IgA on stool analysis

Other indications

Dysbiosis

Supplemental Support

1. Nutrients that heal the intestines
2. Gut healing nutrients and vitamin U
3. Vitamin B complex
4. Pancreatic enzymes

Lifestyle changes

- Please see the handout in the appendix on Foods containing milk or dairy
- Avoid all refined carbohydrates and refined sugar
- Limit the consumption of complex carbohydrates
- Avoid all dairy
- Chew food thoroughly
- Find and eliminate all other food allergies

NOTES:

111. Are there foods you could not give up? (1 = yes, 0 = no)

Many people crave the foods they are allergic to. Having a food that you cannot give up is a strong indication of a hidden, unrecognized food allergy. Most people associate an allergy with a full-blown immediate reaction, like breaking out in hives after eating peanuts. Hidden allergies usually take longer to manifest with a reaction taking place anywhere from 24 to 72 hours later. This makes it very difficult to identify the offending food.

Cravings for certain foods can also be an indication of certain nutritional deficiencies. For instance people who crave chocolate are very often magnesium deficient, craving fatty foods can indicates an essential fatty acid deficiency and it is well known that craving ice or dirt (a condition called pica) can indicate iron deficiency.

People with hidden allergies have many chronic health problems that they probably do not associate with any particular food. But one of the things we have to look at is the reason or cause of the sensitivity or allergy in the first place. The answer lies in the digestive tract.
Functional hypochlorhydria and pancreatic insufficiency causes the maldigestion of carbohydrates, fats and proteins. Large macromolecules are left undigested and form the substrate for bacterial growth leading to a dysbiosis. Over time the villi, the large absorptive surface of the intestines, becomes irritated and inflamed, which causes it to become less dense. The large macromolecules, especially proteins, can then penetrate the intestinal mucous membrane. Once in the bloodstream, the body's immune system will recognize the small protein or part of a protein as foreign, and produces antibodies against it. It is the reaction of the antibody/antigen complex that produces the classic allergy symptoms. A congested liver allows these allergens to circulate freely in the bloodstream, without being identified and destroyed.

Treatment, therefore, needs to address the underlying cause of the allergy by thoroughly assessing the digestive and liver system and beginning therapy to restore the gut, and promote healthy liver function. Treatment also calls for the identification and avoidance of the offending foods. Occasionally when the offending food is avoided, the symptoms can flare-up for 4-5 days. This can last for a short while, but the end result is the client feels better. We can also provide adjunctive nutritional therapy to help the client.

<u>1° Indication</u>
Dysbiosis- abnormal intestinal flora and increased intestinal hyperpermeability

Further assessment	1. Increased urinary indican and sediment levels 2. Stool analysis- either comprehensive digestive analysis or a parasite profile 3. Check for tenderness in the Chapman reflex for the colon located bilaterally along the iliotibial band on the thighs. Palpate the colon for tenderness and tension. 4. Check for tenderness in the Chapman reflex for the small intestine located on the 8th, 9th and 10th intercostal spaces near the tip of the rib. Also palpate four quadrants in a 2" to

	3" radius around the umbilicus for tenderness and tension 5. Decreased secretory IgA on stool analysis

2° Indication

Liver congestion with detoxification problems, especially phase I and II detoxification

Further assessment	1. Check for tenderness in the Chapman reflex for the liver-gallbladder located over the 6th intercostal space on the right side 2. Check for tenderness in the Liver point located on the 3rd rib, 3 " to the right of the sternum, at the costochondral junction. 3. Check for tenderness underneath the right rib cage 4. Assess for Hepato-biliary congestion with the Acoustic Cardiogram (ACG), which will show post-systolic rounding due to increased backpressure on the pulmonic and aortic valve. It may also show through to the tricuspid valve if chronic. 5. Increased SGOT, SGPT on a blood chemistry panel

Other indications

1. Hypochlorhydria
2. Pancreatic insufficiency
3. Adrenal hypofunction
4. Mineral deficiency

Supplemental Support

Multiple herbal anti-histamines

Liver support:

1. Nutrients to support Phase II liver detoxification
2. Herbs that cleanse the liver
3. Glutathione, cysteine, and Glycine
4. Powdered detoxification support formula
5. Plant source molybdenum

Dysbiosis:

1. Micro Emulsified Oregano
2. Nutrients that heal the intestines
3. L-Glutamine
4. Betaine HCL, Pepsin, and pancreatin
5. Water soluble fiber and colon health nutrients
6. Multiple nutrients that support the immune system
7. Lactobacillus acidophilus and Bifidobacterium bifidus

Lifestyle changes

Please refer to the handouts in the appendix on the Dysbiosis diet and Recommendations for keeping the liver healthy

112. Asthma, sinus infections, stuffy nose

The symptoms of asthma, sinus infections and a stuffy nose can all be traced to the digestive system and a series of events that trigger these symptoms and increase the susceptibility to infection.

There is probably a functional hypochlorhydria and pancreatic enzyme deficiency, which causes a maldigestion of carbohydrates, fats and proteins. The maldigestion of food leaves large macromolecules undigested, which form the substrate for dysbiosis formation. Dysbiosis can be described as an abnormal intestinal flora. The intestinal flora, comprising of billions of bacteria, forms a fine film on the inside of the intestines. Everything you eat passes through this bacterial layer, which alters and filters the foodstuffs. When the intestinal flora is not intact, the absorptive ability of the intestinal mucous membranes becomes impaired and you get an abnormally permeable intestinal mucous membrane.

Over time the villi, the large absorptive surface of the intestines, becomes irritated and inflamed by the large macromolecules and the dysbiosis, which causes it to become less dense. The large, incompletely digested macromolecules, especially proteins, start to be able to penetrate the intestinal mucous membrane. With the destruction of the villi comes the reduction of the Gut Associated Lymphoid Tissue (GALT) and the secretory IgA, the body's first line defense against "foreign" invaders. Once in the bloodstream, the body's immune system recognizes the small protein or part of a protein as foreign, and produces antibodies against it. It is the reaction of the antibody/antigen complex that produces the symptoms of allergies that can cause asthma and a stuffy nose.

Sinus infections are a reflection of the dysbiosis in both the small intestine and more importantly in the sinuses themselves. New research has linked a chronic fungal infection with chronic sinus infections. Many people with chronic sinus infections have had numerous courses of antibiotics to treat the infection, with no success. This can also contribute the dysbiosis in the small intestine.

Treatment, therefore, needs to address the underlying cause by thoroughly assessing the digestive system and beginning therapy to restore a healthy gut function.

1° Indication

Dysbiosis

Further assessment	1. Increased urinary indican and sediment levels 2. Stool analysis- either CDSA or a parasite profile 3. Check for tenderness in the Chapman reflex for the colon located bilaterally along the iliotibial band on the thighs. Palpate the colon for tenderness and tension. 4. Check for tenderness in the Chapman reflex for the small intestine located on the 8th, 9th and 10th intercostal spaces near the tip of the rib. Also palpate four quadrants in a 2" to 3" radius around the umbilicus for tenderness and tension 5. Decreased secretory IgA on stool analysis

Other indications

1. Hypochlorhydria and/or pancreatic insufficiency
2. Adrenal hypofunction

3. Mineral deficiency

Supplemental Support

1. Micro Emulsified Oregano
2. Nutrients that heal the intestines
3. Betaine HCL, Pepsin, and pancreatin
4. Water soluble fiber and nutrients to support healthy colon
5. L-Glutamine
6. Multiple nutrients that support the immune system
7. Lactobacillus acidophilus and Bifidobacterium bifidus

Lifestyle changes: Please see the handout in the appendix on the Dysbiosis diet

NOTES:

113. Bizarre vivid or nightmarish dreams

Bizarre, vivid or nightmarish dreams are a sign of increased toxicity within the body. Increased toxicity within the body comes from a heavy body burden, a decreased ability to detoxify or an inability to properly eliminate. The environment is a source of a lot of external toxicity from the air we breathe, the water we drink and the food we eat, which is severely polluted with preservatives and chemical additives.

The altered internal environment of the body is also a source of increased toxicity. Dysbiosis caused by the growth of yeast, bacteria and parasites, produces a lot of metabolic toxins that can cause these symptoms. There may be a need for liver support, as the liver has the main job of detoxifying any toxins, a need to clear up the dysbiosis and a need to support the kidney.

1° Indication

Liver congestion with detoxification problems

Further assessment	1. Check for tenderness in the Chapman reflex for the liver-gallbladder located over the 6th intercostal space on the right. 2. Check for tenderness in the Liver point located on the 3rd rib, 3 " to the right of the sternum, at the costochondral junction. 3. Check for tenderness underneath the right rib cage. 4. Assess for Hepato-biliary congestion with the Acoustic Cardiogram (ACG), which will show post-systolic rounding due to increased backpressure on the pulmonic and aortic valve. It may also show through to the tricuspid valve if chronic. 5. Increased SGOT, SGPT on a blood chemistry panel 6. Various labs do liver detoxification panels

2° Indication

Dysbiosis- abnormal intestinal flora and increased intestinal hyperpermeability

Further assessment	1. Increased urinary indican and sediment levels 2. Stool analysis- either CDSA or a parasite profile 3. Check for tenderness in the Chapman reflex for the colon located bilaterally along the iliotibial band on the thighs. Palpate the colon for tenderness and tension. 4. Check for tenderness in the Chapman reflex for the small intestine located on the 8th, 9th and 10th intercostal spaces near the tip of the rib. Also palpate four quadrants in a 2" to 3" radius around the umbilicus for tenderness and tension. 5. Decreased secretory IgA on stool analysis

3° Indication

Need to support kidney function to promote adequate elimination

Further assessment	1. Check for tenderness in the Chapman reflex for the kidneys located 1" lateral and 1" superior from the umbilicus on the

	medial margin of the Rectus abdominus muscle. Have clients tighten stomach muscles to palpate. 2. Check for an increase in blood pressure when the client goes from standing to supine 3. Routine and functional urinalysis 4. Blood chemistry renal function panel

Supplemental Support

Liver support:
1. Nutrients to support Phase II liver detoxification
2. Herbs that cleanse the liver
3. Glutathione, cysteine, and Glycine
4. Powdered detoxification support formula
5. Plant source molybdenum

Dysbiosis:
1. Micro Emulsified Oregano
2. Nutrients that heal the intestines
3. L-Glutamine
4. Betaine HCL, Pepsin, and pancreatin
5. Water soluble fiber and colon health nutrients
6. Multiple nutrients that support the immune system
7. Lactobacillus acidophilus and Bifidobacterium bifidus

Kidney:

a. Multiple nutrients for supporting renal function
b. Kidney tissue (neonatal bovine)
c. Culture of Beet Juice containing Arginase
d. Magnesium
e. Pyridoxal-5-phosphate
f. Bio AE-Mulsion

Lifestyle changes

Please refer to the handouts in the appendix on the Dysbiosis and Recommendations for keeping the liver healthy

NOTES:

114. Use over-the-counter pain medications

The use of Non-Steroidal Anti Inflammatory drugs (NSAIDs) can cause irritation to the gastrointestinal lining leading to an increased intestinal hyperpermeability, which can lead to an increased sensitivity to certain allergenic foods.

Another problem with NSAID use is the increased stress on the livers detoxification system. The liver is the main organ of detoxification and the constant need to detoxify over the counter pain medications can lead to a dysfunction in either of the two phases of detoxification, and an increase in oxidative stress, which can lead to an increase in pain and inflammation. Clients on these types of medication need extra liver support.

Phase I detoxification involves the oxidation, reduction and/or hydrolysis of a molecule to make it less toxic. Many of the enzymes in this phase require molybdenum.

Phase II detoxification is a process of conjugation, which makes the molecule water-soluble, so that it can be removed from the body. This phase requires adequate levels of glycine and glutathione, along with many other different nutrients for adequate conjugation.

1° Indication

Increased intestinal hyperpermeability

Further assessment	1. Check for tenderness in the Chapman reflex for the small intestine located on the 8th, 9th and 10th intercostal spaces near the tip of the rib. Also palpate four quadrants in a 2" to 3" radius around the umbilicus for tenderness and tension 2. Check for tenderness in the Chapman reflex for the colon located bilaterally along the iliotibial band on the thighs. Palpate the colon for tenderness and tension. 3. Increased urinary indican levels

2° Indication

Increased need for liver support to help with phase I and II detoxification problems

Further assessment	1. Check for tenderness in the Chapman reflex for the liver-gallbladder located over the 6th intercostal space on the right 2. Check for tenderness in the Liver point located on the 3rd rib, 3 " to the right of the sternum, at the costochondral junction. 3. Check for tenderness underneath the right rib cage 4. Increased SGOT, SGPT on a blood chemistry panel 5. Various labs do liver detoxification panels

Other indications

Essential fatty acid need

Supplemental Support

1. Broad spectrum proteolytic enzymes
2. Bromelain
3. Nutrients that heal the intestines
4. Gut healing nutrients and vitamin U
5. Broad spectrum anti-oxidants
6. Glutathione, cysteine, and Glycine
7. Herbs that cleanse the liver
8. Nutrients to support Phase II liver detoxification

115. Feel spacey or unreal

This symptom can be due to many things: food allergies, low adrenal function, low thyroid function or hypoglycemia. One of the main causes is dysbiosis, especially from Candida. An overgrowth of Candida can lead to an enormous amount of toxicity in the body, which can affect the brain causing a spacey, unreal like feeling. It has been shown that toxins with opioid like properties are often released by yeast and bacteria in the digestive system. These travel to the brain and cause symptoms of feeling spacey and unreal. People have often described it as being "out of the body". Working to eliminate the dysbiosis and support the liver can help decrease this symptom.

1° Indication

Dysbiosis from Candida infection

Further assessment	1. Increased urinary indican 2. Stool analysis- either comprehensive digestive analysis or a parasite profile 3. Check for tenderness in the Chapman reflex for the colon located bilaterally along the iliotibial band on the thighs. Palpate the colon for tenderness and tension. 4. Check for tenderness in the Chapman reflex for the small intestine located on the 8th, 9th and 10th intercostal spaces near the tip of the rib. Also palpate four quadrants in a 2" to 3" radius around the umbilicus for tenderness and tension. 5. Decreased secretory IgA on stool analysis

2° Indication

Increased need for liver support

Further assessment	1. Check for tenderness in the Chapman reflex for the liver-gallbladder located over the 6th intercostal space on the right 2. Check for tenderness in the Liver point located on the 3rd rib, 3 " to the right of the sternum, at the costochondral junction. 3. Check for tenderness underneath the right rib cage 4. Increased SGOT, SGPT on a blood chemistry panel 5. Various labs do liver detoxification panels

Other indications

1. Adrenal and thyroid hypofunction
2. Food allergies and Hypoglycemia

Supplemental Support

Dysbiosis:	**Liver support:**
1. Micro Emulsified Oregano 2. Nutrients that heal the intestines 3. Betaine HCL, Pepsin, and pancreatin 4. Water soluble fiber and colon health nutrients 5. nutrients to support the immune system	1. Nutrients to support Phase II liver detoxification 2. Herbs that cleanse the liver 3. Glutathione, cysteine, and Glycine 4. Powdered detoxification support formula 5. Plant source molybdenum

LARGE INTESTINE

116. Anus itches
117. Coated tongue
118. Feel worse in moldy or musty place
119. Taken antibiotics for a combined time of: 1 =< 1 mo., 2 = < 3 mos., 3 = > 3 mos.
120. Fungus or yeast infections
121. Ring worm, "jock itch", "athletes foot", nail fungus
122. Eating sugar, starch or drinking alcohol increases yeast symptoms
123. Stools hard or difficult to pass
124. History of parasites (1 = yes, 0 = no)
125. Less than one bowel movement per day
126. Stools have corners or edges are flat or ribbon shaped
127. Stools are not well formed (loose)
128. Irritable bowel or mucus colitis
129. Blood in stool
130. Mucus in stool
131. Excessive foul smelling lower bowel gas
132. Bad breath or strong body odors
133. Painful to press along outer sides of thighs (Iliotibial Band)
134. Cramping in lower abdominal region
135. Dark circles under eyes

116. Anus itches

Anal itching has a number of possible causes including intestinal parasites, which is especially true if the client has unexplained Diarrhea or has recently returned from foreign travel. It can also be due to a need for bile salts and/or hydrochloric acid

<u>1° Indication</u>

Intestinal parasites

Further assessment	1. CBC- look for elevated eosinophils and basophils 2. A stool test can help detect which parasite, if any, is present. Start with one random stool. If no parasite is found and the index of suspicion is high repeat the stool test, but this time do a purged sample with either a large bolus of vitamin C or magnesium sulfate. Collect the next two stools for testing. 3. Check for tenderness in the Chapman reflex for the colon located bilaterally along the iliotibial band on the thighs. Palpate the colon for tenderness and tension. 4. Decreased secretory IgA on stool analysis

<u>2° Indication</u>

Digestive dysfunction with hydrochloric acid and/or bile salt need

Further assessment	**For HCL need** 1. Check Ridler HCL reflex for tenderness 1 inch below xyphoid and over to the left edge of the rib cage 2. Check for tenderness in the Chapman reflex for the stomach and upper digestion located in 6th intercostal space on the left 3. Check for a positive zinc tally: A client holds a solution of aqueous zinc sulfate in their mouth and tells you if and when they can taste it. Clients who are zinc deficient will report no taste from the solution. 4. Gastric acid assessment using Gastrotest 5. Increased urinary indican levels **For Bile salt need** 1. Check for tenderness underneath the right rib cage 2. Check for tenderness and nodulation on the web between thumb and fore-finger of right hand 3. Check for tenderness in the Chapman reflex for the liver-gallbladder located over the 6th intercostal space on the right

<u>Other indications</u>

1. Vitamin A and Zinc need

Supplemental Support

1. Water soluble fiber and colon health nutrients 2. Nutrients that heal the intestines 3. Betaine HCL, Pepsin, and pancreatin 4. Larch arabinogalactans	5. Micro Emulsified Oregano 6. Beet juice and bile salts 7. Bromelain 8. Lactobacillus acidophilus and Bifidobacterium bifidus

117. Coated tongue

A coated tongue is an indication of some kind of disturbance in the digestive organs. Its main indication is a toxic bowel with dysbiosis and/or increased intestinal hyper-permeability. It may also show a need for digestive enzymes or HCL supplementation.

1° Indication

Toxic bowel with dysbiosis and /or increased intestinal hyperpermeability

Further assessment	1. Increased urinary indican 2. Stool analysis- either comprehensive digestive analysis or a parasite profile 3. Check for tenderness in the Chapman reflex for the colon located bilaterally along the iliotibial band on the thighs. Palpate the colon for tenderness and tension. 4. Check for tenderness in the Chapman reflex for the small intestine located on the 8th, 9th and 10th intercostal spaces near the tip of the rib. Also palpate four quadrants in a 2" to 3" radius around the umbilicus for tenderness and tension

2° Indication

Pancreatic enzyme need or hydrochloric acid

Further assessment	**Pancreatic enzymes** 1. Check Ridler enzyme point for tenderness 1 inch below xyphoid and over to the right edge of the rib cage 2. Check for tenderness in the Chapman reflex for the pancreas located in the 7th intercostal space 3. Increased urinary sediment levels **Hydrochloric acid** 1. Check Ridler HCL reflex for tenderness 1 inch below xyphoid and over to the left edge of the rib cage 2. Check for tenderness in the Chapman reflex for the stomach and upper digestion located in 6th intercostal space on the left 3. Check for a positive zinc tally: A client holds a solution of aqueous zinc sulfate in their mouth and tells you if and when they can taste it. An almost immediate very bitter taste indicates the client does not need zinc. Clients who are zinc deficient will report no taste from the solution.

Supplemental Support

1. Micro Emulsified Oregano
2. Nutrients that heal the intestines
3. Betaine HCL, Pepsin, and pancreatin
4. Water soluble fiber and colon health nutrients
5. Lactobacillus acidophilus and Bifidobacterium bifidus
6. Pancreatic Enzymes, broad spectrum proteolytic enzymes, and Bromelain

Lifestyle changes

Please see the handout in the appendix on the Dysbiosis diet and the Diet to aid digestion

118. Feel worse in moldy or musty place

Feeling worse in moldy and musty places is a strong indication of a dysbiosis in the digestive tract with an overgrowth of yeast (Candida). The body can sometimes be so overburdened with yeast that even the least amount of toxic exposure can precipitate a bad reaction. The body may also need supplemental molybdenum, a trace mineral that acts as a co-factor for the liver's detox pathways.

1° Indication
Dysbiosis with yeast overgrowth

Further assessment	1. Increased urinary indican 2. Stool analysis- either comprehensive digestive analysis or a parasite profile 3. Check for tenderness in the Chapman reflex for the colon located bilaterally along the iliotibial band on the thighs. Palpate the colon for tenderness and tension. 4. Check for tenderness in the Chapman reflex for the small intestine located on the 8th, 9th and 10th intercostal spaces near the tip of the rib. Also palpate four quadrants in a 2" to 3" radius around the umbilicus for tenderness and tension. 5. Decreased secretory IgA on stool analysis

Other indications
Molybdenum need

Supplement Support

1. Micro Emulsified Oregano
2. Nutrients that heal the intestines
3. Betaine HCL, Pepsin, and pancreatin
4. Water soluble fiber and colon health nutrients
5. Multiple nutrients that support the immune system
6. Lactobacillus acidophilus and Bifidobacterium bifidus

Lifestyle changes
Please see the handout in the appendix on the Dysbiosis diet

NOTES:

119. Taken any antibiotic for a combined time of (1 = < 1 mo., 2 = < 3 mos., 3 = > 3 mos.)
120. Fungus or yeast infections
121. Ring worm, "jock itch", "athlete's foot", nail fungus
122. Yeast symptoms increase with sugar, starch or alcohol

The above four questions all indicate a dysbiosis in the intestines with an overgrowth of Candida yeast. The more courses of antibiotics someone has taken, the more severe the dysbiosis in the body. Antibiotics wipe out all the normal, necessary bacteria in the digestive tract. This can lead to an increased intestinal permeability in the lining of the digestive tract and an increased susceptibility to allergies. Yeast infections can flourish in such an environment, especially if the beneficial bacteria are not replaced. Yeast does not have to stay confined to the digestive tract. It will manifest wherever there is a disturbance to the environment of the body. It particularly likes moist and warm places such as the inner thighs, between the toes, in the mouth and under the arms. Yeast also likes sugar, refined starches and alcohol, which form a perfect culture medium for yeast growth throughout the body. A successful anti-yeast protocol involves the client abstaining from all forms of sugar and potentially yeasty food.

One also should consider the possibility of an increased heavy metal body burden. There is some evidence that the body tolerates the Candida overgrowth because Candida, to some extent, helps deal with the heavy metals. One cannot, therefore, get rid of the Candida until the heavy metal body burden has been assessed and removed.

1° Indication

Dysbiosis with yeast overgrowth

Further assessment	1. Increased urinary indican 2. Stool analysis for candida and parasites 3. Check for tenderness in the Chapman reflex for the colon located bilaterally along the iliotibial band on the thighs. Palpate the colon for tenderness and tension. 4. Check for tenderness in the Bennet reflex for the small intestine. Palpate four quadrants in a 2" to 3" radius around the umbilicus for tenderness and tension. 5. Hair analysis. 6. Decreased secretory IgA on stool analysis.

Supplement Support

1. Micro Emulsified Oregano
2. Digestive support: Nutrients to heal the intestines, Betaine HCL, Pepsin, & pancreatin
3. Water soluble fiber and colon health nutrients
4. Multiple nutrients that support the immune system
5. Probiotics: Lactobacillus acidophilus and Bifidobacterium bifidus

Lifestyle changes

Please see the handout in the appendix on the Dysbiosis diet

123. Stools hard or difficult to pass

Stools that are difficult or hard to pass are an indication of constipation. Constipation is a subjective symptom where stools are too hard, too small, too infrequent, difficult to expel, or when the client has a feeling of incomplete evacuation after the bowel movement is over. Other objective signs are fewer than 3-5 stools per week, or more than 3 days without a stool. Average bowel transit time is 50-100 hours. The optimum bowel transit time is 17-30 hours. From a functional perspective a client should be considered constipated if a day passes without a bowel movement. Even if the client has a bowel movement every day, there still may be problems. Any significant, sudden change in bowel habits can be a sign of organic disease and must therefore be pursued.

The most common cause of constipation is a lack of dietary fiber and adequate hydration. Many people do not take their supplementary fiber with adequate amounts of water. This can make the constipation much worse, and cause the stool to be harder and more difficult to pass. Treating constipation is a process of trying one approach, seeing if it works and if it doesn't moving to the next step. The most likely causes of constipation in a functional list is: lack of fiber, lack of adequate hydration, a deficiency in pancreatic enzymes and hydrochloric acid, biliary congestion with a need for bile salts, dysbiosis, food allergies and a low functioning thyroid.

1° Indication

Assess the colon for lack of fiber and adequate hydration.

Further assessment	1. Have a client check their bowel transit time. Give 6 "00" caps of activated charcoal and ask them to record how long it takes for the black to appear and to go completely away. Various dyes, including beets, sweetcorn and un-popped popcorn can also be used. 2. Assess the client's hydration status. Have client stand with hands by their side and check and palpate the veins in the right hand. Have them slowly raise their hand to heart level and see if the veins still stick out. Veins that are only just visible or not visible at all are a sign of dehydration 3. Check for tenderness in the Chapman reflex for the colon located bilaterally along the iliotibial band on the thighs. 4. Palpate the colon for tenderness and tension.

2° Indication

Pancreatic enzyme need or hydrochloric acid

Further assessment	**Pancreatic enzymes** 1. Check Ridler enzyme point for tenderness 1 inch below xyphoid and over to the right edge of the rib cage 2. Check for tenderness in the Chapman reflex for the pancreas located in the 7th intercostal space 3. Increased urinary sediment levels **Hydrochloric acid** 1. Check Ridler HCL reflex for tenderness 1 inch below xyphoid and over to the left edge of the rib cage

	2. Check for tenderness in the Chapman reflex for the stomach and upper digestion located in 6th intercostal space on the left 3. Check for a positive zinc tally: A client holds a solution of aqueous zinc sulfate in their mouth and tells you if and when they can taste it. An almost immediate very bitter taste indicates the client does not need zinc. Clients who are zinc deficient will report no taste from the solution. 4. Gastric acid assessment using Gastrotest 5. Increased urinary indican levels

Other indications

1. Biliary congestion with a need for bile salts
2. Dysbiosis
3. Food allergies
4. Low functioning thyroid
5. Magnesium deficiency

Supplemental Support

1. Micro Emulsified Oregano
2. Water soluble fiber and nutrients to support healthy colon
3. Nutrients that heal the intestines
4. Betaine HCL, Pepsin, and pancreatin
5. Pancreatic enzymes
6. Beet juice, taurine, vitamin C and pancreolipase

Lifestyle changes

- Eat a high fiber, low fat diet. Include bran, seeds and vegetables into your diet.
- Avoid overeating and frequent snacking.
- Avoid refined carbohydrates (white flour), cheese, potatoes and meats, which contribute to constipation.
- Drink plenty of fluids, at least 6-8 glasses per day. Water is best. Avoid coffee, tea and fizzy drinks
- Include grapes, cherries, melons, licorice, spinach, and psyllium seeds and laxative foods such as prunes and pectin containing fruits (apples, figs, pears, bananas).
- **Abdominal massage**: Starting at the lower right side of your belly, massage up to your ribs then across your upper stomach and down the left side making a big circle around your navel. Perform massage after every meal to stimulate the colon and train your bowels to move after each meal.
- **Exercise** is a bowel stimulant. Some type of aerobic exercise at least 30 minutes, three to four times per week is helpful. Wear loose clothes around the waist.
- Hot applications to the abdomen; hot water bottle, hot wet towels

NOTES:

124. History of parasites (1 = yes, 0 = no)

A client may indicate a history of parasites, which may have been treated; yet present no evidence to show that the parasites were effectively eliminated from the body. Parasites are very persistent and can linger for long periods of time. Their presence can contribute to low-grade sickness and often-unrelated symptoms from allergies, and fibromyalgia to Benign Prostatic Hypertrophy and chronic sinusitis. As we continue to use more antibiotics, the environment becomes more toxic, the quality of food continues to decline, and we continue to decrease our aerobic exercise, we will become more susceptible to parasitic infections.

1° Indication

Intestinal parasites

Further assessment	1. CBC to see if eosinophils or basophils are elevated 2. Stool test for ova and parasite can help detect which parasite, if any, is present. Start with one random stool. If no parasite is found and the index of suspicion is high repeat the stool test, but this time do a purged sample with either a large bolus of vitamin C or magnesium sulfate. Collect the next two stools for testing. 3. Check for tenderness in the Chapman reflex for the colon located bilaterally along the iliotibial band on the thighs. Palpate the colon for tenderness and tension. 4. Decreased secretory IgA on stool analysis.

2° Indication

Digestive dysfunction with hydrochloric acid need

Further assessment	1. Check Ridler HCL reflex for tenderness 1 inch below xyphoid and over to the left edge of the rib cage 2. Check for tenderness in the Chapman reflex for the stomach and upper digestion located in 6th intercostal space on the left 3. Check for a positive zinc tally: A client holds a solution of aqueous zinc sulfate in their mouth and tells you if and when they can taste it. An almost immediate very bitter taste indicates the client does not need zinc. Clients who are zinc deficient will report no taste from the solution. 4. Gastric acid assessment using Gastrotest 5. Increased urinary indican levels

Supplemental Support

1. Water soluble fiber and colon health nutrients
2. Digestive support: Nutrients to heal the intestines, Betaine HCL, Pepsin, & pancreatin
3. Larch arabinogalactans
4. Micro Emulsified Oregano
5. Beet juice, taurine, vitamin C and pancreolipase
6. Bromelain, cellulase, lipase, and amylase

Lifestyle changes

Please see the handout in the appendix on the Dysbiosis diet

125. Less than one bowel movement per day

Less than one bowel movement is sign of constipation. Constipation is a subjective symptom where stools are too hard, too small, too infrequent, difficult to expel, or when the client has a feeling of incomplete evacuation after the bowel movement is over. Other objective signs are fewer than *3-5* stools per week, or more than 3 days without a stool. Average bowel transit time is 50-100 hours. The optimum bowel transit time is 17-30 hours. From a functional perspective a client should be considered constipated if a day passes without a bowel movement. Even if the client has a bowel movement every day, there still may be problems. Any significant, sudden change in bowel habits can be a sign of organic disease and must therefore be pursued.

The most common cause of constipation is a lack of dietary fiber and adequate hydration. Many people do not take their supplementary fiber with adequate amounts of water. This can make the constipation much worse, and cause the stool to be harder and more difficult to pass. Treating constipation is a process of trying one approach, seeing if it works and if it doesn't moving to the next step. The most likely causes of constipation in a functional list are: lack of fiber, lack of adequate hydration, a deficiency in pancreatic enzymes and hydrochloric acid, biliary congestion with a need for bile salts, dysbiosis, food allergies and a low functioning thyroid. Constipation is also a sign of magnesium deficiency.

<u>1° Indication</u>
Assess the colon for lack of fiber and adequate hydration.

Further assessment	1. Have a client check their bowel transit time. Give 6 "00" caps of activated charcoal and ask them to record how long it takes for the black to appear and to go completely away. Various dyes, including beets, sweetcorn, and un-popped popcorn can also be used. 2. Assess the client's hydration status. Have client stand with hands by their side and check and palpate the veins in the right hand. Have them slowly raise their hand to heart level and see if the veins still stick out. Veins that are only just visible or not visible at all are a sign of dehydration 3. Check for tenderness in the Chapman reflex for the colon located bilaterally along the iliotibial band on the thighs. 4. Palpate the colon for tenderness and tension. 5. Decreased secretory IgA on stool analysis.

<u>2° Indication</u>
Pancreatic enzyme need or hydrochloric acid

Further assessment	**Pancreatic enzymes** 1. Check Ridler enzyme point for tenderness 1 inch below xyphoid and over to the right edge of the rib cage 2. Check for tenderness in the Chapman reflex for the pancreas located in the 7th intercostal space 3. Increased urinary sediment levels

	Hydrochloric acid 1. Check Ridler HCL reflex for tenderness 1 inch below xyphoid and over to the left edge of the rib cage 2. Check for tenderness in the Chapman reflex for the stomach and upper digestion located in 6th intercostal space on the left 3. Check for a positive zinc tally: A client holds a solution of aqueous zinc sulfate in their mouth and tells you if and when they can taste it. An almost immediate very bitter taste indicates the client does not need zinc. Clients who are zinc deficient will report no taste from the solution. 4. Gastric acid assessment using Gastrotest 5. Increased urinary indican levels

Other indications

1. Biliary congestion with a need for bile salts
2. Dysbiosis
3. Food allergies
4. Low functioning thyroid
5. Magnesium deficiency

Supplemental Support

1. Micro Emulsified Oregano
2. Water soluble fiber and nutrients to support healthy colon
3. Nutrients that heal the intestines
4. Betaine HCL, Pepsin, and pancreatin
5. Pancreatic enzymes
6. Beet juice, taurine, vitamin C and pancreolipase

Lifestyle changes

- Eat a high fiber, low fat diet. Include bran, seeds and vegetables into your diet.
- Avoid overeating and frequent snacking.
- Avoid refined carbohydrates (white flour), cheese, potatoes and meats, which contribute to constipation.
- Drink plenty of fluids, at least 6-8 glasses per day. Water is best. Avoid coffee, tea and fizzy drinks
- Include grapes, cherries, melons, licorice, spinach, and psyllium seeds and laxative foods such as prunes and pectin containing fruits (apples, figs, pears, bananas).
- **Abdominal massage**: Starting at the lower right side of your belly, massage up to your ribs then across your upper stomach and down the left side making a big circle around your navel. Perform massage after every meal to stimulate the colon and train your bowels to move after each meal.
- **Exercise** is a bowel stimulant. Some type of aerobic exercise at least 30 minutes, three to four times per week is helpful. Wear loose clothes around the waist.
- Hot applications to the abdomen; hot water bottle, hot wet towels

NOTES:

126. Stools have corners or edges, are flat or ribbon shaped

A stool that has corners or edges, or is flat or ribbon shaped suggests the possibility of spastic bowel, rectal narrowing or stricture (pencil shaped), decreased elasticity, or partial obstruction (uterus malposition, prostatitis, polyp, and tumor). All of these conditions are serious and should be evaluated by a clinician specializing in colon abnormalities.

If pathology is ruled out consider that a misshapen stool is a sign of long bowel transit time and/or muscular weakness in the colon causing peristaltic changes.

1° Indication

Assess the colon for lack of fiber and adequate hydration.

Further assessment	1. Have a client check their bowel transit time. Give 6 "00" caps of activated charcoal and ask them to record how long it takes for the black to appear and to go completely away. Various dyes, including beets, sweetcorn, and un-popped popcorn can also be used. 2. Assess the client's hydration status. Have client stand with hands by their side and check and palpate the veins in the right hand. Have them slowly raise their hand to heart level and see if the veins still stick out. Veins that are only just visible or not visible at all are a sign of dehydration 3. Check for tenderness in the Chapman reflex for the colon located bilaterally along the iliotibial band on the thighs. 4. Palpate the colon for tenderness and tension. 5. Decreased secretory IgA on stool analysis.

Supplemental Support

1. Micro Emulsified Oregano
2. Water soluble fiber and nutrients to support healthy colon
3. Nutrients that heal the intestines
4. Betaine HCL, Pepsin, and pancreatin
5. Pancreatic enzymes
6. Beet juice, taurine, vitamin C and pancreolipase

Lifestyle changes

- Eat a high fiber, low fat diet. Include bran, seeds and vegetables into your diet.
- Avoid overeating and frequent snacking.
- Avoid refined carbohydrates (white flour), cheese, potatoes and meats, which contribute to constipation.
- Drink plenty of fluids, at least 6-8 glasses/day. Water is best. Avoid coffee, tea & soda
- Include grapes, cherries, melons, licorice, spinach, and psyllium seeds and laxative foods such as prunes and pectin containing fruits (apples, figs, pears, bananas).
- **Abdominal massage**: Starting at the lower right side of your belly, massage up to your ribs then across your upper stomach and down the left side making a big circle around your navel. Perform massage after every meal to stimulate the colon and train your bowels to move after each meal.

- **Exercise** is a bowel stimulant. Some type of aerobic exercise at least 30 minutes, three to four times per week is helpful. Wear loose clothes around the waist.
- Hot applications to the abdomen; hot water bottle, hot wet towels

127. Stools are not well formed (loose)

A stool that is not well formed is a sign of diarrhea. Diarrhea refers to an increased frequency, volume, or fluidity of stool and is a common symptom of many conditions. Diarrhea is usually a mild episode lasting just a few days and is a way for the body to cleanse itself of irritants. However, it can also be an indication of a serious underlying condition. Diarrhea can be due to a variety of causes including infections or overgrowth of bacteria, viruses, or parasites (sometimes secondary to antibiotic use); the use of laxatives or medications causing increased motility; inflammatory bowel disease; malabsorption; emotional stress; and food allergies. The main dangers of diarrhea include dehydration and mineral or electrolyte imbalance, malabsorption, weight loss, or the presence of a more serious underlying condition. Below are some general recommendations to control diarrhea. If diarrhea lasts for more than a few days, is severe and acute, contains blood or pus, or is associated with a high fever, weight loss, listlessness, severe cramping, or vomiting, see your clinician. Its cause must be determined and treated.

Generally, if the cause is in the small intestine, the diarrhea is characterized by large quantities of water and/or fatty stools; if the diarrhea is due to disease in or of the colon, the stool are frequent and often accompanied by blood, mucus or pus; it the disease is rectal in origin, there are often frequent movements of a small amount of stool.

<u>1° Indication</u>

Intestinal parasites and/or dysbiosis

Further assessment	1. CBC to see if eosinophils or basophils are elevated 2. Stool test for ova and parasite can help detect which parasite, if any, is present. Start with one random stool. If no parasite is found and the index of suspicion is high repeat the stool test, but this time do a purged sample with either a large bolus of vitamin C or magnesium sulfate. Collect the next two stools for testing. 3. Decreased secretory IgA on stool analysis.

<u>2° Indication</u>

Malabsorption- assess small and large intestine

Further assessment	1. Check for tenderness in the Chapman reflex for the colon located bilaterally along the iliotibial band on the thighs. Palpate the colon for tenderness and tension. 2. Check for tenderness in the Chapman reflex for the small intestine located on the 8th, 9th and 10th intercostal spaces near the tip of the rib. Also palpate four quadrants in a 2" to 3" radius around the umbilicus for tenderness and tension 3. Increased urinary indican and sediment 4. Decreased bowel transit time. Have a client check their bowel transit time. Give 6 "00" caps of activated charcoal and ask them to record how long it takes for the black to appear and to go completely away. Beets or dye can also be used.

Other indications

1. Too much vitamin C or magnesium can make stool loose
2. Lactose intolerance
3. Consumption of sorbitol, mannitol and other types of insoluble sugars

Supplemental Support

1. Bentonite clay
2. Micro Emulsified Oregano
3. Water soluble fiber and nutrients to support healthy colon
4. Nutrients that heal the intestines
5. Gut healing nutrients and vitamin U
6. Betaine HCL, Pepsin, and pancreatin
7. Pancreatic enzymes
8. Chlorophyllins

Lifestyle changes

Please see the handout in the appendix on recommendations for Diarrhea

NOTES:

128. Irritable bowel or mucus colitis

Irritable bowel syndrome or IBS and mucous colitis are common conditions that present with a combination of any of the following symptoms: abdominal pain, constipation or Diarrhea, hyper secretion of the colonic mucus, flatulence, nausea or anorexia, and varying degrees of anxiety or depression. Many other conditions may mimic the symptoms of IBS and should be ruled out by. The causes for IBS are not completely clear, but physiological, psychological and dietary factors have all been linked to this condition.

1° Indication

Upper digestive assessment needed

Further assessment	**Pancreatic enzymes** 1. Check Ridler enzyme point for tenderness 1 inch below xyphoid and over to the right edge of the rib cage 2. Check for tenderness in the Chapman reflex for the pancreas located in the 7th intercostal space 3. Increased urinary sediment levels **Hydrochloric acid** 1. Check Ridler HCL reflex for tenderness 1 inch below xyphoid and over to the left edge of the rib cage 2. Check for tenderness in the Chapman reflex for the stomach and upper digestion located in 6th intercostal space on the left 3. Check for a positive zinc tally: A client holds a solution of aqueous zinc sulfate in their mouth and tells you if and when they can taste it. An almost immediate very bitter taste indicates the client does not need zinc. Clients who are zinc deficient will report no taste from the solution. 4. Gastric acid assessment using Gastrotest 5. Increased urinary indican levels

2° Indication

Small and large intestine assessment

Further assessment	1. Check for tenderness in the Chapman reflex for the colon located bilaterally along the iliotibial band on the thighs. Palpate the colon for tenderness and tension. 2. Check for tenderness in the Chapman reflex for the small intestine located on the 8th, 9th and 10th intercostal spaces near the tip of the rib. Also palpate four quadrants in a 2" to 3" radius around the umbilicus for tenderness and tension 3. Comprehensive digestive stool analysis

Supplemental Support

1. Betaine HCL, Pepsin, and pancreatin
2. Bentonite clay
3. Water soluble fiber and nutrients to support healthy colon
4. Digestive support: Nutrients to heal the intestines, Betaine HCL, Pepsin, & pancreatin
5. Pancreatic enzymes
6. Chlorophyllins

Lifestyle changes

1. Increase dietary fiber
2. Eliminate allergic/intolerant foods
3. Address psychological components

Foods to Include:

- Baked apples
- Steamed/baked vegetables, all kinds
- Brown rice
- Millet
- Beans, split peas, lentils
- Spelt flour products
- Potatoes
- Oatmeal
- Kidney beans
- Oat bran

Foods to Avoid:

- Raw foods
- All hydrogenated oils
- Spicy foods; peppers (red and black)
- Coffee, black tea
- Alcohol
- Cheese and milk
- Beef, pork
- Wheat flours (includes white flour)
- All refined sugar and sugar desserts
- Vinegar and Mustard

NOTES:

129. Blood in stool

Blood in the stool can be an indication of serious pathology. You need to get information concerning the color of the stool. A black stool is usually a result of bleeding into the upper GI tract. The cause could be ulcer, Crohn's disease, colitis or cancer, iron, bismuth, charcoal or a heavy meat diet. A red stool is usually the result of bleeding from lower GI tract (Hemorrhoids, fissures, colitis, cancer) or even beets.

If you are in doubt as to the cause of the bleeding please refer to a gastroenterologist for further work-up and evaluation.

<u>1° Indication</u>

Assess lower bowel for bleeding

Further assessment	1. Have client perform 3-6 occult blood tests at home to bring into the office for evaluation and assessment 2. Perform a rectal examination to examine the rectal mucosa or refer out to a clinician specialized in such procedures 3. Check CBC for hidden signs of anemia and microscopic bleeding

NOTES:

130. Mucus in stool

Mucus appears in the stool in conditions of parasympathetic excitability. Excessive production can occur from irritation to the gastrointestinal tract as seen in colitis, food sensitivity and pancreatitis. Translucent gelatinous mucus clinging to the surface of formed stool occurs in spastic constipation, mucous colitis, emotionally disturbed clients or excessive straining at stool. Bloody mucus clinging to stool suggests a neoplasm or inflammation of rectal canal. Mucus with pus and blood is seen in ulcerative colitis, bacillary dysentery, ulcerative cancer of colon, or acute diverticulitis

1° Indication

Upper digestive assessment needed

Further assessment	**Pancreatic enzymes** 1. Check Ridler enzyme point for tenderness 1 inch below xyphoid and over to the right edge of the rib cage 2. Check for tenderness in the Chapman reflex for the pancreas located in the 7th intercostal space 3. Increased urinary sediment levels **Hydrochloric acid** 1. Check Ridler HCL reflex for tenderness 1 inch below xyphoid and over to the left edge of the rib cage 2. Check for tenderness in the Chapman reflex for the stomach and upper digestion located in 6th intercostal space on the left 3. Check for a positive zinc tally: A client holds a solution of aqueous zinc sulfate in their mouth and tells you if and when they can taste it. An almost immediate very bitter taste indicates the client does not need zinc. Clients who are zinc deficient will report no taste from the solution. 4. Increased urinary indican levels

2° Indication

Small and large intestine assessment

Further assessment	1. Check for tenderness in the Chapman reflex for the colon located bilaterally along the iliotibial band on the thighs. Palpate the colon for tenderness and tension. 2. Check for tenderness in the Chapman reflex for the small intestine located on the 8th, 9th and 10th intercostal spaces near the tip of the rib. Also palpate four quadrants in a 2" to 3" radius around the umbilicus for tenderness and tension 3. Functional 24-hour digestive urinalysis 4. Comprehensive digestive stool analysis. 5. Decreased secretory IgA on stool analysis.

Supplemental Support

1. Digestive support: Nutrients to heal the intestines, Betaine HCL, Pepsin, & pancreatin
2. Bentonite clay
3. Water soluble fiber and nutrients to support healthy colon
4. Chlorophyllins

131. Excessive foul smelling lower bowel gas

Excessive fouls smelling lower bowel gas is a strong indicator of dysbiosis and a disturbed lower digestive system. There may also be a maldigestion occurring in the upper gastrointestinal tract that leaves partially undigested food that exacerbates the dysbiosis.

1° Indication

Dysbiosis caused by an overgrowth of bacteria or yeast

Further assessment	1. Increased urinary indican levels 2. Stool analysis- either comprehensive digestive analysis or a parasite profile 3. Check for tenderness in the Chapman reflex for the colon located bilaterally along the iliotibial band on the thighs. Palpate the colon for tenderness and tension. 4. Check for tenderness in the Chapman reflex for the small intestine located on the 8th, 9th and 10th intercostal spaces near the tip of the rib. Also palpate four quadrants in a 2" to 3" radius around the umbilicus for tenderness and tension. 5. Decreased secretory IgA on stool analysis.

2° Indication

Pancreatic enzyme need or hydrochloric acid

Further assessment	**Pancreatic enzymes** 1. Check Ridler enzyme point for tenderness 1 inch below xyphoid and over to the right edge of the rib cage 2. Check for tenderness in the Chapman reflex for the pancreas located in the 7th intercostal space 3. Increased urinary sediment levels **Hydrochloric acid** 1. Check Ridler HCL reflex for tenderness 1 inch below xyphoid and over to the left edge of the rib cage 2. Check for tenderness in the Chapman reflex for the stomach and upper digestion located in 6th intercostal space on the left 3. Check for a positive zinc tally: A client holds a solution of aqueous zinc sulfate in their mouth and tells you if and when they can taste it. An almost immediate very bitter taste indicates the client does not need zinc. Clients who are zinc deficient will report no taste from the solution. 4. Gastric acid assessment using Gastrotest 5. Increased urinary indican levels

Other indications

Liver detoxification problems

Supplemental Support

1. Micro Emulsified Oregano
2. Digestive support: Nutrients to heal the intestines, Betaine HCL, Pepsin, & pancreatin

3. Water soluble fiber and colon health nutrients
4. Multiple nutrients that support the immune system
5. Lactobacillus acidophilus and Bifidobacterium bifidus
6. Pancreatic Enzymes
7. Broad spectrum proteolytic enzymes
8. Bromelain

Lifestyle changes

Please see handouts in the appendix on the Dysbiosis diet and the Diet to aid digestion

NOTES:

132. Bad breath or strong body odors

Bad breath or strong body odors are an indication of a disturbed digestive system. If the digestive system is assessed and any dysfunction is corrected, the chances are that the halitosis will go. It can, of course, be caused by poor dental hygiene.

1° Indication

Dysbiosis caused by an overgrowth of bacteria or yeast

Further assessment	1. Increased urinary indican levels 2. Stool analysis- either comprehensive digestive analysis or a parasite profile 3. Check for tenderness in the Chapman reflex for the colon located bilaterally along the iliotibial band on the thighs. Palpate the colon for tenderness and tension. 4. Check for tenderness in the Chapman reflex for the small intestine located on the 8th, 9th and 10th intercostal spaces near the tip of the rib. Also palpate four quadrants in a 2" to 3" radius around the umbilicus for tenderness and tension

2° Indication

Pancreatic enzyme need or hydrochloric acid

Further assessment	**Pancreatic enzymes** 1. Check Ridler enzyme point for tenderness 1 inch below xyphoid and over to the right edge of the rib cage 2. Check for tenderness in the Chapman reflex for the pancreas located in the 7th intercostal space 3. Increased urinary sediment levels **Hydrochloric acid** 1. Check Ridler HCL reflex for tenderness 1 inch below xyphoid and over to the left edge of the rib cage 2. Check for tenderness in the Chapman reflex for the stomach and upper digestion located in 6th intercostal space on the left 3. Check for a positive zinc tally: A client holds a solution of aqueous zinc sulfate in their mouth and tells you if and when they can taste it. An almost immediate very bitter taste indicates the client does not need zinc. Clients who are zinc deficient will report no taste from the solution.

Other indications

Liver detoxification problems

Supplemental Support

1. Micro Emulsified Oregano
2. Digestive support: Nutrients to heal the intestines, Betaine HCL, Pepsin, & pancreatin
3. Water soluble fiber and colon health nutrients
4. Broad spectrum proteolytic and pancreatic enzymes

Lifestyle changes: Please see handouts on the Dysbiosis diet and the Diet to aid digestion

133. Painful to press along outer sides of thighs (Iliotibial Band)

This is a sign of dysfunction in the colon. The colon has a referral zone to the iliotibial band, a group of muscles along the outside of the thigh. Tenderness in that area is referred from the colon. Colon dysfunction can indicate dehydration, dysbiosis, parasites or just a poor diet high in refined foods and low in fiber. It is important to remember that the prostate in men and the uterus in women will have a similar referral area in the middle portion of the iliotibial band bilaterally.

1° Indication

Assess the colon for lack of fiber and adequate hydration.

Further assessment	1. Have a client check their bowel transit time. Give six "00" caps of activated charcoal and ask them to record how long it takes for the black to appear and to go completely away. Various dyes, including beets, sweetcorn, and un-popped popcorn can also be used. 2. Assess the client's hydration status. Have client stand with hands by their side and check and palpate the veins in the right hand. Have them slowly raise their hand to heart level and see if the veins still stick out. Veins that are only just visible or not visible at all are a sign of dehydration 3. Check for tenderness in the Chapman reflex for the colon located bilaterally along the iliotibial band on the thighs. 4. Palpate the colon for tenderness and tension.

2° Indication

Dysbiosis caused by an overgrowth of bacteria or yeast

Further assessment	1. Increased urinary indican levels 2. Stool analysis- either comprehensive digestive analysis or a parasite profile 3. Check for tenderness in the Chapman reflex for the colon located bilaterally along the iliotibial band on the thighs. Palpate the colon for tenderness and tension. 4. Check for tenderness in the Chapman reflex for the small intestine located on the 8th, 9th and 10th intercostal spaces near the tip of the rib. Also palpate four quadrants in a 2" to 3" radius around the umbilicus for tenderness and tension. 5. Decreased secretory IgA on stool analysis.

Supplemental Support

1. Water soluble fiber and colon health nutrients
2. Garlic and chlorophyllins
3. Micro Emulsified Oregano
4. Nutrients that heal the intestines
5. Lactobacillus acidophilus and Bifidobacterium bifidus
6. Butyrate
7. Anti-fungal herbs
8. Bromelain, cellulase, lipase, and amylase

Lifestyle changes

- Eat a high fiber, low fat diet. Include bran, seeds and vegetables into your diet.
- Avoid overeating and frequent snacking.
- Avoid refined carbohydrates (white flour), cheese, potatoes and meats, which contribute to constipation.
- Drink plenty of fluids, at least 6-8 glasses per day. Water is best. Avoid coffee, tea and fizzy drinks
- Include grapes, cherries, melons, licorice, spinach, and psyllium seeds and laxative foods such as prunes and pectin containing fruits (apples, figs, pears, bananas).
- **Abdominal massage**: Starting at the lower right side of your belly, massage up to your ribs then across your upper stomach and down the left side making a big circle around your navel. Perform massage after every meal to stimulate the colon and train your bowels to move after each meal.
- **Exercise** is a bowel stimulant. Some type of aerobic exercise at least 30 minutes, three to four times per week is helpful. Wear loose clothes around the waist.
- Hot applications to the abdomen; hot water bottle, hot wet towels

NOTES:

134. Cramping in lower abdominal region

There are a number of structures to consider when a client is complaining of cramping in the lower abdominal region. The first to come to mind is the appendix. Appendicitis is obviously an emergency issue that should be evaluated thoroughly and referred to the emergency room if it is acute. Other potentially dangerous conditions to consider include intestinal obstruction, salpingitis, ovarian cysts or diverticulitis.

From a functional perspective, the most likely cause of cramping in the lower abdominal region is an ileocecal valve disturbance. The ileocecal valve separates the small from the large intestine and controls the movement of stool from one functional area to the other. Most digestion and assimilation occurs in the small intestine, whereas the primary role of the large intestine is the absorption of water. A dysbiosis in either the small or large intestines can cause ileocecal valve irritation, which can spasm. Cramping in the lower abdominal area needs careful assessment.

1° Indication

Dysbiosis caused by an overgrowth of bacteria or yeast

Further assessment	1. Increased urinary indican levels 2. Stool analysis- either comprehensive digestive analysis or a parasite profile 3. Check for tenderness in the Chapman reflex for the colon located bilaterally along the iliotibial band on the thighs. Palpate the colon for tenderness and tension. 4. Check for tenderness in the Chapman reflex for the small intestine located on the 8th, 9th and 10th intercostal spaces near the tip of the rib. Also palpate four quadrants in a 2" to 3" radius around the umbilicus for tenderness and tension. 5. Decreased secretory IgA on stool analysis.

2° Indication

Colonic and/or small intestine dysfunction with possible constipation

Further assessment	1. Check for tenderness in the Chapman reflex for the colon located bilaterally along the iliotibial band on the thighs. Palpate the colon for tenderness and tension. 2. Check for tenderness in the Chapman reflex for the small intestine located on the 8th, 9th and 10th intercostal spaces near the tip of the rib. Also palpate four quadrants in a 2" to 3" radius around the umbilicus for tenderness and tension 3. Increased urinary indican and sediment 4. Decreased bowel transit time. Have a client check their bowel transit time. Give 6 "00" caps of activated charcoal and ask them to record how long it takes for the black to appear and to go completely away. Various dyes, including beets, sweetcorn, and un-popped popcorn can also be used.

Supplemental Support

1. Water soluble fiber and colon health nutrients
2. Garlic and chlorophyllins
3. Micro Emulsified Oregano
4. Nutrients that heal the intestines
5. Lactobacillus acidophilus and Bifidobacterium bifidus
6. Butyrate
7. Anti-fungal herbs
8. Bromelain, cellulase, lipase, and amylase

Lifestyle changes

Please see the Dysbiosis diet for dietary and lifestyle recommendations

NOTES:

135. Dark circles under eyes

Dark circles under the eyes are a classic sign of food allergies. Allergies are overreactions of the immune system. The immune system is a very complex interconnected network, comprising the various different white blood cells (lymphocytes, granulocytes, macrophages, mast cells), as well as the entire system of mucous membranes throughout the body, but especially in the digestive system, where specialized lymphatic tissue, called Peyer's patches, plays an essential role in the Gut Associated Lymphoid Tissue or GALT. Another essential component of the immune system is the normally present bacterial colonies in the mucous membranes of the digestive system.

An allergy begins long before the manifestation of allergic like symptoms. The body has to be set up to respond to an allergen. This usually begins in early childhood. It takes a severely disturbed intestinal environment, the internal terrain of the body, to react allergenically. Unfortunately this disturbance to the intestinal environment goes unnoticed, since it is chronic, and tends to build up over many years.

The disturbance to the intestinal environment is called dysbiosis. Dysbiosis can be described as an abnormal intestinal flora and an abnormally permeable intestinal mucous membrane. The intestinal flora, comprising of billions of bacteria, forms a fine film on the inside of the intestines. Everything you eat passes through this bacterial layer, which alters and filters the foodstuffs. When the intestinal flora is not intact, the absorptive ability of the intestinal mucous membranes becomes impaired.

Functional hypochlorhydria and pancreatic insufficiency causes the maldigestion of carbohydrates, fats and proteins. Large macromolecules are left undigested and form the substrate for dysbiosis formation. Over time the villi, the large absorptive surface of the intestines, becomes irritated and inflamed, which causes it to become less dense. The large, incompletely digested macromolecules, especially proteins, start to be able to penetrate the intestinal mucous membrane. With the destruction of the villi comes the reduction of the GALT and the secretory IgA, the body's first line defense against "foreign" invaders. Once in the bloodstream, the body's immune system recognizes the small protein or part of a protein as foreign, and produces antibodies against it. It is the reaction of the antibody/antigen complex that produces the classic allergy symptoms.

The body's second layer of defense lies in the liver. The liver normally screens the blood for antigens. On each pass through the body, the blood must pass through the liver for cleaning and detoxification. The liver will normally take these foreign substances and destroy them or get them out of the body. Unfortunately liver dysfunction is a very common occurrence in our society. The destruction of foreign substances will not occur if the liver is not functioning as it should, if there is too much of the substance to get rid of easily or the liver's phase I and II detoxification pathways cannot destroy it.

Over 80% of the human immune system is thus situated alongside the intestines. It is therefore understandable that disturbances of the intestines and the intestinal flora place a tremendous overload on the immune system, which then often reacts "allergically" to otherwise quite innocuous proteins. Allergies are thus usually indirect ailments of the intestinal mucous membrane. Thus, in treating allergy clients, the greatest attention needs to be given to restoring the intestinal flora and the intestinal mucous membrane.

1° Indication

Dysbiosis- abnormal intestinal flora and increased intestinal hyperpermeability

Further assessment	1. Increased urinary indican and sediment levels 2. Stool analysis- either comprehensive digestive analysis or a parasite profile 3. Check for tenderness in the Chapman reflex for the colon located bilaterally along the iliotibial band on the thighs. Palpate the colon for tenderness and tension. 4. Check for tenderness in the Chapman reflex for the small intestine located on the 8th, 9th and 10th intercostal spaces near the tip of the rib. Also palpate four quadrants in a 2" to 3" radius around the umbilicus for tenderness and tension. 5. Decreased secretory IgA on stool analysis.

2° Indication

Liver congestion with detoxification problems, especially phase I and II detoxification

Further assessment	1. Check for tenderness in the Chapman reflex for the liver-gallbladder located over the 6th intercostal space on the right side 2. Check for tenderness in the Liver point located on the 3rd rib, 3" to the right of the sternum, at the costochondral junction. 3. Check for tenderness underneath the right rib cage 4. Assess for Hepato-biliary congestion with the Acoustic Cardiogram (ACG), which will show post-systolic rounding due to increased backpressure on the pulmonic and aortic valve. Increased SGOT, SGPT on a blood chemistry panel 5. Various labs do liver detoxification panels

Other indications

1. Hypochlorhydria and pancreatic insufficiency
2. Adrenal hypofunction
3. Mineral deficiency

Supplemental Support

1. Multiple herbal anti-histamines
2. Nutrients to support Phase II liver detoxification and herbs that cleanse the liver
3. Powdered detoxification support formula with Glutathione, cysteine, and Glycine
4. Plant source molybdenum
5. Micro Emulsified Oregano
6. Digestive support: Nutrients to heal the intestines, Betaine HCL, Pepsin, & pancreatin
7. L-glutamine
8. Colon support: Water soluble fiber, Lactobacillus acidophilus & Bifidobacterium bifidus

Lifestyle changes

Please see the handouts on the Dysbiosis diet and recommendations for a healthy liver

MINERAL NEEDS

136. History of Carpal Tunnel Syndrome (1 = yes, 0 = no)
137. History of lower right abdominal pain or ileocecal valve problems (1 = yes, 0 = no)
138. History of stress fractures (1 = yes, 0 = no)
139. Bone loss (reduced density on bone scan)
140. Are you shorter than you used to be?(1 = yes, 0 = no)
141. Calf, foot or toe cramps at rest
142. Cold sores, fever blisters or herpes lesions
143. Frequent fevers
144. Frequent skin rashes and / or hives
145. Have you ever had a herniated disc? (1 = yes, 0 = no)
146. Excessively flexible joints, "double jointed"
147. Joints pop or click
148. Pain or swelling in joints
149. Bursitis or tendonitis
150. History of bone spurs (1 = yes, 0 = no)
151. Morning stiffness
152. Nausea with vomiting
153. Crave chocolate
154. Feet have a strong odor
155. Tendency to anemia
156. Whites of eyes (sclera) blue tinted
157. Hoarseness
158. Difficulty swallowing
159. Lump in throat
160. Dry mouth, eyes and / or nose
161. Gag easily
162. White spots on fingernails
163. Cuts heal slowly and / or scar easily
164. Decreased sense of taste or smell

136. History of Carpal Tunnel Syndrome 1 = yes, 0 = no)

The carpal tunnel is a circular structure located on the palm side of the wrist. Blood vessels, tendons and the median nerve travel through the carpal tunnel and are susceptible to entrapment when the pressure increases inside this tunnel. The nerve is often the first structure to feel the effects leading to numbness, tingling and burning in the thumb and first three fingers. This is accompanied by stiffness and weakness of the hand and the pain is often worse at night. Other complications are swelling, limited motion of the wrist and fingers and inability to perform simple tasks such as picking up small objects.

There are several causes of carpal tunnel syndrome (CTS) but most cases are due to a reversible nutritional imbalance in Vitamin B6, zinc and magnesium, overuse of the wrist, or injury. These factors contribute to CTS being recognized as the second most common type of occupational disorder. Pregnant women and people taking birth control pills are more susceptible.

1° Indication

B6, Zinc and magnesium deficiency

Further assessment	1. B6 levels can be assessed by running a serum homocysteine or a B6 EGOT (Erythrocyte Glutamine-Oxaloacetate Transaminase) test 2. Assess for mineral deficiency using Tissue mineral assessment test. Place a standard blood pressure cuff around the largest portion of the client's calf muscle (sitting). Instruct the client to let you know when they feel the onset of cramping pain and gradually inflate the cuff. Stop and deflate immediately when threshold has been reached. Less than 200 mmHg is considered deficient in minerals. Use the neurolingual testing to challenge the body with several types of magnesium to see if this increases the threshold above 200mmHg. 3. Check for a positive zinc tally: A client holds a solution of aqueous zinc sulfate in their mouth and tells you if and when they can taste it. An almost immediate very bitter taste indicates the client does not need zinc. Clients who are zinc deficient will report no taste from the solution.

Other indications

1. Occupational stress 2. Hypochlorhydria 3. Wrist, elbow or shoulder dysfunction	4. Tissue alkalinity 5. Hypothyroid

Supplemental Support

1. Multiple nutrient formula with zinc, magnesium and B6 to support the carpal tunnel
2. Multiple nutrients to support bone health
3. Betaine HCL and Pepsin
4. Nutritional zinc and magnesium

Lifestyle changes:

Restrict use of wrist until the CTS has completely resolved

137. History of lower right abdominal pain or ileocecal valve problems (1 = yes, 0 = no)

There are a number of serious conditions to consider when a client is complaining of right abdominal pain. The first to come to mind is the appendix. Appendicitis is obviously an emergency issue that should be evaluated thoroughly and referred to the emergency room if it is acute. Other potentially dangerous conditions to consider include intestinal obstruction, salpingitis, ovarian cysts or diverticulitis. Assess whether or not this is an acute situation. The most likely cause of a history of mild pain or discomfort in the lower abdominal region is an ileocecal valve disturbance. The ileocecal valve separates the small from the large intestine and controls the movement of stool from one functional area to the other. Most digestion and assimilation occurs in the small intestine, whereas the primary role of the large intestine is the absorption of water. Dysbiosis in either the small or large intestines can cause ileocecal valve irritation leading to irritation and discomfort.

<u>1° Indication</u>

Dysbiosis caused by an overgrowth of bacteria or yeast

Further assessment	1. Increased urinary indican and urinary sediment levels 2. Stool analysis for Candida or parasites 3. Check for tenderness in the Chapman reflex for the colon located bilaterally along the iliotibial band on the thighs. Palpate the colon for tenderness and tension. 4. Check for tenderness in the Bennet' reflex for the small intestine.Palpate four quadrants in a 2" to 3" radius around the umbilicus for tenderness and tension. 5. Decreased secretory IgA on stool analysis.

<u>2° Indication</u>

Colonic and/or small intestine dysfunction with possible constipation

Further assessment	1. Check for tenderness in the Chapman reflex for the small intestine located on the 8th, 9th and 10th intercostal spaces near the tip of the rib. Also palpate four quadrants in a 2" to 3" radius around the umbilicus for tenderness and tension 2. Decreased bowel transit time. Have a client check their bowel transit time. Give 6 "00" caps of activated charcoal and ask them to record how long it takes for the black to appear and to go completely away. Beets and dyes can also be used.

Supplemental Support

1. Colon support: Fiber, Lactobacillus acidophilus & Bifidobacterium bifidus
2. Garlic and chlorophyllins
3. Micro Emulsified Oregano
4. Nutrients that heal the intestines
5. Butyrate
6. Anti-fungal herbs
7. Bromelain, cellulase, lipase, and amylase

<u>Lifestyle changes:</u> Please see the handout in the appendix on the Dysbiosis diet

138. History of stress fractures
139. Bone loss (reduced density on bone scan)
140. Are you shorter than you used to be? (1 = yes, 0 = no)

The above three questions are all indicators for poor bone health. A history of stress fractures and bone loss are strong signs of osteoporosis and poor bone integrity. A loss in height is also an indication of osteoporosis and poor bone integrity but could also be due to inadequate hydration. The intervertebral disks need adequate hydration. Without it, they can begin to shrink, causing an overall loss in height.

Osteoporosis is a disease characterized by low bone density and a gradual change in the overall bone structure leading to fragile and brittle bones, susceptible to fractures. Assessing the risk factors for osteoporosis will give a good picture of what is going on, and will allow you to take the best course of action.

Major risk factors for developing osteoporosis include:

1. Having a slight or slender build,
2. Being Caucasian, Asian or other non-black ethnicity,
3. Having a family history of osteoporosis,
4. Being underweight or small muscle mass,
5. Having a low dietary intake of calcium and vitamin D,
6. Early menopause,
7. Late menarche or amenorrhea,
8. Prolonged use of corticosteroids, antacids or diuretics.

There are several nutritional and lifestyle factors that affect overall bone health and the possible development of osteoporosis, they include:

1. Insufficient calcium intake (or from a functional perspective this may have more to do with an inability to utilize dietary calcium),
2. Vitamin D and K deficiencies,
3. High inorganic phosphorous intake (from sodas etc.)
4. Other mineral deficiencies (magnesium, boron, manganese etc.)

The standard Western diet/lifestyle is a set-up for poor bone health and the formation of osteoporosis:

1. Highly refined foods,
2. High intakes of calcium depleting sodas, which contain high levels of inorganic phosphorous,
3. Alcohol and cigarettes,
4. A fairly sedentary lifestyle,
5. Large consumption of sugar,
6. Widespread vitamin and mineral deficiencies.

There is a strong hormonal factor to bone metabolism. Estrogen, DHEA and progesterone are the three main sex hormones that influence bone. Other hormones such as testosterone, parathyroid hormone, growth hormone and insulin all play a role in bone metabolism. Women who are postmenopausal are at an increased risk of osteoporosis.
There are two types of bone: trabecular and cortical. The cortical bone is the hard bony covering and the trabecular bone is the inside part of the bone where the marrow is. Trabecular bone provides the protection from fractures, has a higher rate of turnover than cortical bone and is the type of bone loss that is most impacted by menopause. Cortical bone loss occurs with mineral and vitamin deficiencies.

The following nutrients are important for healthy bones:

Calcium
Women over the age of 35 who ingest less than 1 gram of calcium daily (1.5 grams for postmenopausal women) are often in negative calcium balance. Studies indicate that a high calcium intake during childhood and adolescence may reduce the risk of osteoporosis. It is uncertain whether calcium supplementation reduces bone loss after menopause. The responsiveness may depend on their age. It appears that calcium supplementation in the first 5 years of menopause attenuates but doesn't stop bone loss from the long bones and has little effect on the spine. Calcium supplementation should be combined with vitamin D to increase absorption.

Vitamin K
Osteoporotic clients have a decreased mineralization of bone. A deficiency of vitamin K can lead to impaired mineralization of bone due to inadequate osteocalcin synthesis. Osteoporotic clients generally have low serum vitamin K values. In one study, supplemental vitamin K reduced urinary calcium loss in post-menopausal women with excess urinary calcium excretion.

Zinc
Low serum levels of zinc have been reported in osteoporotic clients. Because Westerners generally eat below the RDA of zinc, supplementation is recommended.

Magnesium
As much as 50% of magnesium is found in the bones. Studies indicate that a magnesium deficiency is common in women with osteoporosis and is associated with abnormal calcification of the bone.

Manganese
Manganese deficiency is common in women with osteoporosis. A deficiency may accelerate bone loss as well as result in defective bone formation. Manganese stimulates production of mucopolysaccharides, which are responsible for providing a structure for calcification to occur.

Potassium
Studies indicate that potassium is important in reducing urinary calcium excretion.

Other important nutrients include:

- Silicon
- Vitamin D
- Vitamin C
- Folic acid
- Vitamin B6
- Boron
- Copper
- Vitamin B12
- Strontium

1° Indication

Poor bone health

Further assessment	1. Have client get some form of bone densiometry to follow the course of treatment and progress of the disease. 2. Assess for mineral deficiency using Tissue mineral assessment test. Place a standard blood pressure cuff around the largest portion of the client's calf muscle (sitting). Instruct the client to let you know when they feel the onset of cramping pain and gradually inflate the cuff. Stop and deflate immediately when threshold has been reached. Less than 200 mmHg is considered deficient in minerals. Use the neurolingual testing to challenge the body with several types of calcium and other co-factors to see if this increases the threshold above 200mmHg. 3. Check client's urine for the loss of type 1 collagen (several labs offer this test often called Bone Resorption Assessment) 4. Check client's urine for calcium loss (Sulkowitch test)

2° Indication

Assess client for hypochlorhydria

Further assessment	1. Check Ridler HCL reflex for tenderness 1 inch below xyphoid and over to the left edge of the rib cage 2. Check for tenderness in the Chapman reflex for the stomach and upper digestion located in 6th intercostal space on the left 3. Check for a positive zinc tally: A client holds a solution of aqueous zinc sulfate in their mouth and tells you if and when they can taste it. An almost immediate very bitter taste indicates the client does not need zinc. Clients who are zinc deficient will report no taste from the solution. 4. Gastric acid assessment using Gastrotest 5. Increased urinary indican levels

Supplemental Support

1. Multiple nutrients to support bone health
2. Alkaline Ash minerals (Calcium, Magnesium,Potassium)
3. Flax Seed Oil
4. Multiple nutrients to support thyroid function with pituitary glandular
5. Betaine HCL, Pepsin, and pancreatin
6. Emulsified Viatmin D drops
7. Potassium iodide

Lifestyle changes: Please see the handout in the appendix on Diet and lifestyle recommendations for healthy bones

141. Calf, foot or toe cramps at rest

Calf, foot or toe cramps at rest are an indication of calcium, magnesium or potassium deficiency. It is often necessary to take these minerals with an effective co-factor, such as supplemental HCl and essential fatty acids which will increase their digestion and/or absorption.

1° Indication

Calcium, magnesium and/or potassium deficiency

Further assessment	1. Assess for mineral deficiency using Tissue mineral assessment test. Place a standard blood pressure cuff around the largest portion of the client's calf muscle (sitting). Instruct the client to let you know when they feel the onset of cramping pain and gradually inflate the cuff. Stop and deflate immediately when threshold has been reached. Less than 200 mmHg is considered deficient in minerals. Use the neurolingual testing to challenge the body with several different minerals and other co-factors to see which combination of minerals and co-factors increases the threshold above 200mmHg. 2. Assess for mineral insufficiency by using Dr. Kane's mineral assessment tests. 3. Assess the impact of mineral deficiencies on the body's acid buffering capacities by using Dr. Bieler's salivary pH acid challenge.

Supplemental Support

1. Alkaline Ash minerals (Calcium, Magnesium,Potassium)
2. Calcium and magnesium with or without parathyroid tissue
3. Emulsified Vitamin E drops
4. Multiple nutrients to support bone health
5. Multiple mineral without iron or copper
6. Calcium
7. Magnesium
8. Betaine HCL, Pepsin, and pancreatin
9. Mixed fatty acids (walnut, hazelnut, sesame, and apricot)

Lifestyle changes

Please see the handout in the appendix on Food sources of calcium and Diet and lifestyle recommendations for healthy bones

NOTES:

142. Cold sores, fever blisters or herpes lesions

Herpes lesions, in the form of cold sores or fever blisters are the external manifestation of the Herpes simplex virus. Herpes is known to be a stress related illness, which causes the virus to migrate from the nerve root, where it lives, and manifest as a blister. Various stressors such as overexposure to sun, illness, physical or emotional stress, medications and certain foods may precipitate the lesions. There seems to be a relationship to the intake of the amino acids lysine to arginine. The lower the lysine intake and the greater the arginine intake the greater the risk of a herpes outbreak.

Herpes lesions are also associated with a decrease availability of calcium in the tissue. Or, put in another way a low calcium level in the tissue can predispose one to developing a herpes outbreak. Calcium deficiency will also increase the likelihood of an outbreak. Stress will cause an increase in adrenal output of mineral corticoids, which can cause calcium to be excreted from the body.

1° Indication

Stress and adrenal overload

Further assessment	1. Check for unilateral tenderness in the inguinal ligament 2. Check for a paradoxical pupillary reflex by shining a light into a client's eye and grading the reaction of the pupil. A pupil that fails to constrict indicates adrenal exhaustion 3. Check for the presence of postural hypotension. A drop of more than 10 points is an indication of adrenal insufficiency. 4. Check for tenderness in the medial knee at the insertion of the sartorius muscle at the Pes Anserine. 5. Check for a chronic short leg due to posterior-inferior ilium 6. Assess for adrenal insufficiency with the Acoustic Cardiogram (ACG), which will show static in both the systolic and diastolic rest phases. You will also see an elevated S2 sound.

2° Indication

Calcium deficiency

Further assessment	1. Assess for mineral deficiency using Tissue mineral assessment test. Place a standard blood pressure cuff around the largest portion of the client's calf muscle (sitting). Instruct the client to let you know when they feel the onset of cramping pain and gradually inflate the cuff. Stop and deflate immediately when threshold has been reached. Less than 200 mmHg is considered deficient in minerals. Use the neurolingual testing to challenge the body with several types of magnesium to see if this increases the threshold above 200mmHg.

Other indications

Essential fatty acid deficiency

Supplemental Support

1. Calcium
2. L-Lysine
3. Flax Oil
4. Adrenal tissue (neonatal bovine)
5. Selenium
6. Buffered vitamin C with bioflavanoids

Lifestyle changes

Please see the handout in the appendix on the Herpes diet

NOTES:

143. Frequent fevers

Fever is not a disease but a symptom of illness. The body is responding to a problem and the body is in the process of eliminating it. Fever is an ally, and, if you are seeing frequent fevers in a child, you need to educate their parents about that. It is extremely rare for fevers to cause brain damage.

Fevers below 102° F are to be considered as "friendly" and of use to the body. The underlying cause should be dealt with, if the fever is consistently above that level.

The fever producing mechanism is as follows:

a. Any type of tissue injury (infection, trauma, tumor) will lead to the production of pyrogenes, which causes an increase in WBCs.
b. Pyrogenes cause the hypothalamus to reset the thermostatic set point of the body higher than the range of 97°-99°.
c. The hypothalamus triggers activities that increase body heat: shivering, vasoconstriction etc.
d. The temperature of the body increases until the new set point is reached.

With frequent fevers there is a possibility of an auto-immune like process in the body, which produces pyrogenes in response to inflammation. Frequent fevers need to be thoroughly assessed with blood chemistry and CBC studies to monitor the various different components of the immune system.

If no apparent cause for frequent fevers exists, then there may be a calcium deficiency, especially in children.

1° Indication

Calcium deficiency

Further assessment	1. Assess for mineral deficiency using Tissue mineral assessment test. Place a standard blood pressure cuff around the largest portion of the client's calf muscle (sitting). Instruct the client to let you know when they feel the onset of cramping pain and gradually inflate the cuff. Stop and deflate immediately when threshold has been reached. Less than 200 mmHg is considered deficient in minerals. Use the neurolingual testing to challenge the body with several types of magnesium to see if this increases the threshold above 200mmHg. 2. Assess calcium status using Dr. Kane's oral mineral tests 3. Run a urine calcium to assess calcium loss through the urine. This is an important test to do with clients taking calcium supplementation

Other indications

1. Immune insufficiency
2. Hypothalamus dysfunction

Supplemental Support

1. Calcium and magnesium with or without parathyroid tissue
2. Multiple mineral without iron or copper
3. Calcium supplementation

Lifestyle changes:

Please see the handout on Food sources of calcium

NOTES:

144. Frequent skin rashes and / or hives

Frequent skin rashes and/or hives are an indication of calcium insufficiency and essential fatty acid needs. It is also an indicator of some sort of allergic response. Hives are a manifestation of immediate or Type 1 hypersensitivity allergic reactions. It is important to thoroughly assess the digestive tract to rule out significant digestive involvement with frequent hives.

1° Indication

Calcium deficiency

Further assessment	1. Assess for mineral deficiency using Tissue mineral assessment test. Place a standard blood pressure cuff around the largest portion of the client's calf muscle (sitting). Instruct the client to let you know when they feel the onset of cramping pain and gradually inflate the cuff. Stop and deflate immediately when threshold has been reached. Less than 200 mmHg is considered deficient in minerals. Use the neurolingual testing to challenge the body with several types of calcium to see if this increases the threshold above 200mmHg. 2. Assess calcium status using Dr. Kane's oral mineral tests 3. Run a urine calcium to assess calcium loss through the urine. This is an important test to do with clients taking calcium supplementation

2° Indication

Essential fatty acid deficiency.

Further assessment	1. Oral pH less that 7.2 indicates essential fatty acid deficiency 2. Repeated muscle challenge. This challenge involves a simple, normal muscle test repeated once per second, 20 times with regular intensity. As in a standard muscle test, the joint is positioned in such a way that the muscle to be tested is shortened. The practitioner applies pressure to the joint to lengthen the muscle, until a "locking" is noted. A positive result occurs when "locking" of the muscle and joint does not occur, indicating deficient free fatty acids. 3. Fatty acid profile via laboratory testing of blood

3° Indication

Digestive dysfunction- with HCL and/or pancreatic enzyme need

Further assessment	**Hydrochloric acid** 1. Check Ridler HCL reflex for tenderness 1 inch below xyphoid and over to the left edge of the rib cage 2. Check for tenderness in the Chapman reflex for the stomach and upper digestion located in 6th intercostal space on the left 3. Check for a positive zinc tally: A client holds a solution of aqueous zinc sulfate in their mouth and tells you if and when

	they can taste it. An almost immediate very bitter taste indicates the client does not need zinc. Clients who are zinc deficient will report no taste from the solution. 4. Gastric acid assessment using Gastrotest 5. Increased urinary indican levels **Pancreatic enzymes** 4. Check Ridler enzyme point for tenderness 1 inch below xyphoid and over to the right edge of the rib cage 5. Check for tenderness in the Chapman reflex for the pancreas located in the 7th intercostal space 6. Increased urinary sediment levels

Other indications

Low adrenal function

Supplemental Support

1. Calcium and magnesium with or without parathyroid tissue 2. Multiple mineral without iron or copper 3. Calcium supplementation 4. Essential fatty acids: Flax seed Oil, EPA and DHA from fish oil, Mixed fatty acids (walnut, hazelnut, sesame, and apricot) 5. Digestive support: Betaine HCL, Pepsin, and Pancreatin, and Pancreatic enzymes

Lifestyle changes

Please see the handout in the appendix on Food sources of calcium

NOTES:

145. Have you ever had a herniated disc? (1 = yes, 0 = no)

A history of herniated discs is an indication of a general need for connective tissue support. Balancing the overall structure of the body is essential and a general protocol for supporting the connective tissue is important.

The following is a list of nutrients that are useful for healing connective tissue:

1. Vitamin B12
2. Glucosamine hydrochloride
3. MSM
4. Vitamin B6
5. Vitamin C complex
6. Calcium and magnesium
7. Essential fatty acids
8. Chondroitin sulfate

1° Indication
Mineral deficiency

Further assessment	1. Assess for mineral deficiency using Tissue mineral assessment test. Place a standard blood pressure cuff around the largest portion of the client's calf muscle (sitting). Instruct the client to let you know when they feel the onset of cramping pain and gradually inflate the cuff. Stop and deflate immediately when threshold has been reached. Less than 200 mmHg is considered deficient in minerals. Use the neurolingual testing to challenge the body with several different types of minerals and other co-factors to see which combination of minerals and co-factors increases the threshold above 200mmHg. 2. Assess for mineral insufficiency by using Dr. Kane's mineral assessment tests. 3. Assess the impact of mineral deficiencies on the body's acid buffering capacities by using Dr. Bieler's salivary pH acid challenge.

Supplemental Support

1. B12
2. Glucosamin hydrochloride
3. Pyridoxal-5-phosphate
4. Chondroitin sulfates and manganese
5. Multiple nutrients to support bone health
6. Broad spectrum proteolytic enzymes
7. Calcium and magnesium with or without parathyroid tissue
8. Essential fatty acids: Mixed fatty acids (walnut, hazelnut, sesame, and apricot), EPA and DHA from fish oil

NOTES:

146. Excessively flexible joints, "double jointed

Excessively flexible joints or being "double jointed" is an indication of increased ligament laxity. From a functional perspective, increased ligament laxity is a strong sign of adrenal insufficiency. This is also seen in people who either do not hold or do not respond to their osseous adjustments. It may also be an indication of a general need for connective tissue support. Balancing the overall structure of the body is essential and a general protocol for supporting the connective tissue is important.

The following is a list of nutrients that are useful for healing connective tissue:

1. Vitamin B12
2. Glucosamine hydrochloride
3. MSM
4. Vitamin B6
5. Vitamin C complex
6. Calcium and magnesium
7. Essential fatty acids
8. Chondroitin sulfate

1° indication

Low adrenal function

Further assessment	1. Check for tenderness in the inguinal ligament bilaterally 2. Check for tenderness at the medial knee bilaterally, at the insertion of the sartorius muscle at the Pes Anserine. 3. Check for a paradoxical pupillary reflex by shining a light into a client's eye and grading the reaction of the pupil. A pupil that fails to constrict indicates adrenal exhaustion 4. Check for the presence of postural hypotension. A drop of more than 10 points is an indication of adrenal insufficiency 5. Check for a chronic short leg due to a posterior-inferior ilium. An adrenal indicator when confirmed with postural hypotension and a paradoxical pupillary response. 6. Check the cortisol/DHEA rhythm with an adrenal stress profile 7. Increased chloride in the urine is a sign of hypoadrenal function 8. Assess for adrenal insufficiency with the Acoustic Cardiogram (ACG), which will show static in both the systolic and diastolic rest phases. You will also see an elevated S2 sound.

2° Indication

Mineral deficiency

Further assessment	1. Assess for mineral deficiency using Tissue mineral assessment test. Place a standard blood pressure cuff around the largest portion of the client's calf muscle (sitting). Instruct the client to let you know when they feel the onset of cramping pain and gradually inflate the cuff. Stop and deflate immediately when threshold has been reached. Less than 200 mmHg is considered deficient in minerals. Use the

	neurolingual testing to challenge the body with several different types of minerals and other co-factors to see which combination of minerals and co-factors increases the threshold above 200mmHg. 2. Assess for mineral insufficiency by using Dr. Kane's mineral assessment tests. 3. Assess the impact of mineral deficiencies on the body's acid buffering capacities by using Dr. Bieler's salivary pH acid challenge.

Supplemental Support

1. Adrenal support: Adrenal tissue (neonatal bovine) and adaptogenic herbs to support adrenal function
2. Vitamin B12
3. Glucosamine hydrochloride
4. Pyridoxal-5-phosphate
5. Chondroitin sulfates and manganese
6. Broad spectrum proteolytic enzymes
7. Calcium and magnesium with or without parathyroid tissue
8. Essential fatty acids: Mixed fatty acids (walnut, hazelnut, sesame, and apricot), EPA and DHA from fish oil
9. Multiple nutrients to support bone health

Lifestyle changes

Please see the handout in the appendix on the Adrenal restoration measures

NOTES:

147. Joints pop or click

Joints that pop or click are associated with a general need for connective tissue support. Balancing the overall structure of the body is essential and a general protocol for supporting the connective tissue is important.

The following is a list of nutrients that are useful for healing connective tissue:

1. Vitamin B12
2. Glucosamine hydrochloride
3. MSM
4. Vitamin B6
5. Vitamin C complex
6. Calcium and magnesium
7. Essential fatty acids
8. Chondroitin sulfate

1° Indication

Mineral deficiency

Further assessment	1. Assess for mineral deficiency using Tissue mineral assessment test. Place a standard blood pressure cuff around the largest portion of the client's calf muscle (sitting). Instruct the client to let you know when they feel the onset of cramping pain and gradually inflate the cuff. Stop and deflate immediately when threshold has been reached. Less than 200 mmHg is considered deficient in minerals. Use the neurolingual testing to challenge the body with several different types of minerals and other co-factors to see which combination of minerals and co-factors increases the threshold above 200mmHg. 2. Assess for mineral insufficiency by using Dr. Kane's mineral assessment tests. 3. Assess the impact of mineral deficiencies on the body's acid buffering capacities by using Dr. Bieler's salivary pH acid challenge.

Supplemental Support

1. Vitamin B12
2. Glucosamine hydrochloride
3. Pyridoxal-5-phosphate
4. Chondroitin sulfates and manganese
5. Multiple nutrients to support bone health
6. Broad spectrum proteolytic enzymes
7. Calcium and magnesium with or without parathyroid tissue
8. Essential fatty acids: Mixed fatty acids (walnut, hazelnut, sesame, and apricot), EPA and DHA from fish oil

NOTES:

148. Pain or swelling in joints

There are many causes for pain and swelling in the joints. One of the most common causes is arthritis, either osteoarthritis or an inflammatory arthritis such as rheumatoid arthritis. Many types of arthritis are associated with dysbiosis and an increased intestinal hyperpermeability. Assessment of the digestive system is important.

Many people with pain or swelling in the joints are helped with B6 supplementation. The supplemental support has some ideas for helping these clients cope with pain, and promote joint healing.

1° Indication

Dysbiosis caused by an overgrowth of bacteria or yeast

Further assessment	1. Increased urinary indican levels 2. Stool analysis- either comprehensive digestive analysis or a parasite profile 3. Check for tenderness in the Chapman reflex for the colon located bilaterally along the iliotibial band on the thighs. Palpate the colon for tenderness and tension. 4. Check for tenderness in the Chapman reflex for the small intestine located on the 8th, 9th and 10th intercostal spaces near the tip of the rib. Also palpate four quadrants in a 2" to 3" radius around the umbilicus for tenderness and tension. 5. Decreased secretory IgA on stool analysis.

2° Indication

B6 deficiency

Further assessment	1. B6 levels can be assessed by running a serum homocysteine or a B6 EGOT (Erythrocyte Glutamine-Oxaloacetate Transaminase) test

Supplemental Support

1. Pyridoxal-5-phosphate
2. Vitamin B complex
3. Colon support: Water soluble fiber and Lactobacillus acidophilus & Bifidobacterium bifidus
4. Garlic and chlorophyllins
5. Micro Emulsified Oregano
6. Digestive support: Nutrients to heal the intestines, Betaine HCL, Pepsin, & pancreatin
7. Chondroitin sulfates and manganese
8. Beet juice, taurine, vitamin C and pancreolipase

Lifestyle changes

Please see the handout in the appendix on the Dysbiosis diet

149. Bursitis or tendonitis

Bursitis:

Bursitis is an acute or chronic inflammation of a bursa. A bursa is a pocket of connective tissue found adjacent to a joint. Lined by a smooth inner surface, it facilitates the gliding movements of muscles and tendons over bony prominences. Bursitis is inflammation of a bursa, which results in pain, tenderness, and stiffness and in some cases, swelling and redness. The inflammatory process can affect any bursa, but bursitis involving the shoulder, elbow, hip and knee are most common.

Although the cause of this condition is unknown, repetitive direct pressure over a bursa can be a predisposing factor. In particular, certain activities or occupations are associated with specific example because of the nature of the physical stress placed on the bursa: e.g. housemaids knee (kneeling), students elbow (leaning). Shoulder bursitis, the most common type, is characterized by an aching pain localized on the outside of the top of the shoulder. Lifting and backwardly rotating the arm intensifies the pain. Typically, there is stiffness in the morning, which diminishes with heat and routine activities.

Tendonitis:

Tendonitis is an Inflammation of the lining of the tendon sheath (tenosynovitis) and of the enclosed tendon (tendinitis). It occurs spontaneously or in association with injury, work and sports activities, certain types of arthritis or infection. As with bursitis, the shoulder is most commonly affected. The attachment of the biceps tendon at the shoulder is especially vulnerable to this condition. Bicipital tendinitis is manifested by aching along the biceps muscle that radiates up to the shoulder and down to the forearm. The pain is worse with movement. Among other common locations for tendinitis are the elbow, wrist, hand, knee, and ankle.

Bursitis and tendonitis are basically due to an over-use and inflammation in the joint with a lack of essential nutrients. Balancing the overall structure of the body is essential and a general protocol for supporting the connective tissue is important.

The following is a list of nutrients that are useful for healing connective tissue:

1. Vitamin B12
2. Glucosamine hydrochloride
3. MSM
4. Vitamin B6
5. Vitamin C complex
6. Calcium and magnesium
7. Essential fatty acids
8. Chondroitin sulfate

1° Indication

Mineral deficiency

Further assessment	1. Assess for mineral deficiency using Tissue mineral assessment test. Place a standard blood pressure cuff around the largest portion of the client's calf muscle (sitting). Instruct the client to let you know when they feel the onset of cramping pain and gradually inflate the cuff. Stop and deflate immediately when threshold has been reached. Less

	than 200 mmHg is considered deficient in minerals. Use the neurolingual testing to challenge the body with several different types of minerals and other co-factors to see which combination of minerals and co-factors increases the threshold above 200mmHg. 2. Assess for mineral insufficiency by using Dr. Kane's mineral assessment tests. 3. Assess the impact of mineral deficiencies on the body's acid buffering capacities by using Dr. Bieler's salivary pH acid challenge.

Supplemental Support

1. B12 Lozenges
2. Glucosamine hydrochloride
3. Pyridoxal-5-phosphate
4. Chondroitin sulfates and manganese
5. Multiple nutrients to support bone health
6. Broad spectrum proteolytic enzymes
7. Calcium and magnesium with or without parathyroid tissue
8. Essential fatty acids: Mixed fatty acids (walnut, hazelnut, sesame, and apricot), EPA and DHA from fish oil

NOTES:

150. History of bone spurs (1 = yes, 0 = no)

Bone spurs are bony projections associated with osteoarthritis. From a functional perspective, they are associated with a primary mineral insufficiency, digestive dysfunction and thyroid hypo-function. Bone spurs may also be a sign of fluoride toxicity, which is associated with a calcium deficiency. Heel spurs respond well to B12 supplementation, with the appropriate digestive support.

Bone spurs are also associated with the deposition of bone into inappropriate tissue. This is a sign of aberrant calcium metabolism and possibly an alkalinity of the blood. Calcium is on of the minerals in the family of alkaline minerals that act as carbonic salts to neutralize acidity. When these salts react with an acid they form an alkaline salt that is easily excreted from the kidney. Calcium, as one of the major buffers of the blood, will begin to precipitate out of solution when the blood pH begins to drift away from optimal. The calcium will cause problems as it settles into the tissues causing not only bone spurs, but also cataracts, kidney stones, and even bursitis.

1° Indication
Mineral dysfunction with digestive dysfunction

Further assessment	1. Assess for mineral deficiency using Tissue mineral assessment test. Place a standard blood pressure cuff around the largest portion of the client's calf muscle (sitting). Instruct the client to let you know when they feel the onset of cramping pain and gradually inflate the cuff. Stop and deflate immediately when threshold has been reached. Less than 200 mmHg is considered deficient in minerals. Use the neurolingual testing to challenge the body with several different types of minerals and other co-factors to see which combination of minerals and co-factors increases the threshold above 200mmHg. 2. Check Ridler HCL reflex for tenderness 1 inch below xyphoid and over to the left edge of the rib cage 3. Check for tenderness in the Chapman reflex for the stomach and upper digestion located in 6th intercostal space on the left 4. Increased urinary indican levels 5. Assess for mineral insufficiency by using Dr. Kane's mineral assessment tests. 6. Assess the impact of mineral deficiencies on the body's acid buffering capacities by using Dr. Bieler's salivary pH acid challenge.

2° Indication
Thyroid dysfunction

Further assessment	1. Check for tenderness in the Chapman reflex for the thyroid located in the second intercostal space near the sternum on the right 2. Check for a delayed Achilles return reflex, which is a strong

	sign of a hypo-functioning thyroid 3. Check for general costochondral tenderness, a thyroid indicator 4. Check for pre-tibial edema, a sign of a hypo-functioning thyroid 5. Iodine test: Use a tincture of 2% iodine solution, and paint a 3" by 3" square on the client's abdomen. The client is to leave the patch unwashed until it disappears. A patch that has disappeared within 24 hours is an indication of iodine need. 6. Have client assess their basal metabolic temperature by taking their axillary temperature first thing in the morning for 5 straight days. An average temperature below 36.6°C is an indication of hypo-thyroidism

Supplemental Support

1. Multiple mineral without iron or copper
2. Calcium and magnesium with or without parathyroid tissue
3. Alkaline Ash minerals (Calcium, Magnesium,Potassium)
4. Multiple nutrients to support bone health
5. Multiple nutrients to support thyroid function with pituitary glandular
6. Potassium iodide

NOTES:

151. Morning stiffness

Morning stiffness can be a sign of vitamin B6 need and/or essential fatty acid supplementation. Vitamin B6 is an essential vitamin that is involved in the following functions in the body: energy metabolism, nervous system function, immune function and homocysteine metabolism. Women on the birth control pill will often be B6 deficient.

1° Indication

B6 and/or essential fatty acid deficiency

Further assessment	1. B6 levels can be assessed by running a serum homocysteine or a B6 EGOT (Erythrocyte Glutamine-Oxaloacetate Transaminase) test 2. Oral pH less that 7.2 indicates essential fatty acid deficiency 3. Repeated muscle challenge. This challenge involves a simple, normal muscle test repeated once per second, 20 times with regular intensity. As in a standard muscle test, the joint is positioned in such a way that the muscle to be tested is shortened. The practitioner applies pressure to the joint to lengthen the muscle, until a "locking" is noted. A positive result occurs when "locking" of the muscle and joint does not occur, indicating deficient free fatty acids. 4. Fatty acid profile via laboratory testing of blood

Supplemental Support

1. Pyridoxal-5-phosphate
2. Vitamin B complex
3. Essential fatty acids: Flax Seed Oil, EPA and DHA from fish oil, black currant seed oil and/or Mixed fatty acids (walnut, hazelnut, sesame, and apricot)

NOTES:

152. Nausea with vomiting

Vomiting and nausea can be a sign of serious pathology, and should be investigated. Frequent vomiting is a sign of phosphorous need. It is often seen with digestive dysfunction. The most common of which is biliary insufficiency or stasis. Other digestive causes include inadequate levels of stomach acid, pancreatic insufficiency and excess stomach acid. An irritated mucosal lining of the digestive tract can also cause nausea. One of the problems with persistent vomiting is the potential irritation of the esophageal sphincter, loss of stomach acid and general pH and electrolyte disturbance in the body. The hypochlorhydria caused by persistent vomiting can create absorption problems, especially for the minerals.

Nausea, with or without vomiting is also a sign of gallbladder dysfunction.

1° Indication

Phosphorous need

Further assessment	1. Assess for mineral deficiency using Tissue mineral assessment test. Place a standard blood pressure cuff around the largest portion of the client's calf muscle (sitting). Instruct the client to let you know when they feel the onset of cramping pain and gradually inflate the cuff. Stop and deflate immediately when threshold has been reached. Less than 200 mmHg is considered deficient in minerals. Use the neurolingual testing to challenge the body with several types of minerals to see if this increases the threshold above 200mmHg. 2. Assess for phosphorous insufficiency by using Dr. Kane's mineral assessment tests.

2° Indication

Biliary insufficiency with possible biliary stasis

Further assessment	1. Check for tenderness underneath the right rib cage 2. Check for tenderness and nodulation on the web between thumb and fore-finger of right hand 3. Check for tenderness in the Chapman reflex for the liver-gallbladder located over the 6th intercostal space on the right 4. Blood chemistry and CBC testing for SGOT, SGPT, GGT

3° Indication

Pancreatic insufficiency and stomach acid deficiency

Further assessment	**Pancreatic enzymes** 1. Check Ridler enzyme point for tenderness 1 inch below xyphoid and over to the right edge of the rib cage 2. Check for tenderness in the Chapman reflex for the pancreas located in the 7th intercostal space 3. Increased urinary sediment levels **Hydrochloric acid** 1. Check Ridler HCL reflex for tenderness 1 inch below

	xyphoid and over to the left edge of the rib cage 2. Check for tenderness in the Chapman reflex for the stomach and upper digestion located in 6th intercostal space on the left 3. Gastric acid assessment using Gastrotest

Other indications

1. Drugs/toxins
2. Pregnancy
3. Mechanical obstruction

Supplemental Support

1. Nutritional phosphorous 2. Beet juice, taurine, vitamin C and pancreolipase with or without bile salts 3. Phosphatidylcholine 4. Betaine HCL, Pepsin, and pancreatin 5. Pancreatic enzymes 6. Gut healing nutrients and vitamin U (to soothe irritated mucosa)

Lifestyle changes

Please see the handout in the appendix on Healthy lifestyle for a healthy gallbladder

NOTES:

153. Crave chocolate

Craving of chocolate is a common sign of magnesium deficiency. Other symptoms of magnesium deficiency include:

1. Being ticklish,
2. Being agoraphobic, they often dislike being in crowds
3. Having insomnia and/or restless leg syndrome.

The chocolate craving may also indicate a blood sugar dysregulation problem and a need to support the adrenals.

1° Indication

Magnesium deficiency

Further assessment	1. Assess for mineral deficiency using Tissue mineral assessment test. Place a standard blood pressure cuff around the largest portion of the client's calf muscle (sitting). Instruct the client to let you know when they feel the onset of cramping pain and gradually inflate the cuff. Stop and deflate immediately when threshold has been reached. Less than 200 mmHg is considered deficient in minerals. Use the neurolingual testing to challenge the body with several different types of magnesium and other co-factors to see which combination of magnesium and co-factors increases the threshold above 200mmHg. 2. Assess for magnesium insufficiency by using Dr. Kane's mineral assessment tests.

2° Indication

Blood sugar dysregulation, hypoglycemia and need for adrenal support.

Further assessment	1. Check for tenderness in the Chapman reflex for the liver-gallbladder located over the 6th intercostal space on the right 2. Check for tenderness in the Liver point located on the 3rd rib, 3 " to the right of the sternum, at the costochondral junction. 3. Check for tenderness underneath the right rib cage 4. Check for tenderness in the Chapman reflex for the pancreas located in the 7th intercostal space on the left 5. Check for tenderness or guarding at the head of the pancreas located in the upper left quadrant of the abdominal region 1/2 to 2/3 of the way between the umbilicus and the angel of the ribs 6. Check for tenderness in the inguinal ligament bilaterally 7. Check for a paradoxical pupillary reflex by shining a light into a client's eye and grading the reaction of the pupil. A pupil that fails to constrict indicates adrenal exhaustion 8. Check for the presence of postural hypotension. A drop of more than 10 points is an indication of adrenal insufficiency

Supplemental Support

1. Magnesium
2. Calcium and magnesium with or without parathyroid tissue
3. Multiple nutrients to support sugar handling problems
4. Adrenal support: Adaptogenic herbs to support adrenal function and Adrenal tissue (neonatal bovine)
5. Beet juice, taurine, vitamin C and pancreolipase

Lifestyle changes

Please see the handout in the appendix on food sources of magnesium

NOTES:

154. Feet have a strong odor

Feet having a strong odor is a common sign of magnesium insufficiency. Other symptoms of magnesium deficiency include:

1. Being ticklish,
2. Being agoraphobic, they often dislike being in crowds
3. and having insomnia and/or restless leg syndrome.

The strong odor of the feet may also indicate a need for liver and/or gallbladder support.

1° Indication
Magnesium deficiency

Further assessment	1. Assess for mineral deficiency using Tissue mineral assessment test. Place a standard blood pressure cuff around the largest portion of the client's calf muscle (sitting). Instruct the client to let you know when they feel the onset of cramping pain and gradually inflate the cuff. Stop and deflate immediately when threshold has been reached. Less than 200 mmHg is considered deficient in minerals. Use the neurolingual testing to challenge the body with several different types of magnesium and other co-factors to see which combination of magnesium and co-factors increases the threshold above 200mmHg. 2. Assess for magnesium insufficiency by using Dr. Kane's mineral assessment tests.

2° Indication
Need for liver and gallbladder support

Further assessment	1. Check for tenderness in the Chapman reflex for the liver-gallbladder located over the 6th intercostal space on the right side. 2. Check for tenderness in the Liver point located on the 3rd rib, 3 " to the right of the sternum, at the costochondral junction. 3. Check for tenderness underneath the right rib cage

Supplemental Support

1. Magnesium
2. Calcium and magnesium with or without parathyroid tissue
3. Nutrients to support Phase II liver detoxification
4. Herbs that cleanse the liver
5. Beet juice, taurine, vitamin C and pancreolipase
6. Glutathione, cysteine, and Glycine
7. Powdered detoxification support formula

Lifestyle changes
Please see the handout in the appendix on Recommendations for keeping your liver healthy and food sources of magnesium

155. Tendency to anemia

Anemia is often treated as if it were due to iron deficiency. There are a number of other nutritional causes for anemia including B12, folic acid, copper and B6 deficiencies. A thorough analysis of a blood chemistry and CBC can uncover the true cause of an anemia.

Often a compromised digestive tract, with a tendency towards hypochlorhydria can cause a persistent anemia, because the minerals and vitamins are not being absorbed properly due to the functional low HCL levels in the stomach. A thorough assessment of the digestive tract is warranted in cases of stubborn anemia.

1° Indication

Assess for true cause of anemia

Further assessment	1. Assess anemia from blood chemistry and CBC for possible nutritional causes

2° Indication

Assess for digestive dysfunction for possible hydrochloric acid need

Further assessment	1. Check Ridler HCL reflex for tenderness 1 inch below xyphoid and over to the left edge of the rib cage 2. Check for tenderness in the Chapman reflex for the stomach and upper digestion located in 6th intercostal space on the left 3. Check for a positive zinc tally: A client holds a solution of aqueous zinc sulfate in their mouth and tells you if and when they can taste it. An almost immediate very bitter taste indicates the client does not need zinc. Clients who are zinc deficient will report no taste from the solution. 4. Gastric acid assessment using Gastrotest 5. Increased urinary indican levels

Supplemental Support

1. Vitamin B12 and folic acid
2. Pyridoxal-5-phosphate
3. Betaine HCL, Pepsin, and pancreatin
4. Nutritional copper
5. Iron
6. Multiple mineral without iron or copper

NOTES:

156. Whites of eyes (sclera) blue tinted

Blue tinted whites of the eye are a fairly specific indicator of iron deficiency anemia. Iron deficiency anemia is a common, though often over treated form of anemia. It is important to thoroughly assess a client with anemia by doing follow-up blood studies.

Often a compromised digestive tract, with a tendency towards hypochlorhydria can cause a persistent anemia, because the minerals and vitamins are not being absorbed properly due to the functional low HCL levels in the stomach. A thorough assessment of the digestive tract is warranted in cases of stubborn anemia.

1° Indication

Assess for true cause of anemia

Further assessment	1. Assess anemia from blood chemistry and CBC for possible nutritional causes

2° Indication

Assess for digestive dysfunction for possible hydrochloric acid need

Further assessment	1. Check Ridler HCL reflex for tenderness 1 inch below xyphoid and over to the left edge of the rib cage 2. Check for tenderness in the Chapman reflex for the stomach and upper digestion located in 6th intercostal space on the left 3. Betaine HCL and pepsin 4. Gastric acid assessment using Gastrotest 5. Increased urinary indican levels

Supplemental Support

1. Iron 2. Betaine HCL, Pepsin, and pancreatin

NOTES:

157. Hoarseness

Frequent hoarseness is a sign of parathyroid dysfunction. The parathyroid glands are a pair of small glands, located in the throat near the thyroid. The parathyroid produces a hormone called parathyroid hormone or PTH. PTH causes an increase in the resorption of calcium from the bone and the intestines. Therefore, PTH is one of the major factors in the regulation of calcium concentration in extra-cellular fluid.

A decrease in the level of ionized calcium is the primary stimulus for PTH secretion, while an increase in serum calcium inhibits PTH secretion. Parathyroid dysfunction may be a serious metabolic problem that should be evaluated by a doctor qualified to diagnose and treat parathyroid dysfunction.

1° Indication

Parathyroid dysfunction

Further assessment	1. Assess parathyroid by running blood chemistry screen. Look for signs of abnormal calcium metabolism: low Alk phos and serum calcium, high phosphorous 2. Check client's urine for increased calcium excretion, which is a sign of potential hyper-parathyroid dysfunction

Supplemental Support

1. Calcium and magnesium with or without parathyroid tissue
2. Multiple mineral without iron or copper
3. Appropriate calcium supplementation
4. Emulsified Viatmin D drops
5. Beet juice, taurine, vitamin C and pancreolipase

NOTES:

158. Difficulty swallowing

A difficulty swallowing may be serious and needs to be assessed. Possible causes of a difficulty in swallowing include: neurological deficit, obstruction of the esophagus or a motor disorder.

Assess whether the difficulty in swallowing occurs with solids or liquids or both:

Solids only: indicates an obstructive lesion
Liquids and solids: indicates a motor disorder
Difficulty initiating swallowing: a neurological deficit.

If all the above causes are ruled out, look to a parathyroid dysfunction and/or biliary stasis. The parathyroid glands are a pair of small glands, located in the throat near the thyroid. The parathyroid produces a hormone called parathyroid hormone or PTH. PTH causes an increase in the resorption of calcium from the bone and the intestines. Therefore, PTH is one of the major factors in the regulation of calcium concentration in extra-cellular fluid. A decrease in the level of ionized calcium is the primary stimulus for PTH secretion, while an increase in serum calcium inhibits PTH secretion.

Parathyroid dysfunction may be a serious metabolic problem that should be evaluated by a doctor qualified to diagnose and treat parathyroid dysfunction.

1° Indication
Parathyroid dysfunction

Further assessment	1. Assess parathyroid by running blood chemistry screen. Look for signs of abnormal calcium metabolism: low Alk phos and serum calcium, high phosphorous 2. Check client's urine for increased calcium excretion, which is a sign of potential hyper-parathyroid dysfunction

2° Indication
Gallbladder dysfunction with biliary stasis

Further assessment	1. Check for tenderness underneath the right rib cage 2. Check for tenderness and nodulation on the web between thumb and fore-finger of right hand 3. Check for tenderness in the Chapman reflex for the liver-gallbladder located over the 6th intercostal space on the right 4. Assess for Hepato-biliary congestion with the Acoustic Cardiogram (ACG), which will show post-systolic rounding due to increased backpressure on the pulmonic and aortic valve. It may also show through to the tricuspid valve if chronic.

Supplemental Support

1. Calcium and magnesium with or without parathyroid tissue
2. Multiple mineral without iron or copper
3. Emulsified Viatmin D drops
4. Beet juice, taurine, vitamin C and pancreolipase

159. Lump in throat

A lump in the throat is associated with potassium insufficiency and/or biliary stasis.

1° Indication
Potassium insufficiency

Further assessment	1. Assess for mineral deficiency using Tissue mineral assessment test. Place a standard blood pressure cuff around the largest portion of the client's calf muscle (sitting). Instruct the client to let you know when they feel the onset of cramping pain and gradually inflate the cuff. Stop and deflate immediately when threshold has been reached. Less than 200 mmHg is considered deficient in minerals. Use the neurolingual testing to challenge the body with several different types of minerals and other co-factors to see which combination of minerals and co-factors increases the threshold above 200mmHg. 2. Check potassium levels on blood chemistry. 3. Assess for potassium insufficiency by using Dr. Kane's mineral assessment tests. 4. Assess the impact of mineral deficiencies on the body's acid buffering capacities by using Dr. Bieler's salivary pH acid challenge.

2° Indication
Gallbladder dysfunction with biliary stasis

Further assessment	1. Check for tenderness underneath the right rib cage 2. Check for tenderness and nodulation on the web between thumb and fore-finger of right hand 3. Check for tenderness in the Chapman reflex for the liver-gallbladder located over the 6th intercostal space on the right side 4. Assess for Hepato-biliary congestion with the Acoustic Cardiogram (ACG), which will show post-systolic rounding due to increased backpressure on the pulmonic and aortic valve. It may also show through to the tricuspid valve if chronic.

Supplemental Support

1.	Alkaline ash minerals (calcium, magnesium and potassium)
2.	Potassium
3.	Multiple mineral without iron or copper
4.	Beet juice, taurine, vitamin C and pancreolipase

Lifestyle changes
Please see the handout in the appendix on Food sources of potassium

160. Dry mouth, eyes and / or nose

Dry mouth, eyes and/or nose are signs of potassium insufficiency and general mineral deficiency. The tissue mineral test is a great way to help uncover mineral deficiencies.

1° Indication

Potassium insufficiency and general mineral deficiency

Further assessment	1. Assess for mineral deficiency using Tissue mineral assessment test. Place a standard blood pressure cuff around the largest portion of the client's calf muscle (sitting). Instruct the client to let you know when they feel the onset of cramping pain and gradually inflate the cuff. Stop and deflate immediately when threshold has been reached. Less than 200 mmHg is considered deficient in minerals. Use the neurolingual testing to challenge the body with several different types of minerals and other co-factors to see which combination of minerals and co-factors increases the threshold above 200mmHg. 2. Assess for mineral insufficiency using Dr. Kane's mineral assessment tests. 3. Check potassium and calcium levels in the blood 4. Assess the impact of mineral deficiencies on the body's acid buffering capacities by using Dr. Bieler's salivary pH acid challenge.

Supplemental Support

1. Alkaline ash minerals (calcium, magnesium and potassium)
2. Potassium
3. Calcium and magnesium with or without parathyroid tissue
4. Multiple mineral without iron or copper
5. Beet juice, taurine, vitamin C and pancreolipase

Lifestyle changes

Please see the handout in the appendix on Food sources of potassium

NOTES:

161. Gag easily

A person who gags easily is in a state of parasympathetic stress. Too much potassium in relation to calcium can cause "parasympathetic dominance," which causes a general systemic shift toward alkalinity in the body resulting in tendencies toward lethargy, apathy, depression, loss of muscle tone, drive, concentration and emotion. Potassium tends to stimulate the parasympathetic system and therefore the body should be assessed for the correct minerals that can help balance the system.

<u>1° Indication</u>

Mineral imbalance with imbalanced potassium to calcium ratio

Further assessment	1. Assess for mineral deficiency using Tissue mineral assessment test. Place a standard blood pressure cuff around the largest portion of the client's calf muscle (sitting). Instruct the client to let you know when they feel the onset of cramping pain and gradually inflate the cuff. Stop and deflate immediately when threshold has been reached. Less than 200 mmHg is considered deficient in minerals. Use the neurolingual testing to challenge the body with several different types of minerals and other co-factors to see which combination of minerals and co-factors increases the threshold above 200mmHg. 2. Assess for mineral insufficiency by using Dr. Kane's mineral assessment tests. 3. Assess the impact of mineral deficiencies on the body's acid buffering capacities by using Dr. Bieler's salivary pH acid challenge.

Supplemental Support

1. Calcium and magnesium with or without parathyroid tissue 2. Multiple mineral without iron or copper 3. Beet juice, taurine, vitamin C and pancreolipase

NOTES:

162. White spots on fingernails
163. Cuts heal slowly and / or scar easily
164. Decreased sense of taste or smell

These are all symptoms of zinc deficiency. Zinc is an essential mineral to the body and is involved in the following functions in the body:

1. Wound healing,
2. Enhancing immune function,
3. Anti-inflammatory
4. Promoting conversion of thyroxine to triiodothyronine.

Zinc should be supplemented along with a general multiple mineral supplement deficiency is often accompanied by deficiencies in other minerals, including magnesium, selenium and potassium.

1° Indication
Zinc deficiency

Further assessment	1. Positive zinc tally: A client holds a solution of aqueous zinc sulfate in their mouth and tells you if and when they can taste it. An almost immediate very bitter taste indicates the client does not need zinc. Clients who are zinc deficient will report no taste from the solution. 2. Assess for mineral insufficiency by using Dr. Kane's mineral assessment tests. 3. Assess the impact of mineral deficiencies on the body's acid buffering capacities by using Dr. Bieler's salivary pH acid challenge.

Supplemental Support

1. Nutritional zinc
2. Multiple mineral without iron or copper

Lifestyle changes
Please see the handout in the appendix on Food sources of zinc

NOTES:

ESSENTIAL FATTY ACIDS

165. Experience pain relief with aspirin (1 = yes, 0 = no)
166. Crave fatty or greasy foods
167. Low or reduced fat diet (past or present)
168. Tension headaches at base of skull
169. Headaches when out in the hot sun
170. Sunburn easily or suffer sun poisoning
171. Muscles easily fatigued
172. Dry flaky skin and or dandruff

165. Experience pain relief with aspirin (1 = yes, 0 = no)

Aspirin is a non-steroidal anti-inflammatory drug that works to control pain by inhibiting prostaglandin synthesis. Prostaglandins are derivatives of essential fatty acids, and can be either pro-inflammatory (PG2) or anti-inflammatory (PG1 and PG3) in their properties. Pain occurs when an essential fatty acid called arachadonic acid is stripped from the cellular membrane and is converted, via various enzymatic pathways, into a pain causing prostaglandin called prostaglandin-2. Aspirin works by interfering with these pathways. Arachadonic acid is found in commercially raised meat and animal products.

If the client is suffering from pain and inflammation, it might not be a bad idea to decrease the source of arachadonic acid in the body, and increase the precursors of the anti-inflammatory prostaglandins: black currant seed or borage oil, evening primrose oil, flax seed oil and the oils from cold water fish, which include EPA and DHA.
An assessment of essential fatty acid status is important for people in pain.

1° Indication

Essential fatty acid assessment.

Further assessment	1. Oral pH less that 7.2 indicates essential fatty acid deficiency 2. Repeated muscle challenge. This challenge involves a simple, normal muscle test repeated once per second, 20 times with regular intensity. As in a standard muscle test, the joint is positioned in such a way that the muscle to be tested is shortened. The practitioner applies pressure to the joint to lengthen the muscle, until a “locking” is noted. A positive result occurs when ”locking” of the muscle and joint does not occur, indicating deficient free fatty acids. 3. Fatty acid profile via laboratory testing of blood

Supplemental Support

1. Flax seed oil
2. Black currant seed oil
3. Mixed fatty acids (walnut, hazelnut, sesame, and apricot)
4. EPA and DHA from fish oil

Lifestyle changes

Avoid all sources of hydrogenated oils and deep fried foods, which rob the body of essential fatty acids

NOTES:

166. Crave fatty or greasy foods

Craving fatty, greasy food is a sign of essential fatty acid deficiency and a need for bile salts.

1° Indication
Essential fatty acid insufficiency.

Further assessment	1. Oral pH less that 7.2 indicates essential fatty acid deficiency 2. Repeated muscle challenge. This challenge involves a simple, normal muscle test repeated once per second, 20 times with regular intensity. As in a standard muscle test, the joint is positioned in such a way that the muscle to be tested is shortened. The practitioner applies pressure to the joint to lengthen the muscle, until a "locking" is noted. A positive result occurs when "locking" of the muscle and joint does not occur, indicating deficient free fatty acids. 3. Fatty acid profile via laboratory testing of blood

2° Indication
Liver and gallbladder congestion

Further assessment	1. Check for tenderness in the Chapman reflex for the liver-gallbladder located over the 6th intercostal space on the right side 2. Check for tenderness in the Liver point located on the 3rd rib, 3" to the right of the sternum, at the costochondral junction. 3. Check for tenderness underneath the right rib cage 4. Check for tenderness and nodulation on the web between thumb and fore-finger of right hand 5. Assess for Hepato-biliary congestion with the Acoustic Cardiogram (ACG), which will show post-systolic rounding due to increased backpressure on the pulmonic and aortic valve. It may also show through to the tricuspid valve if chronic.

Supplemental Support

1. Flax seed oil
2. Blackcurrant seed oil
3. EPA and DHA from fish oil
4. Mixed fatty acids (walnut, hazelnut, sesame, and apricot)
5. Beet juice and bile salts
6. Phosphatidylcholine
7. Beet juice, taurine, vitamin C and pancreolipase

Lifestyle changes
Avoid all sources of hydrogenated fats and deep fried foods

NOTES:

167. Low or reduced fat diet (past or present)

Low fat diets are a very good way to become deficient in essential fatty acids. Assess this client for essential fatty acid deficiency, and supplement them with the correct essential fatty acids and co-factors for optimal absorption and utilization.

1° Indication

Essential fatty acid insufficiency.

Further assessment	1. Oral pH less that 7.2 indicates essential fatty acid deficiency 2. Repeated muscle challenge. This challenge involves a simple, normal muscle test repeated once per second, 20 times with regular intensity. As in a standard muscle test, the joint is positioned in such a way that the muscle to be tested is shortened. The practitioner applies pressure to the joint to lengthen the muscle, until a "locking" is noted. A positive result occurs when "locking" of the muscle and joint does not occur, indicating deficient free fatty acids. 3. Fatty acid profile via laboratory testing of blood

Other indications

Deficient in fat soluble vitamins: Vitamin A, D and E

Supplemental Support

1. Flax seed oil
2. Blackcurrant seed oil
3. EPA and DHA from fish oil
4. Mixed fatty acids (walnut, hazelnut, sesame, and apricot)
5. Phosphatidylcholine
6. Beet juice, taurine, vitamin C and pancreolipase with or without bile salts

Lifestyle changes

Avoid all sources of hydrogenated oils and deep fried foods, which rob the body of essential fatty acids

NOTES:

168. Tension headaches at base of skull
169. Headaches when out in the hot sun

Tension headaches at the base of the skull and headaches when out in the hot sun are symptoms of essential fatty acid deficiency. Obviously, it is important to assess the most likely causes first. For instance, chronic tension headaches need to be assessed for correct structural alignment, and the workspace needs to be looked into to make sure the ergonomics and work position are not putting too much stress on the client.

Essential fatty acid deficiency is often due to a biliary dysfunction, leading to incomplete emulsification of fatty acids, and is often accompanied by a mineral deficiency, especially calcium.

1° Indication
Essential fatty acid insufficiency.

Further assessment	1. Oral pH less that 7.2 indicates essential fatty acid deficiency 2. Repeated muscle challenge. This challenge involves a simple, normal muscle test repeated once per second, 20 times with regular intensity. As in a standard muscle test, the joint is positioned in such a way that the muscle to be tested is shortened. The practitioner applies pressure to the joint to lengthen the muscle, until a "locking" is noted. A positive result occurs when "locking" of the muscle and joint does not occur, indicating deficient free fatty acids. 3. Fatty acid profile via laboratory testing of blood

2° Indication
Biliary dysfunction

Further assessment	1. Check for tenderness underneath the right rib cage 2. Check for tenderness and nodulation on the web between thumb and fore-finger of right hand 3. Check for tenderness in the Chapman reflex for the liver-gallbladder located over the 6th intercostal space on the right side 4. Assess for Hepato-biliary congestion with the Acoustic Cardiogram (ACG), which will show post-systolic rounding due to increased backpressure on the pulmonic and aortic valve. It may also show through to the tricuspid valve if chronic. 5. Blood chemistry and CBC testing for SGOT, SGPT, GGT

3° Indication
Mineral deficiency

Further assessment	1. Assess for mineral deficiency using Tissue mineral assessment test. Place a standard blood pressure cuff around the largest portion of the client's calf muscle (sitting). Instruct the client to let you know when they feel the onset of

	cramping pain and gradually inflate the cuff. Stop and deflate immediately when threshold has been reached. Less than 200 mmHg is considered deficient in minerals. Use the neurolingual testing to challenge the body with several types of minerals to see if this increases the threshold above 200mmHg. 2. Check for a positive zinc tally: A client holds a solution of aqueous zinc sulfate in their mouth and tells you if and when they can taste it. An almost immediate very bitter taste indicates the client does not need zinc. Clients who are zinc deficient will report no taste from the solution. 3. Assess for mineral insufficiency by using Dr. Kane's mineral assessment tests. 4. Assess the impact of mineral deficiencies on the body's acid buffering capacities by using Dr. Bieler's salivary pH acid challenge.

Other indications

Deficient in fat soluble vitamins: Vitamin A, D and E

Supplemental Support

1. Flax seed oil
2. Blackcurrant seed oil
3. EPA and DHA from fish oil
4. Mixed fatty acids (walnut, hazelnut, sesame, and apricot)
5. Phosphatidylcholine
6. Beet juice, taurine, vitamin C and pancreolipase with or without bile salts

Lifestyle changes

Avoid all sources of hydrogenated fats and deep fried foods

NOTES:

170. Sunburn easily or suffer sun poisoning
171. Muscles easily fatigued

Getting sunburned easily or suffering from sun poisoning, and easily fatigued muscles are a sign of essential fatty acid deficiency. Essential fatty acid deficiency is often due to a biliary dysfunction, leading to incomplete emulsification of fatty acids.

1° Indication

Essential fatty acid insufficiency.

Further assessment	1. Oral pH less that 7.2 indicates essential fatty acid deficiency 2. Repeated muscle challenge. This challenge involves a simple, normal muscle test repeated once per second, 20 times with regular intensity. As in a standard muscle test, the joint is positioned in such a way that the muscle to be tested is shortened. The practitioner applies pressure to the joint to lengthen the muscle, until a "locking" is noted. A positive result occurs when "locking" of the muscle and joint does not occur, indicating deficient free fatty acids. 3. Fatty acid profile via laboratory testing of blood

2° Indication

Calcium deficiency

Further assessment	1. Assess for calcium deficiency using Tissue mineral assessment test. Place a standard blood pressure cuff around the largest portion of the client's calf muscle (sitting). Instruct the client to let you know when they feel the onset of cramping pain and gradually inflate the cuff. Stop and deflate immediately when threshold has been reached. Less than 200 mmHg is considered deficient in minerals. Use the neurolingual testing to challenge the body with several types of calcium to see if this increases the threshold above 200mmHg.

3° Indication

Biliary dysfunction

Further assessment	1. Check for tenderness underneath the right rib cage 2. Check for tenderness and nodulation on the web between thumb and fore-finger of right hand 3. Check for tenderness in the Chapman reflex for the liver-gallbladder located over the 6th intercostal space on the right 4. Assess for Hepato-biliary congestion with the Acoustic Cardiogram (ACG), which will show post-systolic rounding due to increased backpressure on the pulmonic and aortic valve. It may also show through to the tricuspid valve if chronic. 5. Blood chemistry and CBC testing for SGOT, SGPT, GGT

Other indications

Deficient in fat soluble vitamins: Vitamin A, D and E

Supplemental Support

1. Flax seed oil
2. Blackcurrant Seed Oil
3. EPA and DHA from fish oil
4. Mixed fatty acids (walnut, hazelnut, sesame, and apricot)
5. Phosphatidylcholine
6. Beet juice, taurine, vitamin C and pancreolipase with or without bile salts
7. Calcium and Magnesium formula with or without parathyroid tissue
8. RNA/DNA

Lifestyle changes

Avoid all sources of hydrogenated fats and deep fried foods

NOTES:

172. Dry flaky skin and or dandruff

Dry, flaky skin is one of the first indications of an essential fatty acid deficiency. It is important to enquire whether or not your clients are using hydrating lotions. This question refers to dry and flaky skin that occurs without the use of such lotions. Many people take it for granted that they need to use moisturizing lotions in order to have moist skin.

Essential fatty acid deficiency is often due to a biliary dysfunction, leading to incomplete emulsification of fatty acids, and is often accompanied by a mineral deficiency, especially calcium.

1° Indication

Essential fatty acid insufficiency.

Further assessment	1. Oral pH less that 7.2 indicates essential fatty acid deficiency 2. Repeated muscle challenge. This challenge involves a simple, normal muscle test repeated once per second, 20 times with regular intensity. As in a standard muscle test, the joint is positioned in such a way that the muscle to be tested is shortened. The practitioner applies pressure to the joint to lengthen the muscle, until a "locking" is noted. A positive result occurs when "locking" of the muscle and joint does not occur, indicating deficient free fatty acids. 3. Fatty acid profile via laboratory testing of blood

2° Indication

Mineral deficiency

Further assessment	1. Assess for mineral deficiency using Tissue mineral assessment test. Place a standard blood pressure cuff around the largest portion of the client's calf muscle (sitting). Instruct the client to let you know when they feel the onset of cramping pain and gradually inflate the cuff. Stop and deflate immediately when threshold has been reached. Less than 200 mmHg is considered deficient in minerals. Use the neurolingual testing to challenge the body with several types of minerals to see if this increases the threshold above 200mmHg. 2. Check for a positive zinc tally: A client holds a solution of aqueous zinc sulfate in their mouth and tells you if and when they can taste it. An almost immediate very bitter taste indicates the client does not need zinc. Clients who are zinc deficient will report no taste from the solution. 3. Assess for mineral insufficiency by using Dr. Kane's mineral assessment tests. 4. Assess the impact of mineral deficiencies on the body's acid buffering capacities by using Dr. Bieler's salivary pH acid challenge.

Other indications

Deficient in fat soluble vitamins: Vitamin A, D and E

Supplemental Support

1. Flax seed oil
2. Blackcurrant seed oil
3. EPA and DHA from fish oil
4. Mixed fatty acids (walnut, hazelnut, sesame, and apricot)
5. Phosphotidyl choline
6. Beet juice, taurine, vitamin C and pancreolipase with or without bile salts
7. Calcium and Magnesium formula with or without parathyroid tissue
8. Multiple mineral without iron or copper

Lifestyle changes

Avoid all sources of hydrogenated fats and deep fried foods

NOTES:

BLOOD SUGAR DYSREGULATION

173. Awaken a few hours after falling asleep, hard to get back to sleep
174. Crave sweets
175. Binge or uncontrolled eating
176. Excessive appetite
177. Crave coffee or sugar in the afternoon
178. Sleepy in afternoon
179. Fatigue that is relieved by eating
180. Headache if meals are skipped or delayed
181. Irritable before meals
182. Shaky if meals delayed
183. Family members with diabetes (0 = none, 1= 2 or less, 2 =Between 2-4, 3 = More than 4)
184. Frequent thirst
185. Frequent urination

173. Awaken a few hours after falling asleep, hard to get back to sleep

This is a classic symptom of low blood sugar. At night the blood sugar begins to drop, especially at around 1.00 AM in the morning. This client needs to have their blood sugar regulation assessed for hypoglycemia. A diet diary will also indicate the kind of meal they ate that night. Sometimes a little juice or snack right before going to bed can help with the low blood sugar. This is, of course, only a temporary solution. Blood sugar regulation needs to be assessed and the client needs to start on a protocol that will help address this issue.

1° Indication

Blood sugar dysregulation and hypoglycemia.

Further assessment	1. Check for tenderness in the Chapman reflex for the liver-gallbladder located over the 6th intercostal space on the right 2. Check for tenderness in the Liver point located on the 3rd rib, 3 " to the right of the sternum, at the costochondral junction. 3. Check for tenderness underneath the right rib cage 4. Check for tenderness or nodularity in the right thenar pad. 5. Check for tenderness in the Chapman reflex for the pancreas located in the 7th intercostal space on the left 6. Check for tenderness or guarding at the head of the pancreas located in the upper left quadrant of the abdominal region 1/2 to 2/3 of the way between the umbilicus and the angel of the ribs 7. Check fasting blood glucose 8. Run a six hour glucose-insulin tolerance test.

2° Indication

Low adrenal function

Further assessment	1. Check for tenderness in the inguinal ligament bilaterally 2. Check for tenderness at the medial knee bilaterally, at the insertion of the sartorius muscle at the Pes Anserine. 3. Check for a paradoxical pupillary reflex by shining a light into a client's eye and grading the reaction of the pupil. A pupil that fails to constrict indicates adrenal exhaustion 4. Check for the presence of postural hypotension. A drop of more than 10 points is an indication of adrenal insufficiency 5. Check for a chronic short leg due to a posterior-inferior ilium. 6. Assess for adrenal insufficiency with the Acoustic Cardiogram (ACG), which will show static in both the systolic and diastolic rest phases. You will also see an elevated S2 sound.

Other indications

1. B vitamin deficiency
2. Serotonin/melatonin imbalance

Supplemental Support

1. Multiple nutrients to support sugar handling problems
2. Adaptogenic herbs to support adrenal function
3. Adrenal tissue (neonatal bovine)
4. Beet juice, taurine, vitamin C and pancreolipase
5. Pancreatic tissue (neonatal bovine)
6. Herbs that cleanse the liver

Lifestyle changes

Please see the handout in the appendix on Recommendations for controlling blood sugar

NOTES:

174. Crave sweets

The reasons for craving sweets are many, and are often assuaged by eating desserts and sugary snacks. Blood sugar abnormalities, such as reactive hypoglycemia, a deficiency in B vitamins, an overgrowth of yeast in the digestive tract, a deficiency in HCL and/or pancreatic enzymes and hidden food allergies, are all causes of sugar cravings.

The more sugar you eat, the more you will crave it. Sugar is very addictive, and hooks into the primeval need for something sweet. Sweet breast milk was often the taste we first associated with nurturing. The cycle of sweets and sugar craving is a merry-go-round we should all get off. It takes at least 3-4 days to clear the residue of sweets and sugar from the body. It may take a lot longer than that to get rid of the craving. Assessing for blood sugar dysregulation and for yeast overgrowth in the GI is a good place to start. If these do not help, then try assessing the digestive tract for HCL and pancreatic enzyme insufficiency.
Sugar also increases our needs for B vitamins and Vitamin C. The body has to rob its stores of B vitamins to handle the nutrient-devoid sugar. Sugar also places an unnecessary burden on the adrenal glands, another organ essential for blood sugar control. The adrenals respond to sugar by putting out cortisol, which can lead to mineral deficiencies by causing the body to dump minerals.

<u>1° Indication</u>
Blood sugar dysregulation

Further assessment	1. Check for tenderness in the Chapman reflex for the liver-gallbladder located over the 6th intercostal space on the right 2. Check for tenderness in the Liver point located on the 3rd rib, 3 " to the right of the sternum, at the costochondral junction. 3. Check for tenderness underneath the right rib cage 4. Check for tenderness or nodularity in the right thenar pad, which is a pancreas indicator if tender 5. Check for tenderness in the Chapman reflex for the pancreas located in the 7th intercostal space on the left 6. Check for tenderness or guarding at the head of the pancreas located in the upper left quadrant of the abdominal region 1/2 to 2/3 of the way between the umbilicus and the angel of the ribs 7. Check fasting blood glucose 8. Run a six hour glucose-insulin tolerance test.

<u>2° Indication</u>
Low adrenal function

Further assessment	1. Check for tenderness in the inguinal ligament bilaterally 2. Check for tenderness at the medial knee bilaterally, at the insertion of the sartorius muscle at the Pes Anserine. 3. Check for a paradoxical pupillary reflex by shining a light into a client's eye and grading the reaction of the pupil. A pupil that fails to constrict indicates adrenal exhaustion 4. Check for the presence of postural hypotension. A drop of

	more than 10 points is an indication of adrenal insufficiency 5. Check for a chronic short leg due to a posterior-inferior ilium. 6. Assess for adrenal insufficiency with the Acoustic Cardiogram (ACG), which will show static in both the systolic and diastolic rest phases. You will also see an elevated S2 sound.

3° Indication

Dysbiosis with yeast overgrowth

Further assessment	1. Increased urinary indican and sediment levels 2. Stool analysis- either comprehensive digestive analysis or a parasite profile 3. Check for tenderness in the Chapman reflex for the colon located bilaterally along the iliotibial band on the thighs. Palpate the colon for tenderness and tension. 4. Check for tenderness in the Chapman reflex for the small intestine located on the 8th, 9th and 10th intercostal spaces near the tip of the rib. Also palpate four quadrants in a 2" to 3" radius around the umbilicus for tenderness and tension. 5. Decreased secretory IgA on stool analysis.

Other indications

1. Digestive dysfunction with HCL and pancreatic enzyme need
2. Mineral deficiency
3. Hidden food allergies
4. B vitamin need

Supplemental Support

Sugar handling: 1. Multiple nutrients to support sugar handling problems 2. Adaptogenic herbs to support adrenal function 3. Adrenal tissue (neonatal bovine) 4. Beet juice, taurine, vitamin C and pancreolipase 5. Pancreatic tissue (neonatal bovine) 6. Herbs that cleanse the liver **Dysbiosis:** 1. Micro Emulsified Oregano 2. Digestive support: Nutrients to heal the intestines, Betaine HCL, Pepsin, & pancreatin 3. L-Glutamine 4. Water soluble fiber and colon health nutrients 5. Lactobacillus acidophilus and Bifidobacterium bifidus

Lifestyle changes

Please see the handout in the appendix on Recommendations for controlling blood sugar

175. Binge or uncontrolled eating

Binge or uncontrolled eating is a sign of hydrochloric acid or digestive enzyme need. It is also associated with blood sugar dysregulation and hidden food allergies.

1° Indication

Digestive dysfunction with hydrochloric acid need

Further assessment	1. Check Ridler HCL reflex for tenderness 1 inch below xyphoid and over to the left edge of the rib cage 2. Check for tenderness in the Chapman reflex for the stomach and upper digestion located in 6th intercostal space on the left 3. Check for a positive zinc tally: A client holds a solution of aqueous zinc sulfate in their mouth and tells you if and when they can taste it. An almost immediate very bitter taste indicates the client does not need zinc. Clients who are zinc deficient will report no taste from the solution. 4. Gastric acid assessment using the Gastrotest 5. Increased urinary indican levels

2° Indication

Blood sugar dysregulation

Further assessment	1. Check for tenderness in the Chapman reflex for the liver-gallbladder located over the 6th intercostal space on the right 2. Check for tenderness in the Liver point located on the 3rd rib, 3 " to the right of the sternum, at the costochondral junction. 3. Check for tenderness in the Chapman reflex for the pancreas located in the 7th intercostal space on the left 4. Check for tenderness or guarding at the head of the pancreas located in the upper left quadrant of the abdominal region 1/2 to 2/3 of the way between the umbilicus and the angel of the ribs 5. Check fasting blood glucose and 6. Run a six hour glucose-insulin tolerance test.

3° Indication

Low adrenal function

Further assessment	1. Check for tenderness in the inguinal ligament bilaterally 2. Check for tenderness at the medial knee bilaterally, at the insertion of the sartorius muscle at the Pes Anserine. 3. Check for a paradoxical pupillary reflex by shining a light into a client's eye and grading the reaction of the pupil. A pupil that fails to constrict indicates adrenal exhaustion 4. Check for the presence of postural hypotension. A drop of more than 10 points is an indication of adrenal insufficiency 5. Check for a chronic short leg due to a posterior-inferior ilium. 6. Assess for adrenal insufficiency with the Acoustic Cardiogram (ACG), which will show static in both the systolic and diastolic rest phases. You will also see an elevated S2 sound.

Other indications

Hidden food allergies

Supplemental Support

1. Multiple nutrients to support sugar handling problems
2. Adaptogenic herbs to support adrenal function
3. Adrenal tissue (neonatal bovine)
4. Beet juice, taurine, vitamin C and pancreolipase
5. Pancreatic tissue (neonatal bovine)
6. Herbs that cleanse the liver
7. Betaine HCL, Pepsin, and pancreatin
8. Pancreatic Enzymes

Lifestyle changes

Please see the handout in the appendix on Diet and digestion, and recommendations for controlling blood sugar.

NOTES:

176. Excessive appetite

An excessive appetite is often sign of yeast or bacteria overgrowth in the digestive system, or even intestinal parasites. With a severe candidiasis large portions of the food are consumed to keep the overgrowth alive. Poor digestion or blood sugar dysregulation can also contribute to an excessive appetite. A client has to eat more food in order to get a small amount digested and absorbed.

1° Indication

Dysbiosis with yeast overgrowth

Further assessment	1. Increased urinary indican and sediment levels 2. Stool analysis- either comprehensive digestive analysis or a parasite profile 3. Check for tenderness in the Chapman reflex for the colon located bilaterally along the iliotibial band on the thighs. Palpate the colon for tenderness and tension. 4. Check for tenderness in the Chapman reflex for the small intestine located on the 8th, 9th and 10th intercostal spaces near the tip of the rib. Also palpate four quadrants in a 2" to 3" radius around the umbilicus for tenderness and tension. 5. Decreased secretory IgA on stool analysis.

2° Indication

Digestive dysfunction with hydrochloric acid need

Further assessment	1. Check Ridler HCL reflex for tenderness 1 inch below xyphoid and over to the left edge of the rib cage 2. Check for tenderness in the Chapman reflex for the stomach and upper digestion located in 6th intercostal space on the left 3. Check for a positive zinc tally: A client holds a solution of aqueous zinc sulfate in their mouth and tells you if and when they can taste it. An almost immediate very bitter taste indicates the client does not need zinc. Clients who are zinc deficient will report no taste from the solution. 4. Gastric acid assessment using Gastrotest 5. Increased urinary indican levels

Other indications

Blood sugar dysregulation

Supplemental Support

Dysbiosis:	**HCl and pancreatic enzyme need:**
1. Micro Emulsified Oregano 2. Nutrients that heal the intestines 3. Betaine HCL, Pepsin, and pancreatin 4. Water soluble fiber 5. Nutrients to support the immune system 6. Lactobacillus acidophilus and Bifidobacterium bifidus	1. Betaine HCL, Pepsin, and pancreatin 2. Pancreatic Enzymes 3. Broad spectrum proteolytic enzymes 4. Bromelain

177. Crave coffee or sugar in the afternoon
178. Sleepy in afternoon
179. Fatigue that is relieved by eating
180. Headache if meals are skipped or delayed
181. Irritable before meals
182. Shaky if meals delayed

All of the above questions are dealing with low blood sugar and a tendency towards hypoglycemia. Hypoglycemia is a syndrome that involves the complex interrelations between the pancreas, liver and adrenal glands. The liver helps with short-term blood sugar control due to its store of glycogen and its ability to raise blood sugar when it begins to drop. The adrenal glands, due to the cortisol and other stress hormones, will help raise blood sugar in a crisis. Unfortunately, our bodies have learned to perceive much of the modern stresses of life as a crisis, leading to low adrenal function and blood sugar problems. The adrenals usually compensate for a weak pancreas.

There are a couple of different patterns of hypoglycemia to think about:

1. The first type wakes in the morning absolutely ravenous, needs to eat every 2 hours and craves carbohydrates and refined sugars. They cannot deal without eating every few hours. This picture is your typical reactive hypoglycemic. They do well with a high protein or a high complex carbohydrate diet. This type has more to do with an inability to store glycogen in the liver. The reserves of glucose overnight are very small and the client wakes hungry in the night and/or needs to eat first thing upon arising.

2. The second type wakes up groggy, needs 3 cups of coffee to get started and can then go for hours without eating. They can get by with coffee and an occasional donut for lunch. In the evening they eat a huge meal and collapse asleep. They feel lousy on the weekends and cannot tolerate vacation because they feel terrible. Ultimately they have to have some type of stress in their lives to keep going. This pattern is suggestive of a difficulty releasing glycogen from the liver until the liver is stimulated by cortisol. Cortisol stimulation stimulates the liver to release the stored glycogen. Without it clients cannot keep up.

Hypoglycemia is very debilitating, and causes many people onto a refined carbohydrate roller coaster, which they use to cope with the symptoms of low blood sugar. It is our job to help them control their blood sugar in more appropriate, and life-sustaining ways.

<u>1° Indication</u>

Blood sugar dysregulation and hypoglycemia.

Further assessment	1. Check for tenderness in the Chapman reflex for the liver-gallbladder located over the 6th intercostal space on the right 2. Check for tenderness in the Liver point located on the 3rd rib, 3 " to the right of the sternum, at the costochondral junction.

	3. Check for tenderness or nodularity in the right thenar pad 4. Check for tenderness in the Chapman reflex for the pancreas located in the 7th intercostal space on the left 5. Check for tenderness or guarding at the head of the pancreas located in the upper left quadrant of the abdominal region 1/2 to 2/3 of the way between the umbilicus and the angel of the ribs 6. Check fasting blood glucose, triglycerides and LDH levels on a blood chemistry screen 7. Run a six hour glucose-insulin tolerance test.

2° indication

Low adrenal function

Further assessment	1. Check for tenderness in the inguinal ligament bilaterally, an adrenal indicator 2. Check for tenderness at the medial knee bilaterally, at the insertion of the sartorius muscle at the Pes Anserine. This is an adrenal indicator. 3. Check for a paradoxical pupillary reflex by shining a light into a client's eye and grading the reaction of the pupil. A pupil that fails to constrict indicates adrenal exhaustion 4. Check for the presence of postural hypotension. A drop of more than 10 points is an indication of adrenal insufficiency 5. Check for a chronic short leg due to a posterior-inferior ilium. An adrenal indicator when confirmed with postural hypotension and a paradoxical pupillary response. 6. Assess for adrenal insufficiency with the Acoustic Cardiogram (ACG), which will show static in both the systolic and diastolic rest phases. You will also see an elevated S2 sound.

Supplemental support

1. Multiple nutrients to support sugar handling problems
2. Adaptogenic herbs to support adrenal function
3. Adrenal tissue (neonatal bovine)
4. Beet juice, taurine, vitamin C and pancreolipase
5. Pancreatic tissue (neonatal bovine)
6. Herbs that cleanse the liver

Lifestyle changes

Please see the handout in the appendix on Recommendations for controlling blood sugar

NOTES:

183. Family members with diabetes (0 = none, 1 = 2 or less, 2 = between 2 - 4, 3 = More than 4)
184. Frequent thirst
185. Frequent urination

The above questions are all indications of a trend towards higher than optimal blood sugar levels and Diabetes. Diabetes has a very strong genetic tendency, and often runs in families. Frequent thirst and urination, along with itching of the skin, frequent infections and loss of sensation in the lower extremities are some of the symptoms of diabetes.

Diabetes can be split into two categories: Insulin-dependent diabetes and non-insulin dependent diabetes. For insulin dependent diabetics insulin is a necessity. There is overwhelming evidence that adult onset diabetes is responsive to dietary changes and nutritional supplementation. Dietary regulation and awareness are important in all cases of diabetes, and in some cases diet alone may control the disease.

A whole food diet that is moderate in high quality protein, moderate in complex carbohydrates, moderate in fat, low in refined and concentrated sugars is recommended. If your client is overweight, a diet low in calories is also suggested. The avoidance of processed, commercial, empty-calorie foods, which are deficient in essential vitamins and minerals, will help the body regenerate those organs that may be damaged. Studies show that treating food sensitivities reduces dependence on insulin and helps regulate blood glucose levels.

Studies have also shown that a diet high in fiber helps reduce insulin or oral hypoglycemic drugs used to maintain blood glucose levels. Up to 100 grams of fiber are recommended per day.

The use of appropriate labs and functional testing will allow you to individualize a client's supplement, diet and lifestyle program. Many clients with diabetes are on some kind of medication, which should be continued unless you are the prescribing clinician. Be aware that some of the nutritional treatments for diabetes, along with diabetic medication, can push a diabetic client into a hypoglycemic like situation. Make sure that the client is carefully monitoring their blood glucose levels throughout the day. Start with one supplement at a time and use low dosages initially. Following these simple guidelines should prevent any side effects.

<u>1° Indication</u>

Assess for diabetes

Further assessment	1. Follow client with appropriate lab work: a. Fasting glucose levels b. Glucose readings throughout the day, charted c. Hemoglobin A1C levels for long term glucose control d. Thyroid panel- TSH, T4, T3, T3-uptake, Free T3 e. Lipid assessment- Cholesterol, HDL, LDL, Triglycerides

It is beyond the scope of this manual to outline a full, in-depth treatment protocol for diabetes. Please see the handout in the appendix on Diabetes for some dietary information for clients.

Supplemental Support

1. High potency multiple nutrients for sugar handling
2. Broad spectrum anti-oxidants
3. Nutrients to normalize cholesterol and triglycerides
4. Multiple nutrients for supporting renal function
5. L-Carnitine
6. Chromium
7. Nutrients to support eye function
8. Buffered vitamin C with bioflavanoids

Lifestyle changes

Please see the handout in the appendix on Recommendations for controlling blood sugar

NOTES:

VITAMIN NEED

186. Muscles become easily fatigued
187. Feel exhausted or sore after moderate exercise
188. Vulnerable to insect bites
189. Loss of muscle tone, heaviness in arms / legs
190. Enlarged heart, or congestive heart failure
191. Pulse slow / below 65 (1 = yes, 0 = no)
192. Ringing in the ears (Tinnitus)
193. Numbness, tingling or itching in hands or feet
194. Depressed
195. Fear of impending doom
196. Worrier, apprehensive, anxious
197. Nervous or agitated
198. Feelings of insecurity
199. Heart races
200. Can hear heart beat on pillow at night
201. Whole body or limb jerk as falling asleep
202. Night sweats
203. Restless leg syndrome
204. Cracks at corner of mouth (Cheilosis)
205. Fragile skin, easily chaffed, as in shaving
206. Polyps or warts
207. MSG sensitivity
208. Wake up without remembering dreams
209. Small bumps on back of arms
210. Strong light at night irritates eyes
211. Nose bleeds and / or tend to bruise easily
212. Bleeding gums especially when brushing teeth

186. Muscles become easily fatigued

Muscles that become easily fatigued are a sign of essential fatty acid deficiency and/or Vitamin B1 (thiamine). Most people take their B vitamins in a vitamin B complex. Dr. Royal Lee considered the B complex to be two distinct vitamin complexes, with different physiological actions. According to Dr. Lee, Vitamin B was thiamine based and contained the other B vitamins that were soluble in alcohol including B12, B5 and B4. Vitamin G, on the other hand, was riboflavin based and contained the B vitamins that were not soluble in alcohol.

People who have muscles that are easily fatigued should be assessed for essential fatty acid deficiency, and the B complex they should be on is *Naturally occurring thiamine*. This symptom could also be due to gallbladder dysfunction and lack of tissue oxygenation requiring supplemental vitamin E.

1° Indication

Essential fatty acid insufficiency.

Further assessment	1. Oral pH less that 7.2 indicates essential fatty acid deficiency 2. Repeated muscle challenge. This challenge involves a simple, normal muscle test repeated once per second, 20 times with regular intensity. As in a standard muscle test, the joint is positioned in such a way that the muscle to be tested is shortened. The practitioner applies pressure to the joint to lengthen the muscle, until a "locking" is noted. A positive result occurs when "locking" of the muscle and joint does not occur, indicating deficient free fatty acids.

2° Indication

Vitamin B1 (Thiamine) deficiency

Further assessment	An excellent way to assess for Thiamine (vitamin B1) deficiency is with the Acoustic Cardiogram (ACG), which will show a depressed S1 heart sound reading. There will not be enough amplitude in the graph. An increased Anion gap and a decreased CO_2 on a chem. screen is indicative of low thiamine levels.

Other indications

1. Gallbladder dysfunction
2. Lack of tissue oxygenation

Supplemental support

1. Essential fatty acids: Flax Seed Oil, Blackcurrant Seed Oil, EPA and DHA from fish oil, Mixed fatty acids (walnut, hazelnut, sesame, and apricot)
2. Naturally occurring thiamine
3. Phosphatidylcholine
4. Beet juice, taurine, vitamin C and pancreolipase with or without bile salts
5. Emulsified vitamin E drops

187. Feel worse, sore after moderate exercise

Feeling worse and sore after moderate exercise is an indication of low thyroid function and a vitamin B1 (thiamine) need.

1° Indication
Low thyroid function

Further assessment	1. Check for tenderness in the Chapman reflex for the thyroid located in the second intercostal space near the sternum on the right 2. Check for a delayed Achilles return reflex, which is a strong sign of a hypo-functioning thyroid 3. Check for general costochondral tenderness, which is a thyroid indicator 4. Check for pre-tibial edema, which is a sign of a hypo-functioning thyroid 5. Iodine test: Use a tincture of 2% iodine solution, and paint a 3" by 3" square on the client's abdomen. The client is to leave the patch unwashed until it disappears. The square should still be there in 24 hours. If it has disappeared, there is an indication of iodine need 6. Have client assess their basal metabolic temperature by taking their axillary temperature first thing in the morning for 5 straight days. An average temperature below 36.6°C is an indication of hypo-thyroidism

2° Indication
Vitamin B1 (Thiamine) deficiency

Further assessment	1. An excellent way to assess for Thiamine (vitamin B1) deficiency is with the Acoustic Cardiogram (ACG), which will show a depressed S1 heart sound reading. There will not be enough amplitude in the graph. 2. An increased Anion gap and a decreased CO_2 on a chem. screen is indicative of low thiamine levels.

Supplemental support

1. Multiple nutrients to support thyroid function with pituitary glandular
2. Potassium iodide
3. Pituitary/hypothalamus tissue (neonatal bovine)
4. Nutrients to support thyroid function
5. Flax seed oil
6. Naturally occurring thiamine

Lifestyle changes
Please see the handout in the appendix on recommendations for dealing with low thyroid function

188. Vulnerable to insect bites

Being vulnerable to insect bites is a classic sign of B complex need. For some reason people with low B vitamins in their body are very susceptible to mosquito and fleabites. It has been hypothesized that the B vitamins put out a certain odor that biting insects do not like, or that we still get bitten but the bites go unnoticed and away very quickly. Whatever the reason, advise your clients to take a low dose naturally occurring B complex before going on that summer camping trip.

1° Indication

B complex need

Further assessment	1. An excellent way to assess for B vitamin need is with the Acoustic Cardiogram (ACG). By analyzing the graphical output of the heart sounds one can determine the type of B vitamins that are deficient. For instance thiamine (vitamin B1) deficiency will show a depressed S1 heart sound reading. There will not be enough amplitude in the graph. Riboflavin (vitamin B2) will show an elongated S1 heart sound reading due to weak aortic and pulmonic valve closure.

Supplemental support

1. Low dose naturally occurring B Vitamin Complex
2. Riboflavin and the associated B vitamins
3. Naturally occurring thiamine

NOTES:

189. Loss of muscle tone, heaviness in arms / legs

Loss of muscle tone and heaviness in the arms and legs are signs of either a vitamin B1 (thiamine) deficiency or amino acid needs. For some people there is a compromise in the digestive system that prevents adequate digestion of protein. Hypochlorhydria and or pancreatic insufficiency will cause incomplete breakdown of protein, and prevent the release of amino acids from the proteins. Certain amino acids including Tryptophan, arginine, and lysine are very vulnerable to certain cooking methods e.g. high heat baking, which destroys the basic structure of the amino acid, rendering them unusable by the body.

1° Indication

Vitamin B1 (thiamine) need

Further assessment	1. An excellent way to assess for Thiamine (vitamin B1) deficiency is with the Acoustic Cardiogram (ACG), which will show a depressed S1 heart sound reading. There will not be enough amplitude in the graph. 2. An increased Anion gap and a decreased CO_2 on a chem. screen is indicative of low thiamine levels.

2° Indication

Amino acid need secondary to a pancreatic insufficiency and hypochlorhydria

Further assessment	**Pancreatic enzymes** 1. Check Ridler enzyme point for tenderness 1 inch below xyphoid and over to the right edge of the rib cage 2. Check for tenderness in the Chapman reflex for the pancreas located in the 7th intercostal space 3. Increased urinary sediment levels. Look for high uric acid sediment. **Hydrochloric acid** 1. Check Ridler HCL reflex for tenderness 1 inch below xyphoid and over to the left edge of the rib cage 2. Check for tenderness in the Chapman reflex for the stomach and upper digestion located in 6th intercostal space on the left 3. Check for a positive zinc tally: A client holds a solution of aqueous zinc sulfate in their mouth and tells you if and when they can taste it. An almost immediate very bitter taste indicates the client does not need zinc. Clients who are zinc deficient will report no taste from the solution. 4. Gastric acid assessment using Gastrotest

Supplement support

1. Digestive support: Nutrients to heal the intestines, Betaine HCL, Pepsin, & pancreatin
2. Pancreatic Enzymes, Bromelain, cellulase, lipase, and amylase
3. Nutritional zinc
4. Naturally occurring thiamine
5. Liquid amino acids

Lifestyle changes: Please see the handout in the appendix on diet to aid digestion

190. Enlarged heart or heart failure

This is obviously a serious medical condition that needs to be dealt with by a cardiovascular specialist. Nutritional therapies such as diet changes and supplements work well with the more traditional approaches to cardiovascular disease such as surgery or drug treatment. An enlarged heart or heart failure is a sign of a congestive type of heart disease. The congestive type of heart disease responds to vitamin B1 (thiamine) in the form of naturally occurring thiamine.
Most people take their B vitamins in a vitamin B complex. Dr. Royal Lee considered the B complex to be two distinct vitamin complexes, with different physiological actions. According to Dr. Lee, Vitamin B was thiamine based and contained the other B vitamins that were soluble in alcohol including B12, B5 and B4. Vitamin G, on the other hand, was riboflavin based and contained the B vitamins that were not soluble in alcohol.

People with the congestive types of heart disease tend to be hypotensive, crave sugar, feel bad or run down, are often sick and, as mentioned above, respond well to Naturally occurring thiamine. It is important to remember that heart disease is a mirror for the rest of the body, which is often overloaded with over consumption of processed and refined foods. Other possible causes are biliary dysfunction and mineral needs.

<u>1° Indication</u>
Vitamin B1 (thiamine) need

Further assessment	1. An excellent way to assess for Thiamine (vitamin B1) deficiency is with the Acoustic Cardiogram (ACG), which will show a depressed S1 heart sound reading. There will not be enough amplitude in the graph. 2. An increased Anion gap and a decreased CO_2 on a chem. screen is indicative of low thiamine levels.

<u>2° Indication</u>
Gallbladder dysfunction

Further assessment	1. Check for tenderness underneath the right rib cage 2. Check for tenderness and nodulation on the web between thumb and fore-finger of right hand 3. Check for tenderness in the Chapman reflex for the liver-gallbladder located over the 6th intercostal space on the right 4. Assess for Hepato-biliary congestion with the Acoustic Cardiogram (ACG), which will show post-systolic rounding due to increased backpressure on the pulmonic and aortic valve. It may also show through to the tricuspid valve if chronic. 5. Blood chemistry and CBC testing for SGOT, SGPT, GGT

<u>3° Indication</u>
Mineral deficiency

Further assessment	1. Assess for mineral deficiency using Tissue mineral assessment test. Place a standard blood pressure cuff around

	the largest portion of the client's calf muscle (sitting). Instruct the client to let you know when they feel the onset of cramping pain and gradually inflate the cuff. Stop and deflate immediately when threshold has been reached. Less than 200 mmHg is considered deficient in minerals. Use the neurolingual testing to challenge the body with several different types of minerals and other co-factors to see which combination of minerals and co-factors increases the threshold above 200mmHg. 2. Positive zinc tally: A client holds a solution of aqueous zinc sulfate in their mouth and tells you if and when they can taste it. An almost immediate very bitter taste indicates the client does not need zinc. Clients who are zinc deficient will report no taste from the solution. 3. Assess for mineral insufficiency by using Dr. Kane's mineral assessment tests. 4. Assess the impact of mineral deficiencies on the body's acid buffering capacities by using Dr. Bieler's salivary pH acid challenge.

Supplemental support

1. Naturally occurring thiamine
2. Beet juice, taurine, vitamin C and pancreolipase with or without bile salts
3. Herbs that cleanse the liver
4. Calcium and magnesium with or without parathyroid tissue
5. Multiple mineral without iron or copper

Lifestyle changes

Please see the handout in the appendix on recommendations for a healthy heart

NOTES:

191. Pulse slow / below 65 (1 = yes, 0 = no)

When the pulse is below 65 the following possible causes of the problem should be considered:

1. A need for vitamin B1 (thiamine),
2. Hypercalcemia (excess calcium in the blood),
3. Adrenal hypofunction,
4. Parasympathetic dominance,
5. Endocrine hypofunction,
6. and/or food/environmental sensitivities.

It is important to remember that a person who exercises regularly may have a pulse below 65. This is physiologically normal.

1° Indication

Vitamin B1 (thiamine) need

Further assessment	1. An excellent way to assess for Thiamine (vitamin B1) deficiency is with the Acoustic Cardiogram (ACG), which will show a depressed S1 heart sound reading. There will not be enough amplitude in the graph. 2. An increased Anion gap and a decreased CO_2 on a chem. screen is indicative of low thiamine levels.

2° indication

Low adrenal function

Further assessment	1. Check for tenderness in the inguinal ligament bilaterally 2. Check for tenderness at the medial knee bilaterally, at the insertion of the sartorius muscle at the Pes Anserine. 3. Check for a paradoxical pupillary reflex by shining a light into a client's eye and grading the reaction of the pupil. A pupil that fails to constrict indicates adrenal exhaustion 4. Check for the presence of postural hypotension. A drop of more than 10 points is an indication of adrenal insufficiency. 5. Check for a chronic short leg due to a posterior-inferior ilium. An adrenal indicator when confirmed with postural hypotension and a paradoxical pupillary response. 6. Check the cortisol/DHEA rhythm with a salivary adrenal profile 7. Increased chloride in the urine is a sign of hypoadrenal function. 8. Assess for adrenal insufficiency with the Acoustic Cardiogram (ACG), which will show static in both the systolic and diastolic rest phases. You will also see an elevated S2 sound.

3° indication

Excess calcium in the blood

Further assessment	1. Check the urine for excess calcium excretion 2. Check serum levels of calcium

Supplemental support

1. Naturally occurring thiamine
2. Adrenal tissue (neonatal bovine)
3. Pituitary/hypothalamus tissue (neonatal bovine)
4. Magnesium

Lifestyle changes: Please see the handout on recommendations for a healthy heart

NOTES:

192. Ringing in the ears / Tinnitus

Tinnitus is the perception of sound in the absence of an acoustic stimulus. It is more common in the elderly population yet it can occur in a client of any age. Unfortunately the cause is often not determined in every client. The most common causes of tinnitus are noise-induced damage and age-related hearing loss. It is important to remember that tinnitus is not a disease but a symptom, and it often serves as an important marker for other conditions. Causes include spine, cranial, or TMJ dysfunction, hyper or hypo-tension, damage or reduced circulation resulting in nerve damage, infection with resulting mucous, adrenal hypo-function, thiamine deficiency and food allergies/sensitivities. People with an overactive thyroid, which leads to an increased heart rate, often suffer from tinnitus due to the consequent increased blood flow through the ear causing the ringing. Tinnitus is also one of the symptoms of Meniere's disease. Some people may experience tinnitus for a week or so after a cold or flu, this is annoying but usually subsides after the infection has gone.

There are a number of substances that can exacerbate tinnitus, due to their vasoconstricting properties. These include nicotine and caffeine. Clenching or grinding the teeth, a sign of increased stress, will often trigger ringing in the ears. Reducing stress and relieving TMJ dysfunction improves the tinnitus.

One of the theories for the mechanics of tinnitus suggests that damage to the fine hair cells of the inner ear from loud noise etc. causes them to remain in a constant state of irritation. Any type of stimulation of the auditory nerve is random and spontaneous instead of occurring as a direct consequence of sound waves transmitted to the inner ear. These random electrical impulses are interpreted as noise, usually perceived as high-frequency ringing because the hair cells that are most frequently damaged respond in the high-frequency range. The distress can be minimized by putting the client on an individualized nutritional protocol and by avoiding aggravating factors, such as nicotine and caffeine.

1° Indication

A thorough assessment of the body is needed to find any dysfunction

Supplemental support

1. Gingko Biloba
2. Magnesium
3. Vitamin B12 and folic acid

NOTES:

193. Numbness, tingling or itching in extremities

There are many possible causes of numbness, tingling or itching in the extremities including disc problems, carpal tunnel syndrome, diabetes and any type of nerve entrapment or impingement. A thorough orthopedic and neurological examination should be performed to rule out any of the above structural causes. In the elderly population, who are often achlorhydric, B12 deficiency is very common. B12 deficiency can have long-term irreversible neurological complications. Assess for the presence of hypochlorhydria and treat what you find, to increase the absorption of B12 in these clients. For those who are very deficient consider injectible B12. Consider additional supplementation of folic acid, another vitamin that can have neurological complications when deficient.

1° Indication

Digestive dysfunction with hydrochloric acid need

Further assessment	1. Check Ridler HCL reflex for tenderness 1 inch below xyphoid and over to the left edge of the rib cage 2. Check for tenderness in the Chapman reflex for the stomach and upper digestion located in 6th intercostal space on the left 3. Check for a positive zinc tally: A client holds a solution of aqueous zinc sulfate in their mouth and tells you if and when they can taste it. An almost immediate very bitter taste indicates the client does not need zinc. Clients who are zinc deficient will report no taste from the solution. 4. Gastric acid assessment using Gastrotest 5. Increased urinary indican levels 6. Check the CBC for signs of B12 deficiency: MCV > 90, ↓ RBCs

2° Indication

Vitamin B1 (thiamine) or B complex need

Further assessment	1. An excellent way to assess for Thiamine (vitamin B1) deficiency is with the Acoustic Cardiogram (ACG), which will show a depressed S1 heart sound reading. There will not be enough amplitude in the graph. 2. An increased Anion gap and a decreased CO_2 on a chem. screen is indicative of low thiamine levels.

Supplemental support

1. Betaine HCL, Pepsin, and pancreatin
2. Vitamin B12 and folic acid
3. Naturally occurring thiamine
4. Vitamin B complex

194. Depressed
195. Fear of impending doom

There are many different causes of depression and the symptoms of depression: fear of impending doom, worry, apprehension and anxiety. Lifestyle and core health issues have a very large role to play. Smoking, drinking, alcohol abuse, drugs, prescription medications, and nutritional deficiencies can all play into depression.

Some of the common causes of depression include:

1. Dysbiosis, which robs the body of many essential nutrients,
2. Low thyroid function,
3. Low blood sugar, allergies,
4. Intolerances,
5. Poor adrenal health,
6. Hypochlorhydria, which prevents the digestion of many nutrients and a poor diet.

Many traditional clinicians use antidepressants to treat depression. Most of the modern antidepressants work by increasing the activity of certain chemicals in the brain called neurotransmitters. They act to keep the neurotransmitters around longer by preventing their destruction or recycling. Most of the neurotransmitters in the brain are formed from amino acids, which are found in protein. Serotonin, for instance, is formed from the amino acid Tryptophan.

Nutritional approaches to treating depression are as effective as using anti-depressants for many people, without the many side effects of drug treatment. Many of the nutritional supplements provide the necessary vitamins and minerals that act as co-factors in the metabolic pathways that form the neurotransmitters. These include Vitamin B3, B6, C, iron, copper, 5-hydroxytryptophan, and folic acid.

1° Indication

Dysbiosis with yeast overgrowth

Further assessment	1. Increased urinary indican 2. Stool analysis- either comprehensive digestive analysis or a parasite profile 3. Check for tenderness in the Chapman reflex for the colon located bilaterally along the iliotibial band on the thighs. Palpate the colon for tenderness and tension. 4. Check for tenderness in the Chapman reflex for the small intestine located on the 8th, 9th and 10th intercostal spaces near the tip of the rib. Also palpate four quadrants in a 2" to 3" radius around the umbilicus for tenderness and tension. 5. Decreased secretory IgA on stool analysis.

2° Indication

Low thyroid function

Further assessment	1. Check for tenderness in the Chapman reflex for the thyroid

	located in the second intercostal space near the sternum 2. Check for a delayed Achilles return reflex, which is a strong sign of a hypo-functioning thyroid 3. Check for general costochondral tenderness, which is a thyroid indicator 4. Check for pre-tibial edema, which is a sign of a hypo-functioning thyroid 5. Iodine test: Use a tincture of 2% iodine solution, and paint a 3" by 3" square on the client's abdomen. The client is to leave the patch unwashed until it disappears. The square should still be there in 24 hours. If it has disappeared, there is an indication of iodine need 6. Have client assess their basal metabolic temperature by taking their axillary temperature first thing in the morning for 5 straight days. An average temperature below 36.6°C is an indication of hypo-thyroidism

3° Indication

B vitamin need- especially B1 (thiamine)

Further assessment	1. An excellent way to assess for B vitamin need is with the Acoustic Cardiogram (ACG). By analyzing the graphical output of the heart sounds one can determine the type of B vitamins that are deficient. For instance thiamine (vitamin B1) deficiency will show a depressed S1 heart sound reading. There will not be enough amplitude in the graph. Riboflavin (vitamin B2) will show an elongated S1 heart sound reading due to weak aortic and pulmonic valve closure.

Other indications

1. Low blood sugar
2. Biliary dysfunction
3. Mineral need
4. Low adrenal function
5. Hyperadrenalism
6. Hypochlorhydria
7. Poor diet

Supplemental support

1. Anxiolytic peptides from milk
2. Naturally occurring thiamine
3. High dose synthetic vitamin B complex
4. Pyridoxal-5-phosphate
5. Multiple nutrients to support thyroid function with pituitary glandular
6. Micro Emulsified Oregano
7. Nutrients that heal the intestines
8. Lactobacillus acidophilus
9. Potassium iodide

196. Worrier, apprehensive, anxious
197. Nervous or agitated

Being worried, apprehensive, anxious, nervous or agitated may be signs of an overactive thyroid or adrenal glands, which can produce symptoms of being jittery and wound up. Thyroid hormone acts as an accelerator to the body's metabolism. Too much hormone can cause the metabolism and all its components to work faster and harder, giving the classic high blood pressure type symptoms. Over production of adrenal hormones can cause the symptoms of anxiety and agitation. It is important to ask clients for the consumption of caffeine containing foods and drinks, and other stimulants. Caffeine can cause all of the above symptoms.

1° Indication

Increased thyroid function

Further assessment	1. Check for tenderness in the Chapman reflex for the thyroid located in the second intercostal space near the sternum on the right 2. Check for a delayed Achilles return reflex, which is a strong sign of a hypo-functioning thyroid 3. Check for general costochondral tenderness, which is a thyroid indicator 4. Check for pre-tibial edema, which is a sign of a hypo-functioning thyroid 5. Have client assess their basal metabolic temperature by taking their axillary temperature first thing in the morning for 5 straight days. An average temperature below 36.6°C is an indication of hypo-thyroidism

2° indication

Hyper adrenal output

Further assessment	1. Check for tenderness in the inguinal ligament bilaterally, an adrenal indicator 2. Check for tenderness at the medial knee bilaterally, at the insertion of the sartorius muscle at the Pes Anserine. This is an adrenal indicator. 3. Check for a paradoxical pupillary reflex by shining a light into a client's eye and grading the reaction of the pupil. A pupil that fails to constrict indicates adrenal exhaustion 4. Check for the presence of postural hypotension. A drop of more than 10 points is an indication of adrenal insufficiency. 5. Check for a chronic short leg due to a posterior-inferior ilium. An adrenal indicator when confirmed with postural hypotension and a paradoxical pupillary response. 6. Check the cortisol/DHEA rhythm with a salivary adrenal stress index

Supplemental Support

1. Anxiolytic peptides from milk
2. Lithium
3. Thymus glandular
4. Naturally occurring thiamine
5. Emulsified vitamin A drops
6. Flax Seed Oil
7. Adaptogenic herbs to support adrenal function

NOTES:

198. Feelings of insecurity

There can be psychological reasons for this symptom. But some of the functional problems would include hypo-functioning of the adrenal glands and/or a deficiency in folic acid and other B vitamins.

1° indication

Low adrenal function

Further assessment	1. Check for tenderness in the inguinal ligament bilaterally, an adrenal indicator 2. Check for tenderness at the medial knee bilaterally, at the insertion of the sartorius muscle at the Pes Anserine. This is an adrenal indicator. 3. Check for a paradoxical pupillary reflex by shining a light into a client's eye and grading the reaction of the pupil. A pupil that fails to constrict indicates adrenal exhaustion 4. Check for the presence of postural hypotension. A drop of more than 10 points is an indication of adrenal insufficiency 5. Check for a chronic short leg due to a posterior-inferior ilium. An adrenal indicator when confirmed with postural hypotension and a paradoxical pupillary response. 6. Check the cortisol/DHEA rhythm with a salivary adrenal stress profile e.g. ASI 7. Increased chloride in the urine is a sign of hypoadrenal function 8. Assess for adrenal insufficiency with the Acoustic Cardiogram (ACG), which will show static in both the systolic and diastolic rest phases. You will also see an elevated S2 sound.

2° Indication

Need for folic acid and other B vitamins

Further assessment	1. Check the CBC for signs of B12 and folic acid deficiency: MCV > 90, ↓ RBCs 2. Hyper segmented neutrophils seen on a peripheral blood smear is a microscopic sign for folate deficiency 3. An excellent way to assess for B vitamin need is with the Acoustic Cardiogram (ACG). By analyzing the graphical output of the heart sounds one can determine the type of B vitamins that are deficient. For instance thiamine (vitamin B1) deficiency will show a depressed S1 heart sound reading. There will not be enough amplitude in the graph. Riboflavin (vitamin B2) will show an elongated S1 heart sound reading due to weak aortic and pulmonic valve closure.

Supplemental support

1. Adrenal support: Adrenal tissue (neonatal bovine) & adaptogenic herbs for adrenals
2. Multiple nutrients for blood sugar handling problems
3. B complex: with Riboflavin and/or naturally occurring thiamine
4. Vitamin B12 and folic acid

199. Heart races

This is a symptom that should be checked out by a specialist in cardiovascular medicine. It is important to rule out pathology because heart racing or arrhythmias can have dire consequences if not treated properly. There are, on the other hand, some simple nutritional approaches that can have significant impact on this symptom. For instance many clients with arrhythmias respond very well to magnesium, which often brings the symptoms of heart racing under control.

1° Indication

Assess cardiovascular system

Further assessment	1. Check for tenderness in the Chapman reflex for the heart located in the second intercostal space near the sternum on the left 2. Check for tenderness in the Chapman reflex for the kidney located 1" lateral and 1" superior from the umbilicus on the medial margin of the Rectus abdominus muscle (have client tighten stomach muscle to palpate. 3. Assess for tenderness over the transverse processes at T1 for the MI type, and T2 for the myocardium and the congestive type, 4. Assess blood pressure 5. An excellent way to assess the heart from a functional perspective is with the Acoustic Cardiogram (ACG). By analyzing the graphical output of the heart sounds one can determine many functional disturbances that can be assessed and corrected using nutrition.

2° Indication

Magnesium deficiency

Further assessment	1. Assess for mineral deficiency using Tissue mineral assessment test. Place a standard blood pressure cuff around the largest portion of the client's calf muscle (sitting). Instruct the client to let you know when they feel the onset of cramping pain and gradually inflate the cuff. Stop and deflate immediately when threshold has been reached. Less than 200 mmHg is considered deficient in minerals. Use the neurolingual testing to challenge the body with several different types of magnesium and other co-factors to see which combination of magnesium and co-factors increases the threshold above 200mmHg. 2. Assess for magnesium insufficiency by using Dr. Kane's mineral assessment tests. 3. Assess the impact of mineral deficiencies on the body's acid buffering capacities by using Dr. Bieler's salivary pH acid challenge.

Other indications

1. Hyper-functioning thyroid
2. Hidden food allergies

Supplemental support

1. Multiple nutrients to support heart function
2. Heart tissue (neonatal bovine)
3. CoQ10
4. Magnesium

Lifestyle changes

See the handout in the appendix on recommendations for a healthy heart

NOTES:

200. Can hear heart beat on pillow at night

Being able to hear one's pulse beat on the pillow at night is a sign of circulatory stress. Circulation of blood through the arteries, veins and capillaries is dependent on the health of these vessels. Bioflavonoids are essential nutrients for the health of the linings of blood vessels. Clients who are deficient in calcium and/or Vitamin B1 (thiamine) may also experience this symptom.

1° Indication

Circulatory stress with bioflavonoid need

Further assessment	1. An excellent way to assess the heart from a functional perspective is with the Acoustic Cardiogram (ACG). By analyzing the graphical output of the heart sounds one can determine many functional disturbances that can be assessed and corrected using nutrition.

2° Indication

Thiamine need

Further assessment	1. An excellent way to assess for Thiamine (vitamin B1) deficiency is with the Acoustic Cardiogram (ACG), which will show a depressed S1 heart sound reading. There will not be enough amplitude in the graph. 2. An increased Anion gap and a decreased CO_2 on a chem. screen is indicative of low thiamine levels.

3° Indication

Calcium need

Further assessment	1. Assess for mineral deficiency using Tissue mineral assessment test. Place a standard blood pressure cuff around the largest portion of the client's calf muscle (sitting). Instruct the client to let you know when they feel the onset of cramping pain and gradually inflate the cuff. Stop and deflate immediately when threshold has been reached. Less than 200 mmHg is considered deficient in minerals. Use the neurolingual testing to challenge the body with several different types of minerals and other co-factors to see which combination of minerals and co-factors increases the threshold above 200mmHg. 2. Assess for calcium insufficiency by using Dr. Kane's mineral assessment tests. 3. Assess the impact of mineral deficiencies on the body's acid buffering capacities by using Dr. Bieler's salivary pH acid challenge.

Supplemental support

1. Broad spectrum bioflavanoids, vitamin C, thymus and spleen
2. Multiple vitamins and Minerals
3. Naturally occurring thiamine
4. Calcium and magnesium with or without parathyroid tissue

201. Whole body or limb jerks as falling asleep

This is a sign of calcium, magnesium or potassium need with a possible digestive dysfunction that causes a decreased absorption of minerals. Vitamin E may be needed as a co-factor.

1° Indication
Mineral deficiencies

Further assessment	1. Assess for mineral deficiency using Tissue mineral assessment test. Place a standard blood pressure cuff around the largest portion of the client's calf muscle (sitting). Instruct the client to let you know when they feel the onset of cramping pain and gradually inflate the cuff. Stop and deflate immediately when threshold has been reached. Less than 200 mmHg is considered deficient in minerals. Use the neurolingual testing to challenge the body with several different types of minerals and other co-factors to see which combination of minerals and co-factors increases the threshold above 200mmHg. 2. Positive zinc tally: A client holds a solution of aqueous zinc sulfate in their mouth and tells you if and when they can taste it. An almost immediate very bitter taste indicates the client does not need zinc. Clients who are zinc deficient will report no taste from the solution. 3. Assess for mineral insufficiency by using Dr. Kane's mineral assessment tests. 4. Assess the impact of mineral deficiencies on the body's acid buffering capacities by using Dr. Bieler's salivary pH acid challenge.

2° Indication
Digestive dysfunction

Further assessment	1. Check Ridler HCL reflex for tenderness 1 inch below xyphoid and over to the left edge of the rib cage 2. Check for tenderness in the Chapman reflex for the stomach and upper digestion located in 6th intercostal space on the left 3. Gastric acid assessment using Gastrotest 4. Increased urinary indican levels

Other indications
B vitamin need

Supplemental Support

1. Multiple mineral without iron or copper
2. Calcium and magnesium with or without parathyroid tissue
3. Alkaline Ash minerals (Calcium, Magnesium,Potassium)
4. Multiple nutrients to support bone health
5. Emulsified Vitamin E drops

202. Night sweats

Night sweats may be an indication of an infection or other pathology, which should be ruled out. A common functional cause of night sweats includes a need for liver and kidney support and a deficiency in riboflavin.

1° Indication

Liver congestion with detoxification problems, especially phase I and II detoxification

Further assessment	1. Check for tenderness in the Chapman reflex for the liver-gallbladder located over the 6th intercostal space on the right side 2. Check for tenderness in the Liver point located on the 3rd rib, 3 " to the right of the sternum, at the costochondral junction. 3. Check for tenderness underneath the right rib cage 4. Increased SGOT, SGPT on a blood chemistry panel 5. Various labs do liver detoxification panels 6. Assess for Hepato-biliary congestion with the Acoustic Cardiogram (ACG), which will show post-systolic rounding due to increased backpressure on the pulmonic and aortic valve. It may also show through to the tricuspid valve if chronic.

2° Indication

Need to support kidney function to promote adequate elimination

Further assessment	1. Check for tenderness in the Chapman reflex for the kidneys located 1" lateral and 1" superior from the umbilicus on the medial margin of the Rectus abdominus muscle. Have clients tighten stomach muscles to palpate. 2. Check for tenderness with Murphy's punch to the lower back 3. Check for an increase in blood pressure when the client goes from standing to supine 4. Check BUN and Creatinine levels on a blood chemistry panel

3° Indication

Vitamin B2 (riboflavin) need

Further assessment	1. An excellent way to assess for Riboflavin (vitamin B2) deficiency is with the Acoustic Cardiogram (ACG), which will show an elongated S1 heart sound reading due to weak aortic and pulmonic valve closure.

Supplemental Support

1. Nutrients to support Phase II liver detoxification and herbs that cleanse the liver
2. Glutathione, cysteine, and Glycine
3. Powdered detoxification support formula
4. Multiple nutrients for supporting renal function
5. Kidney tissue (neonatal bovine)
6. Culture of Beet Juice containing Arginase
7. Vitamin B complex with riboflavin

203. Restless leg syndrome

Restless leg syndrome is a sign of calcium, magnesium or potassium need with a possible digestive dysfunction that causes a decreased absorption of minerals. Vitamin E and folic acid may be needed as a co-factor.

1° Indication

Mineral deficiencies

Further assessment	1. Assess for mineral deficiency using Tissue mineral assessment test. Place a standard blood pressure cuff around the largest portion of the client's calf muscle (sitting). Instruct the client to let you know when they feel the onset of cramping pain and gradually inflate the cuff. Stop and deflate immediately when threshold has been reached. Less than 200 mmHg is considered deficient in minerals. Use the neurolingual testing to challenge the body with several different types of minerals and other co-factors to see which combination of minerals and co-factors increases the threshold above 200mmHg. 2. Positive zinc tally: A client holds a solution of aqueous zinc sulfate in their mouth and tells you if and when they can taste it. An almost immediate very bitter taste indicates the client does not need zinc. Clients who are zinc deficient will report no taste from the solution. 3. Assess for mineral insufficiency by using Dr. Kane's mineral assessment tests. 4. Assess the impact of mineral deficiencies on the body's acid buffering capacities by using Dr. Bieler's salivary pH challenge. 5. Assess RBC levels of calcium and potassium

2° Indication

Digestive dysfunction

Further assessment	1. Check Ridler HCL reflex for tenderness 1 inch below xyphoid and over to the left edge of the rib cage 2. Check for tenderness in the Chapman reflex for the stomach and upper digestion located in 6th intercostal space on the left 3. Gastric acid assessment using Gastrotest 4. Increased urinary indican levels

Other indications

1. Vitamin E need
2. B vitamin need

Supplemental Support

1. Multiple mineral without iron or copper
2. Calcium and magnesium with or without parathyroid tissue
3. Alkaline Ash minerals (Calcium, Magnesium,Potassium)
4. Multiple nutrients to support bone health
5. Emulsified vitamin E drops

204. Cracks at corner of mouth (Cheilosis)

Cheilosis can be a sign of digestive dysfunction, especially the colon. Increased toxins in the colon from constipation can cause the corners of the mouth to split and crack. Another cause is calcium and/or thiamine need.

1° Indication

Colonic and/or small intestine dysfunction with possible constipation

Further assessment	1. Check for tenderness in the Chapman reflex for the colon located bilaterally along the iliotibial band on the thighs. Palpate the colon for tenderness and tension. 2. Check for tenderness in the Chapman reflex for the small intestine located on the 8th, 9th and 10th intercostal spaces near the tip of the rib. Also palpate four quadrants in a 2" to 3" radius around the umbilicus for tenderness and tension 3. Increased urinary indican and sediment 4. Decreased bowel transit time. Have a client check their bowel transit time. Give 6 "00" caps of activated charcoal and ask them to record how long it takes for the black to appear and to go completely away. Beets and un-popped popcorn can be used. 5. Decreased secretory IgA on stool analysis.

2° Indication

Thiamine need

Further assessment	1. An excellent way to assess for Thiamine (vitamin B1) deficiency is with the Acoustic Cardiogram (ACG), which will show a depressed S1 heart sound reading. There will not be enough amplitude in the graph. 2. An increased Anion gap and a decreased CO_2 on a chem. Screen is indicative of low thiamine levels.

3° Indication

Calcium need

Further assessment	1. Assess for mineral deficiency using Tissue mineral assessment test. Place a standard blood pressure cuff around the largest portion of the client's calf muscle (sitting). Instruct the client to let you know when they feel the onset of cramping pain and gradually inflate the cuff. Stop and deflate immediately when threshold has been reached. Less than 200 mmHg is considered deficient in minerals. Use the neurolingual testing to challenge the body with several different types of minerals and other co-factors to see which combination of minerals and co-factors increases the threshold above 200mmHg. 2. Assess for calcium insufficiency by using Dr. Kane's mineral assessment tests. 3. Assess the impact of mineral deficiencies on the body's acid buffering capacities by using Dr. Bieler's salivary pH acid challenge.

Supplemental support

1. Water soluble fiber and colon health nutrients
2. Garlic and chlorophyllins
3. Micro Emulsified Oregano
4. Nutrients that heal the intestines
5. Lactobacillus acidophilus and Bifidobacterium bifidus
6. Buffered vitamin C plus bioflavanoids
7. Naturally occurring thiamine
8. Calcium and magnesium with or without parathyroid tissue

NOTES:

205. Fragile skin, easily chaffed, as in shaving

Fragile and friable skin is a common sign of bioflavonoid deficiency, liver congestion and thiamine need. In Chinese medicine the skin is an expression of the liver. Treating the liver congestion and providing the correct nutrients can go a long way to helping clients with this complaint.

1° Indication
Bioflavonoid need

2° Indication
Vitamin B1 (Thiamine) deficiency

Further assessment	1. An excellent way to assess for Thiamine (vitamin B1) deficiency is with the Acoustic Cardiogram (ACG), which will show a depressed S1 heart sound reading. There will not be enough amplitude in the graph. 2. An increased Anion gap and a decreased CO_2 on a chem. Screen is indicative of low thiamine levels.

3° Indication
Liver congestion

Further assessment	1. Check for tenderness in the Chapman reflex for the liver-gallbladder located over the 6th intercostal space on the right 2. Check for tenderness in the Liver point located on the 3rd rib, 3 " to the right of the sternum, at the costochondral junction. 3. Check for tenderness underneath the right rib cage 4. Check for tenderness and nodulation on the web between thumb and fore-finger of right hand 5. Assess for Hepato-biliary congestion with the Acoustic Cardiogram (ACG), which will show post-systolic rounding due to increased backpressure on the pulmonic and aortic valve. It may also show through to the tricuspid valve if chronic.

Supplemental support

1. Broad spectrum bioflavanoids 2. Buffered vitamin C with bioflavanoids 3. Nutrients to support Phase II liver detoxification 4. Beet juice, taurine, vitamin C and pancreolipase 5. Broad spectrum antioxidants 6. Herbs that cleanse the liver

NOTES:

206. Polyps or warts

The presence of polyps or warts is a sign of folic acid need and other B vitamins. Warts are also an indication of an increased viral load in the body, which constantly has to deal with the virus. The virus is walled off in a growth and will stay around as long as the environment of the body supports it.

1° Indication
Need for folic acid and other B vitamins

Further assessment	1. Check the CBC for signs of B12 and folic acid deficiency: MCV > 90, ↓ RBCs 2. Hyper segmented neutrophils on a peripheral blood smear is a microscopic sign for folate deficiency 3. An excellent way to assess for B vitamin need is with the Acoustic Cardiogram (ACG). By analyzing the graphical output of the heart sounds one can determine the type of B vitamins that are deficient. For instance thiamine (vitamin B1) deficiency will show a depressed S1 heart sound reading. There will not be enough amplitude in the graph. Riboflavin (vitamin B2) will show an elongated S1 heart sound reading due to weak aortic and pulmonic valve closure.

2° Indication
Need for immune support

Further assessment	1. Check for tenderness in the Chapman reflex for the thymus located in the 5th intercostal space on the right near the sternum 2. Check for tenderness in the Chapman reflex for the lungs located bilaterally in the 3rd and 4th intercostal space near the sternum 3. Check for tenderness in the histamine point located at five o'clock on the pectoralis muscle in the intercostal space between the 5th and 6th rib on the right side only 4. Assess the client for allergic tension. Take a full one-minute pulse sitting, then stand, wait 15 seconds and take another full minute pulse. If the standing pulse goes up by more than six beats, this is an indication of "allergic tension" 5. Assess the client's vitamin C status with the lingual and urinary ascorbic acid tests

Supplemental support

1. Vitamin B12 and folic acid 2. High dose B vitamin complex

207. MSG sensitivity

MSG is used as a flavor enhancer, especially in Chinese food. Sensitivity to MSG is an indication of a need to support phase II liver detoxification, and an increased need for methyl donors, which help with the metabolic conversion of MSG in the body, especially if there is an increased sensitivity to perfumes, smoke and diesel fumes. Phase II detoxification is a process of conjugation, which makes the toxin water-soluble, so that it can be removed from the body. This phase requires adequate levels of glycine and glutathione, along with many other different nutrients for adequate conjugation.

MSG sensitivity is also an indication of B6 need. A study of 27 students showed that supplementation of B6 in those that were previously sensitive to MSG, at a dose of 200mmHg/day for 12 weeks, produced no MSG sensitivity in 90% of the supplemented students. (Biochem Biophys Res Commun 100:972-7, 1981).

1° Indication

Liver detoxification problems, especially phase II detoxification

Further assessment	1. Check for tenderness in the Chapman reflex for the liver-gallbladder located over the 6th intercostal space on the right side 2. Check for tenderness in the Liver point located on the 3rd rib, 3 " to the right of the sternum, at the costochondral junction. 3. Check for tenderness underneath the right rib cage 4. Increased SGOT, SGPT on a blood chemistry panel

2° Indication

Need for vitamin B6

Further assessment	1. B6 levels can be assessed by running a serum homocysteine or a B6 EGOT (Erythrocyte Glutamine-Oxaloacetate Transaminase) test.

Supplemental Support

1. Plant source of molybdenum
2. Nutrients to support Phase II liver detoxification
3. Herbs that cleanse the liver
4. DL- Methylglycine
5. Glutathione, cysteine, and Glycine
6. Powdered detoxification support formula
7. Pyridoxal-5-phosphate

208. Wake up without remembering dreams

Waking up without remembering dreams is a classic sign of Thiamine (Vitamin B1) deficiency. There may also be sleep disturbance issues, especially if the client is not able to enter REM sleep. During REM sleep the whole body enters a deep state of relaxation and it provides the deepest sleep we can get the. Without REM sleep we do not dream. An increased cortisol output at night and low blood sugar may interfere with sleep patterns. Also consider the possibility of sleep apnea, a condition of brief stoppages of breathing during the night. Please refer to a specialist if sleep apnea is suspected.

1° Indication

Vitamin B1 (Thiamine) deficiency

Further assessment	1. An excellent way to assess for Thiamine (vitamin B1) deficiency is with the Acoustic Cardiogram (ACG), which will show a depressed S1 heart sound reading. There will not be enough amplitude in the graph. 2. An increased Anion gap and a decreased CO_2 on a chem. Screen is indicative of low thiamine levels.

2° Indication

Blood sugar dysregulation.

Further assessment	1. Check for tenderness in the Chapman reflex for the liver-gallbladder located over the 6th intercostal space on the right 2. Check for tenderness in the Liver point located on the 3rd rib, 3 " to the right of the sternum, at the costochondral junction. 3. Check for tenderness underneath the right rib cage 4. Check for tenderness or nodularity in the right thenar pad, which is a pancreas indicator if tender 5. Check for tenderness in the Chapman reflex for the pancreas located in the 7th intercostal space on the left 6. Check for tenderness or guarding at the head of the pancreas located in the upper left quadrant of the abdominal region 1/2 to 2/3 of the way between the umbilicus and the angel of the ribs 7. Check fasting blood glucose 8. Run a six hour glucose-insulin tolerance test.

3° Indication

Low adrenal function

Further assessment	1. Check for tenderness in the inguinal ligament bilaterally 2. Check for tenderness at the medial knee bilaterally, at the insertion of the sartorius muscle at the Pes Anserine. 3. Check for a paradoxical pupillary reflex by shining a light into a client's eye and grading the reaction of the pupil. A pupil that fails to constrict indicates adrenal exhaustion 4. Check for the presence of postural hypotension. A drop of more than 10 points is an indication of adrenal insufficiency

	5. Check for a chronic short leg due to a posterior-inferior ilium. 6. Assess for adrenal insufficiency with the Acoustic Cardiogram (ACG), which will show static in both the systolic and diastolic rest phases. You will also see an elevated S2 sound.

Supplemental Support

1. Naturally occurring thiamine
2. Multiple nutrients to support sugar handling problems
3. Adaptogenic herbs to support adrenal function
4. Adrenal tissue (neonatal bovine)
5. Pancreatic tissue (neonatal bovine)
6. Herbs that cleanse the liver

Lifestyle changes

Please see the handout in the appendix on recommendations for controlling blood sugar

NOTES:

209. Small bumps on back of arms
210. Strong light at night irritates eyes

These symptoms are associated with a deficiency in vitamin A. Small bumps on the back have been called "vitamin A bumps", and are known as hyperkeratosis in dermatology texts. Vitamin A is essential for vision, growth and bone development, growth of the epithelial cells, the immune system, reproduction and has anti-cancer properties. Deficiency of vitamin A can result from low intake, problems with absorption and storage in the body, and interference in the conversion of beta carotene into active vitamin A. Symptoms of deficiency include night blindness, respiratory infections, keratinization of the hair follicles (Vitamin A bumps), reduced immunity, Diarrhea, loss of tooth enamel, loss of bone mass and loss of both taste and smell.

Unfortunately Vitamin A can be toxic in large doses. The toxicity varies from person to person, and the strength of the liver. For some people a dose as low as 20,000 ius/day will be toxic. Typical symptoms of toxicity include fatigue, irritability, vomiting, bone pain, headaches, dry scaly skin, brittle nails, hair loss, enlarged liver and spleen and visual disturbances. The greatest concern for toxicity is in pregnancy, people who have liver problems, alcoholics who are still drinking and someone with gout. Therapeutic doses are generally between 25,000-50,000IU/day. Higher doses can be given short term. It is recommended to keep the dose of Vitamin A below 10,000 IU during pregnancy.

Vitamin A is a fat-soluble vitamin, and a deficiency may be due to an inability to adequately emulsify fats, which is a sign of biliary dysfunction. This may have an impact on not only vitamin A, but also all fat-soluble vitamins (E and D) and essential fatty acids.

1° Indication
Vitamin A deficiency

2° Indication
Gallbladder dysfunction with possible biliary stasis

Further assessment	1. Check for tenderness underneath the right rib cage 2. Check for tenderness and nodulation on the web between thumb and fore-finger of right hand 3. Check for tenderness in the Chapman reflex for the liver-gallbladder located over the 6th intercostal space on the right side 4. Assess for Hepato-biliary congestion with the Acoustic Cardiogram (ACG), which will show post-systolic rounding due to increased backpressure on the pulmonic and aortic valve. It may also show through to the tricuspid valve if chronic. 5. Iodine test: Use a tincture of 2% iodine solution, and paint a 3" by 3" square on the client's abdomen. The client is to leave the patch unwashed until it disappears. The square should still be there in 24 hours. If it has disappeared, there is an indication of iodine need 6. Blood chemistry and CBC testing for SGOT, SGPT, GGT

Supplemental support

1. Emulsified vitamin A drops
2. Beet juice, taurine, vitamin C and pancreolipase with or without bile salts

Lifestyle changes

Please see the handouts in the appendix on Healthy lifestyle for a healthy gallbladder

NOTES:

211. Nose bleeds and / or tend to bruise easily
212. Bleeding gums especially when brushing teeth

Nose bleeds, bleeding gums and bruising easily are all signs of bioflavonoid deficiency. Bioflavonoids are a class of compounds found in brightly colored fruits and vegetables. They serve to stabilize membranes in the body, especially the blood vessel membranes. Bioflavonoids have antioxidant properties, are essential for collagen cross linking (which provides the strength to collagen fibers), they act as an adjuvant to vitamin C and will help re-charge vitamin C in the body. They have anti-inflammatory activity by stabilizing the cell membranes and making them less likely to release their fatty acids and thus preventing the eicosanoid cascade.

<u>1° Indication</u>

Bioflavonoid deficiency and vitamin C need

Further assessment	1. Vitamin C levels can be assessed with the lingual or urinary vitamin C test.

<u>Other indications</u>

Vitamin K need

Supplemental Support

1. Broad spectrum bioflavanoids
2. Buffered Vitamin C with bioflavanoids
3. Broad spectrum anti-oxidants
4. Chlorophyllins

NOTES:

ADRENAL

213. Tend to be a "night person"
214. Difficulty falling asleep
215. Slow starter in the morning
216. Tend to be keyed up, trouble calming down
217. Blood pressure above 120/80
218. Headache after exercising
219. Feeling wired or jittery after drinking coffee
220. Clench or grind teeth
221. Calm on the outside, troubled on the inside
222. Chronic low back pain, worse with fatigue
223. Become dizzy when standing up suddenly
224. Difficult maintaining manipulative correction
225. Pain after manipulative correction
226. Arthritic tendencies
227. Crave salty foods
228. Salt foods before tasting
229. Perspire easily
230. Chronic fatigue, or get drowsy often
231. Afternoon yawning
232. Afternoon headache
233. Asthma, wheezing or difficulty breathing
234. Pain on the medial or inner side of the knee
235. Tendency to sprain ankles or "shin splints"
236. Tendency to need to need sunglasses
237. Allergies and / or hives
238. Weakness, dizziness

213. Tend to be a "night person"
214. Difficulty falling asleep
215. Slow starter in the morning

Being a "night person" or having difficulty falling asleep at night are indications of a need for adrenal support. Cortisol output should gradually decline over the course of the day, and be at its lowest around midnight. In many people the cortisol rhythm is out of balance, causing an increased cortisol output at night.

Cortisol should be highest in the morning. For people who have difficulty in getting up in the morning the cortisol levels can be at its lowest.

All these symptoms are indicative of a person needing adrenal support.

<u>1° indication</u>

Need for adrenal support

Further assessment	1. Check for tenderness in the inguinal ligament bilaterally, an adrenal indicator 2. Check for tenderness at the medial knee bilaterally, at the insertion of the sartorius muscle at the Pes Anserine. This is an adrenal indicator. 3. Check for a paradoxical pupillary reflex by shining a light into a client's eye and grading the reaction of the pupil. A pupil that fails to constrict indicates adrenal exhaustion 4. Check for the presence of postural hypotension. A drop of more than 10 points is an indication of adrenal insufficiency. 5. Check for a chronic short leg due to a posterior-inferior ilium. An adrenal indicator when confirmed with postural hypotension and a paradoxical pupillary response. 6. Check the cortisol/DHEA rhythm with a salivary adrenal stress index e.g. ASI 7. Assess for adrenal insufficiency with the Acoustic Cardiogram (ACG), which will show static in both the systolic and diastolic rest phases. You will also see an elevated S2 sound. 8. Increased chloride in the urine is a sign of low adrenal function

<u>Other indications</u>

Low serotonin or melatonin levels

<u>Supplemental Support</u>

1. Adrenal tissue (neonatal bovine)
2. Adaptogenic herbs to support adrenal function
3. Multiple nutrients for blood sugar handling problems
4. Naturally occurring thiamine

<u>Lifestyle changes</u>

Please see the handout in the appendix on Adrenal restoration measures

216. Tend to be keyed up, trouble calming down

Being keyed up all the time, and having difficulty calming down is a sign of increased adrenal output, or hyperadrenalism. Increased cortisol with a concomitant low DHEA can cause these symptoms. In the beginning stages of adrenal decompensation the body's response to stress is to increase the cortisol output from the adrenal glands.

1° indication

Hyper adrenal output

Further assessment	1. Check for tenderness in the inguinal ligament bilaterally, an adrenal indicator 2. Check for tenderness at the medial knee bilaterally, at the insertion of the sartorius muscle at the Pes Anserine. This is an adrenal indicator. 3. Check for a paradoxical pupillary reflex by shining a light into a client's eye and grading the reaction of the pupil. A pupil that fails to constrict indicates adrenal exhaustion 4. Check for the presence of postural hypotension. A drop of more than 10 points is an indication of adrenal insufficiency 5. Check for a chronic short leg due to a posterior-inferior ilium. An adrenal indicator when confirmed with postural hypotension and a paradoxical pupillary response. 6. Check the cortisol/DHEA rhythm with a salivary adrenal stress index 7. Assess for adrenal insufficiency with the Acoustic Cardiogram (ACG), which will show static in both the systolic and diastolic rest phases. You will also see an elevated S2 sound.

Supplemental support

1. Adaptogenic herbs to support adrenal function

Lifestyle changes

Please see the handout in the appendix on Adrenal restoration measures

NOTES:

217. Blood pressure above 120/80

A differentiation must be made between elevated blood pressure with no obvious medical cause (primary or essential hypertension), and that due to an underlying pathology such as kidney, endocrinological or cerebral disease (secondary hypertension). This question is dealing primarily with essential hypertension. Even though there may be no medical cause for the high blood pressure there are many factors that influence it, including blood sugar abnormalities, liver congestion, renal/adrenal dysfunction, increased blood fats, excess sodium, decreased potassium, deficiency of fiber, excess sucrose, hidden food allergies, hypothyroidism or hyperthyroidism, essential fatty acid deficiency, obesity, deficiency of calcium and magnesium, cadmium toxicity, lead toxicity, and smoking.

1° Indication
Blood sugar dysregulation

Further assessment	1. Check for tenderness in the Chapman reflex for the liver-gallbladder located over the 6th intercostal space on the right side 2. Check for tenderness in the Liver point located on the 3rd rib, 3 " to the right of the sternum, at the costochondral junction. 3. Check for tenderness underneath the right rib cage 4. Check for tenderness or nodularity in the right thenar pad, which is a pancreas indicator if tender 5. Check for tenderness in the Chapman reflex for the pancreas located in the 7th intercostal space on the left 6. Check for tenderness or guarding at the head of the pancreas located in the upper left quadrant of the abdominal region 1/2 to 2/3 of the way between the umbilicus and the angel of the ribs 7. Run a 6 hour glucose-insulin tolerance test

2° Indication
Liver/portal congestion

Further assessment	1. Check for tenderness in the Chapman reflex for the liver-gallbladder located over the 6th intercostal space on the right side 2. Check for tenderness in the Liver point located on the 3rd rib, 3 " to the right of the sternum, at the costochondral junction. 3. Check for tenderness underneath the right rib cage 4. Check for tenderness and nodulation on the web between thumb and fore-finger of right hand 5. Assess for Hepato-biliary congestion with the Acoustic Cardiogram (ACG), which will show post-systolic rounding due to increased backpressure on the pulmonic and aortic valve. It may also show through to the tricuspid valve if chronic.

3° Indication

Renal/adrenal dysfunction

Further assessment	1. Check for tenderness in the Chapman reflex for the kidneys located 1" lateral and 1" superior from the umbilicus on the medial margin of the Rectus abdominus muscle. Have clients tighten stomach muscles to palpate. 2. Check for an increase in blood pressure when the client goes from standing to supine 3. Routine and functional 24-hour urinalysis 4. Blood chemistry renal function panel

Supplemental Support

1. High potency multiple nutrients for sugar handling problems
2. Herbs that cleanse the liver
3. Beet juice, taurine, vitamin C and pancreolipase
4. Nutrients to support Phase II liver detoxification
5. Multiple nutrients for supporting renal function
6. Adaptogenic herbs to support adrenal function
7. Kidney tissue (neonatal bovine)

Lifestyle changes

Please see the handout in the appendix on Recommendations for controlling blood sugar

NOTES:

218. Headache after exercising

A headache after exercise is associated with hypoadrenal functioning. You may want to run an Adrenal stress profile test for cortisol/DHEA ratios to find out the actual stage of decompensation the client is in. Chronic stress will cause the cortisol levels to drop leading to a decreased ability to control the blood sugar, which leads to hypoglycemia, irritability, headaches etc. Headaches after exercise are a strong indicator of the above scenario. Exercise will cause the blood sugar to drop. If the cortisol output is not sufficient, the blood sugar will not be able to be regulated properly leading to all the symptoms of hypoglycemia.

1° indication

Hypo-adrenal output

Further assessment	1. Check for tenderness in the inguinal ligament bilaterally, an adrenal indicator 2. Check for tenderness at the medial knee bilaterally, at the insertion of the sartorius muscle at the Pes Anserine. This is an adrenal indicator. 3. Check for a paradoxical pupillary reflex by shining a light into a client's eye and grading the reaction of the pupil. A pupil that fails to constrict indicates adrenal exhaustion 4. Check for the presence of postural hypotension. A drop of more than 10 points is an indication of adrenal insufficiency 5. Check for a chronic short leg due to a posterior-inferior ilium. An adrenal indicator when confirmed with postural hypotension and a paradoxical pupillary response. 6. Check the cortisol/DHEA rhythm with a salivary adrenal stress profile 7. Increased chloride in the urine is a sign of hypoadrenal function 8. Assess for adrenal insufficiency with the Acoustic Cardiogram (ACG), which will show static in both the systolic and diastolic rest phases. You will also see an elevated S2 sound.

2° Indication

Blood sugar dysregulation

Further assessment	1. Check for tenderness in the Chapman reflex for the liver-gallbladder located over the 6th intercostal space on the right 2. Check for tenderness in the Liver point located on the 3rd rib, 3 " to the right of the sternum, at the costochondral junction. 3. Check for tenderness underneath the right rib cage 4. Check for tenderness or nodularity in the right thenar pad, which is a pancreas indicator if tender 5. Check for tenderness in the Chapman reflex for the pancreas located in the 7th intercostal space on the left

	6. Check for tenderness or guarding at the head of the pancreas located in the upper left quadrant of the abdominal region 1/2 to 2/3 of the way between the umbilicus and the angel of the ribs 7. Run a 6 hour glucose-insulin tolerance test

Supplemental Support

1. Adrenal tissue (neonatal bovine)
2. Adaptogenic herbs to support adrenal function
3. Multiple nutrients for blood sugar handling problems
4. Beet juice, taurine, vitamin C and pancreolipase

Lifestyle changes

Please see the handout in the appendix on Adrenal restoration measures

NOTES:

219. Feeling wired or jittery after drinking coffee

Feeling wired or jittery after drinking coffee is a sign of increased adrenal output, or hyperadrenalism, a need for liver support or insensitivity to coffee. Increased cortisol with a concomitant low DHEA causes symptoms of being wired and jittery. When you add caffeine, an adrenal stimulant, into the body, you will get an exacerbation of the hyperadrenal symptoms. Caffeine is a drug that needs to be detoxified by the liver. If a client does not handle caffeine very well, it is a sign of liver support, especially the phase I detoxification. In the beginning stages of adrenal decompensation the body's response to stress is to increase the cortisol output from the adrenal glands. An insensitivity to coffee and caffeine in general can cause a client to be wired and jittery after coffee.

1° indication

Hyper adrenal output

Further assessment	1. Check for tenderness in the inguinal ligament bilaterally, an adrenal indicator 2. Check for tenderness at the medial knee bilaterally, at the insertion of the sartorius muscle at the Pes Anserine. 3. Check for a paradoxical pupillary reflex by shining a light into a client's eye and grading the reaction of the pupil. A pupil that fails to constrict indicates adrenal exhaustion 4. Check for the presence of postural hypotension. A drop of more than 10 points is an indication of adrenal insufficiency 5. Check for a chronic short leg due to a posterior-inferior ilium. An adrenal indicator when confirmed with postural hypotension and a paradoxical pupillary response 6. Check the cortisol/DHEA rhythm with an adrenal stress index 7. Decreased chloride in the urine is a sign of hyperadrenalism

2° Indication

Need for Liver detoxification support, especially phase I detoxification

Further assessment	1. Check for tenderness in the Chapman reflex for the liver-gallbladder located over the 6th intercostal space on the right 2. Check for tenderness in the Liver point located on the 3rd rib, 3 " to the right of the sternum, at the costochondral junction. 3. Check for tenderness underneath the right rib cage. 4. Increased SGOT, SGPT on a blood chemistry panel 5. Various labs do liver detoxification panels

Other indications

1. Blood sugar dysregulation
2. B6 need

Supplemental Support

1. Adaptogenic herbs to support adrenal function
2. Nutrients to support Phase II liver detoxification
3. Herbs that cleanse the liver
4. Powdered detoxification support formula with Glutathione, cysteine, and Glycine

220. Clench or grind teeth

Clenching or grinding of the teeth can be a serious problem, with a need for expert cranial and TMJ structural balancing. It is also a classic sign of increased stress in a client's life. Elevated stressors on the body will lead to increased sympathetic nervous system activity. The body responds by increasing the hormones Norepinephrine and epinephrine, which leads to a dramatic increase in ACTH. ACTH will act on the adrenal cortex to increase total and free cortisol, which leads to high cortisol levels and all the problems associated with that.
If the stress is not resolved, the body begins its downward spiral into adrenal decompensation and adrenal exhaustion. Treating the adrenals and working on removing the stress in a client's life are essential.

1° indication
Hyper adrenal output

Further assessment	1. Check for tenderness in the inguinal ligament bilaterally, an adrenal indicator 2. Check for tenderness at the medial knee bilaterally, at the insertion of the sartorius muscle at the Pes Anserine. This is an adrenal indicator. 3. Check for a paradoxical pupillary reflex by shining a light into a client's eye and grading the reaction of the pupil. A pupil that fails to constrict indicates adrenal exhaustion 4. Check for the presence of postural hypotension. A drop of more than 10 points is an indication of adrenal insufficiency 5. Check for a chronic short leg due to a posterior-inferior ilium. An adrenal indicator when confirmed with postural hypotension and a paradoxical pupillary response. 6. Check the cortisol/DHEA rhythm with a salivary adrenal stress index e.g. ASI

Supplemental Support

1. Adaptogenic herbs to support adrenal function
2. Buffered vitamin C plus bioflavanoids
3. Pyridoxal-5-phosphate
4. High dose B vitamin complex

Lifestyle changes
Please see the handout in the appendix on Adrenal restoration measures

NOTES:

221. Calm on the outside, troubled on the inside

Being calm on the outside and troubled inside can have psychological reasons. From a functional perspective it points to a need for adrenal support. Blood sugar regulation is so closely tied in with the adrenals that anything that affects the adrenals will have an impact on blood sugar regulation.

1° indication

Need for adrenal support

Further assessment	1. Check for tenderness in the inguinal ligament bilaterally, an adrenal indicator 2. Check for tenderness at the medial knee bilaterally, at the insertion of the sartorius muscle at the Pes Anserine. This is an adrenal indicator. 3. Check for a paradoxical pupillary reflex by shining a light into a client's eye and grading the reaction of the pupil. A pupil that fails to constrict indicates adrenal exhaustion 4. Check for the presence of postural hypotension. A drop of more than 10 points is an indication of adrenal insufficiency 5. Check for a chronic short leg due to a posterior-inferior ilium. An adrenal indicator when confirmed with postural hypotension and a paradoxical pupillary response. 6. Check cortisol/DHEA rhythm with an adrenal stress profile 7. Assess for adrenal insufficiency with the Acoustic Cardiogram (ACG), which will show static in both the systolic and diastolic rest phases. You will also see an elevated S2 sound.

2° Indication

Blood sugar dysregulation

Further assessment	1. Check for tenderness in the Chapman reflex for the liver-gallbladder located over 6th intercostal space on right side 2. Check for tenderness in the Liver point located on the 3rd rib, 3 " to the right of the sternum, at the costochondral junction. 3. Check for tenderness underneath the right rib cage 4. Check for tenderness or nodularity in the right thenar pad, which is a pancreas indicator if tender 5. Check for tenderness in the Chapman reflex for the pancreas located in the 7th intercostal space on the left 6. Check for tenderness or guarding at the head of the pancreas located in the upper left quadrant of the abdominal region 1/2 to 2/3 of the way between the umbilicus and the angel of the ribs 7. Run a 6 hour glucose-insulin tolerance test

Supplemental Support

1. Adrenal support: Adrenal tissue (neonatal bovine) and adrenal adaptogenic herbs 2. Multiple nutrients for blood sugar handling problems 3. Beet juice, taurine, vitamin C and pancreolipase

222. Chronic low back pain, worse with fatigue

Chronic low back pain that is worse with fatigue is a sign of adrenal insufficiency. In applied Kinesiology the pelvic supportive muscles are neurologically related to the adrenal glands. There may also be a need for connective tissue support. Balancing the overall structure of the body is essential and a general protocol for supporting the connective tissue is important.

The following is a list of nutrients that are useful for healing connective tissue:

1. Vitamin B12
2. Glucosamine hydrochloride
3. MSM
4. Vitamin B6
5. Vitamin C complex
6. Calcium and magnesium
7. Essential fatty acids
8. Chondroitin sulfate

1° indication

Low adrenal function

Further assessment	1. Check for tenderness in the inguinal ligament bilaterally 2. Check for tenderness at the medial knee bilaterally, at the insertion of the sartorius muscle at the Pes Anserine. 3. Check for a paradoxical pupillary reflex by shining a light into a client's eye and grading the reaction of the pupil. A pupil that fails to constrict indicates adrenal exhaustion 4. Check for the presence of postural hypotension. A drop of more than 10 points is an indication of adrenal insufficiency 5. Check for a chronic short leg due to a posterior-inferior ilium. An adrenal indicator when confirmed with postural hypotension and a paradoxical pupillary response. 6. Check the cortisol/DHEA rhythm with an adrenal stress profile e.g. ASI 7. Assess for adrenal insufficiency with the Acoustic Cardiogram (ACG), which will show static in both the systolic and diastolic rest phases. You will also see an elevated S2 sound.

2° Indication

Mineral deficiency

Further assessment	1. Assess for mineral deficiency using Tissue mineral assessment test. Place a standard blood pressure cuff around the largest portion of the client's calf muscle (sitting). Instruct the client to let you know when they feel the onset of cramping pain and gradually inflate the cuff. Stop and deflate immediately when threshold has been reached. Less than 200 mmHg is considered deficient in minerals. Use the neurolingual testing to challenge the body with several different types of minerals and other co-factors to see which combination of minerals and co-factors increases the threshold above 200mmHg.

	2. Assess for mineral insufficiency by using Dr. Kane's mineral assessment tests. 3. Assess the impact of mineral deficiencies on the body's acid buffering capacities by using Dr. Bieler's salivary pH acid challenge.

Supplemental Support

1. Adrenal tissue (neonatal bovine)
2. Adaptogenic herbs to support adrenal function
3. Vitamin B12
4. Glucosamine hydrochloride
5. Pyridoxal-5-phosphate
6. Chondroitin sulfates and manganese
7. Broad spectrum proteolytic enzymes
8. Calcium and magnesium with or without parathyroid tissue
9. Essential fatty acids: Mixed fatty acids (walnut, hazelnut, sesame, and apricot), EPA and DHA from fish oil
10. Multiple nutrients to support bone health

Lifestyle changes

Please see the handout in the appendix on the Adrenal restoration measures

NOTES:

223. Become dizzy when standing up suddenly

Becoming dizzy when standing up is a classic sign of low adrenal function. The adrenal glands are responsible for keeping the blood pressure in the normal range for the few seconds of compensation after moving from a recumbent to a standing position. Weakness in the adrenal glands can cause dizziness when standing, known as orthostatic hypotension. A drop of 10 or more points in the systolic blood pressure reading when taken recumbent and standing is a sign of adrenal insufficiency.

1° indication

Low adrenal function

Further assessment	1. Check for tenderness in the inguinal ligament bilaterally 2. Check for tenderness at the medial knee bilaterally, at the insertion of the sartorius muscle at the Pes Anserine. 3. Check for a paradoxical pupillary reflex by shining a light into a client's eye and grading the reaction of the pupil. A pupil that fails to constrict indicates adrenal exhaustion 4. Check for the presence of postural hypotension. A drop of more than 10 points is an indication of adrenal insufficiency 5. Check for a chronic short leg due to a posterior-inferior ilium. An adrenal indicator when confirmed with postural hypotension and a paradoxical pupillary response. 6. Check the cortisol/DHEA rhythm with an adrenal stress profile e.g. ASI 7. Increased chloride in the urine is a sign of hypoadrenal function 8. Assess for adrenal insufficiency with the Acoustic Cardiogram (ACG), which will show static in both the systolic and diastolic rest phases. You will also see an elevated S2 sound.

Supplemental Support

1. Adrenal tissue (bovine neonatal)
2. Multiple nutrients for blood sugar handling problems
3. Adaptogenic herbs to support adrenal function

Lifestyle changes

Please see the handout in the appendix on the Adrenal restoration measures

NOTES:

224. Difficulty maintaining manipulative correction
225. Pain after manipulative correction

A difficulty maintaining manipulative correction or pain after manipulative correction are signs of ligament laxity. From a functional perspective, increased ligament laxity is a strong sign of adrenal insufficiency. It may also be an indication of a general need for connective tissue support. Balancing the overall structure of the body is essential and a general protocol for supporting the connective tissue is important.

The following is a list of nutrients that are useful for healing connective tissue:

1. Vitamin B12
2. Glucosamine hydrochloride
3. MSM
4. Vitamin B6
5. Vitamin C complex
6. Calcium and magnesium
7. Essential fatty acids
8. Chondroitin sulfate

<u>1° indication</u>

Low adrenal function

Further assessment	1. Check for tenderness in the inguinal ligament bilaterally 2. Check for tenderness at the medial knee bilaterally, at the insertion of the sartorius muscle at the Pes Anserine. 3. Check for a paradoxical pupillary reflex by shining a light into a client's eye and grading the reaction of the pupil. A pupil that fails to constrict indicates adrenal exhaustion 4. Check for the presence of postural hypotension. A drop of more than 10 points is an indication of adrenal insufficiency 5. Check for a chronic short leg due to a posterior-inferior ilium. An adrenal indicator when confirmed with postural hypotension and a paradoxical pupillary response. 6. Check the cortisol/DHEA rhythm with an adrenal stress profile e.g. ASI 7. Assess for adrenal insufficiency with the Acoustic Cardiogram (ACG), which will show static in both the systolic and diastolic rest phases. You will also see an elevated S2 sound.

<u>2° Indication</u>

Mineral deficiency

Further assessment	1. Assess for mineral deficiency using Tissue mineral assessment test. Place a standard blood pressure cuff around the largest portion of the client's calf muscle (sitting). Instruct the client to let you know when they feel the onset of cramping pain and gradually inflate the cuff. Stop and deflate immediately when threshold has been reached. Less than 200 mmHg is considered deficient in minerals. Use the neurolingual testing to challenge the body with several different types of minerals and other co-factors to see which combination of minerals and co- 2. Assess the impact of mineral deficiencies on the body's acid buffering capacities by using Dr. Bieler's salivary pH acid challenge.

Supplemental Support

1. Adrenal tissue (neonatal bovine)
2. Adaptogenic herbs to support adrenal function
3. Vitamin B12
4. Glucosamine hydrochloride
5. Pyridoxal-5-phosphate
6. Chondroitin sulfates and manganese
7. Broad spectrum proteolytic enzymes
8. Calcium and magnesium with or without parathyroid tissue
9. Essential fatty acids: Mixed fatty acids (walnut, hazelnut, sesame, and apricot), EPA and DHA from fish oil
10. Multiple nutrients to support bone health

Lifestyle changes

Please see the handout in the appendix on the Adrenal restoration measures

NOTES:

226. Arthritic tendencies

Arthritic tendencies are often a sign of adrenal insufficiency. It is, of course, important to check out osteoarthritis and other kinds of inflammatory arthritis before jumping to the conclusion that the adrenals are under functioning. Many types of arthritis are associated with dysbiosis and an increased intestinal hyperpermeability, therefore assessment of the digestive system is important.

1° indication

Hypo-adrenal output

Further assessment	1. Check for tenderness in the inguinal ligament bilaterally 2. Check for tenderness at the medial knee bilaterally, at the insertion of the sartorius muscle at the Pes Anserine. 3. Check for a paradoxical pupillary reflex by shining a light into a client's eye and grading the reaction of the pupil. A pupil that fails to constrict indicates adrenal exhaustion 4. Check for the presence of postural hypotension. A drop of more than 10 points is an indication of adrenal insufficiency 5. Check for a chronic short leg due to a posterior-inferior ilium. An adrenal indicator when confirmed with postural hypotension and a paradoxical pupillary response. 6. Check cortisol/DHEA rhythm with a salivary adrenal stress 7. Assess for adrenal insufficiency with the Acoustic Cardiogram (ACG), which will show static in both the systolic and diastolic rest phases. You will also see an elevated S2 sound.

2° Indication

Dysbiosis caused by an overgrowth of bacteria or yeast

Further assessment	1. Increased urinary indican levels 2. Stool analysis- either comprehensive digestive analysis or a parasite profile 3. Check for tenderness in the Chapman reflex for the colon located bilaterally along the iliotibial band on the thighs. Palpate the colon for tenderness and tension. 4. Check for tenderness in the Chapman reflex for the small intestine located on the 8th, 9th and 10th intercostal spaces near the tip of the rib. Also palpate four quadrants in a 2" to 3" radius around the umbilicus for tenderness and tension. 5. Decreased secretory IgA on stool analysis.

Supplemental Support

1. Adrenal support: Adrenal tissue (neonatal bovine) and adrenal adaptogenic herbs
2. Colon support: Fiber & Lactobacillus acidophilus and Bifidobacterium bifidus
3. Garlic and chlorophyllins
4. Micro Emulsified Oregano
5. Digestive support: Nutrients to heal the intestines, Betaine HCL, Pepsin, & pancreatin
6. Multiple nutrients for blood sugar handling problems
7. Beet juice, taurine, vitamin C and pancreolipase

227. Crave salty foods
228. Salt foods before tasting

Craving salty foods and salting foods before tasting them are classic signs of adrenal insufficiency and a possible need for electrolytes. The adrenal glands are not only important for a healthy stress response, but also help with mineral balancing in the body via the mineral corticoids. Aldosterone is one such hormone. Aldosterone causes the re-absorption of sodium and chloride. In an adrenal insufficiency the levels of aldosterone in the body may be compromised. This causes a larger excretion of sodium and chloride than is necessary, hence the salt craving.

1° indication

Adrenal insufficiency

Further assessment	1. Check for tenderness in the inguinal ligament bilaterally 2. Check for tenderness at the medial knee bilaterally, at the insertion of the sartorius muscle at the Pes Anserine. 3. Check for a paradoxical pupillary reflex by shining a light into a client's eye and grading the reaction of the pupil. A pupil that fails to constrict indicates adrenal exhaustion 4. Check for the presence of postural hypotension. A drop of more than 10 points is an indication of adrenal insufficiency 5. Check for a chronic short leg due to a posterior-inferior ilium. An adrenal indicator when confirmed with postural hypotension and a paradoxical pupillary response. 6. Check the cortisol/DHEA rhythm with a salivary adrenal stress profile e.g. ASI

2° Indication

Electrolyte balance

Further assessment	1. Assess for mineral insufficiency by using Dr. Kane's mineral assessment tests. 2. Assess the impact of mineral deficiencies on the body's acid buffering capacities by using Dr. Bieler's salivary pH acid challenge. 3. Assess the client's hydration status. Have client stand with hands by their side and check and palpate the veins in the right hand. Have them slowly raise their hand to heart level and see if the veins still stick out. Veins that are only just visible or not visible at all are a sign of dehydration

Supplemental Support

1. Adrenal support: Adrenal tissue (neonatal bovine) & adrenal adaptogenic herbs
2. Multiple nutrients for blood sugar handling problems
3. Beet juice, taurine, vitamin C and pancreolipase

Lifestyle changes

Please see the handout in the appendix on Adrenal restoration measures

229. Perspire easily

A person who perspires easily either has hypo-functioning adrenal glands or has a mineral/ electrolyte deficiency. Easy perspiration should not be confused with excessive perspiration, which is an indication of liver and renal dysfunction.

1° indication

Hypo-adrenal output

Further assessment	1. Check for tenderness in the inguinal ligament bilaterally 2. Check for tenderness at the medial knee bilaterally, at the insertion of the sartorius muscle at the Pes Anserine. 3. Check for a paradoxical pupillary reflex by shining a light into a client's eye and grading the reaction of the pupil. A pupil that fails to constrict indicates adrenal exhaustion 4. Check for the presence of postural hypotension. A drop of more than 10 points is an indication of adrenal insufficiency 5. Check for a chronic short leg due to a posterior-inferior ilium. An adrenal indicator when confirmed with postural hypotension and a paradoxical pupillary response. 6. Check the cortisol/DHEA rhythm with a salivary adrenal stress profile e.g. ASI 7. Assess for adrenal insufficiency with the Acoustic Cardiogram (ACG), which will show static in both the systolic and diastolic rest phases. You will also see an elevated S2 sound.

2° Indication

Mineral and electrolyte deficiency

Further assessment	1. Assess for mineral deficiency using Tissue mineral assessment test. Place a standard blood pressure cuff around the largest portion of the client's calf muscle (sitting). Instruct the client to let you know when they feel the onset of cramping pain and gradually inflate the cuff. Stop and deflate immediately when threshold has been reached. Less than 200 mmHg is considered deficient in minerals. Use the neurolingual testing to challenge the body with several different minerals and other co-factors to see which combination of minerals and co-factors increases the threshold above 200mmHg. 2. Assess for mineral insufficiency by using Dr. Kane's mineral assessment tests. 3. Assess the impact of mineral deficiencies on the body's acid buffering capacities by using Dr. Bieler's salivary pH acid challenge. 4. Assess the client's hydration status. Have client stand with hands by their side and check and palpate the veins in the right hand. Have them slowly raise their hand to heart level and see if the veins still stick out. Veins that are only just visible or not visible at all are a sign of dehydration

Supplemental Support

1. Adrenal tissue (neonatal bovine)
2. Adaptogenic herbs to support adrenal function
3. Bioglycozyme AD
4. Alkaline Ash minerals (Calcium, Magnesium,Potassium)
5. Calcium and magnesium with or without parathyroid tissue
6. Multiple nutrients to support bone health
7. Multiple mineral without iron or copper
8. Betaine HCL, Pepsin, and pancreatin
9. Mixed fatty acids (walnut, hazelnut, sesame, and apricot)

Lifestyle changes

Please see the handout in the appendix on Adrenal restoration measures

NOTES:

230. Chronic fatigue, or get drowsy often

There are many causes of chronic fatigue. It is important to assess whether or not the client is getting enough sleep. There are a number of dietary causes of fatigue including a diet that is too high in refined sugars, multiple mineral and vitamin deficiencies and a person who is consuming the standard Western diet with too much coffee, alcohol and processed foods.
Other causes include low adrenal function, low thyroid function, food allergies and/or digestive dysfunction.

1° indication
Low adrenal function

Further assessment	1. Check for tenderness in the inguinal ligament bilaterally 2. Check for tenderness at the medial knee bilaterally, at the insertion of the sartorius muscle at the Pes Anserine. 3. Check for a paradoxical pupillary reflex by shining a light into a client's eye and grading the reaction of the pupil. A pupil that fails to constrict indicates adrenal exhaustion 4. Check for the presence of postural hypotension. A drop of more than 10 points is an indication of adrenal insufficiency 5. Check for a chronic short leg due to a posterior-inferior ilium. An adrenal indicator when confirmed with postural hypotension and a paradoxical pupillary response. 6. Check the cortisol/DHEA rhythm with a salivary adrenal stress profile e.g. ASI 7. Assess for adrenal insufficiency with the Acoustic Cardiogram (ACG), which will show static in both the systolic and diastolic rest phases. You will also see an elevated S2 sound.

2° Indication
Low thyroid function

Further assessment	1. Check for tenderness in the Chapman reflex for the thyroid located in the second intercostal space near the sternum on the right 2. Check for a delayed Achilles return reflex, which is a strong sign of a hypo-functioning thyroid 3. Check for general costochondral tenderness, which is a thyroid indicator 4. Check for pre-tibial edema, which is a sign of a hypo-functioning thyroid 5. Iodine test: Use a tincture of 2% iodine solution, and paint a 3" by 3" square on the client's abdomen. The client is to leave the patch unwashed until it disappears. The square should still be there in 24 hours. If it has disappeared, there is an indication of iodine need 6. Have client assess their basal metabolic temperature by taking their axillary temperature first thing in the morning for 5 straight days. An average temperature below 36.6° is an indication of hypo-thyroidism

Other indications

1. Food allergies or intolerances
2. Digestive dysfunction
3. Virus: Epstein Barr

Supplemental Support

1. Adrenal tissue (neonatal bovine)
2. Adaptogenic herbs to support adrenal function
3. Multiple nutrients for blood sugar handling problems
4. Pyridoxal-5-phosphate
5. Multiple nutrients to support thyroid function with pituitary glandular
6. Potassium iodide

Lifestyle changes

Please see the handout in the appendix on Adrenal restoration measures

NOTES:

231. Afternoon yawning

Afternoon yawning is a symptom of adrenal insufficiency and hypo-functioning adrenal glands. It is also a sign of needing vitamin B1, thiamine and a low thyroid indicator.

1° indication
Adrenal insufficiency

Further assessment	1. Check for tenderness in the inguinal ligament bilaterally 2. Check for tenderness at the medial knee bilaterally, at the insertion of the sartorius muscle at the Pes Anserine. 3. Check for a paradoxical pupillary reflex by shining a light into a client's eye and grading the reaction of the pupil. A pupil that fails to constrict indicates adrenal exhaustion 4. Check for the presence of postural hypotension. A drop of more than 10 points is an indication of adrenal insufficiency 5. Check for a chronic short leg due to a posterior-inferior ilium. An adrenal indicator when confirmed with postural hypotension and a paradoxical pupillary response. 6. Check the cortisol/DHEA rhythm with a salivary adrenal stress profile e.g. ASI 7. Assess for adrenal insufficiency with the Acoustic Cardiogram (ACG), which will show static in both the systolic and diastolic rest phases. You will also see an elevated S2 sound.

Supplemental Support

1. Adrenal tissue (neonatal bovine)
2. Adaptogenic herbs to support adrenal function
3. Multiple nutrients for blood sugar handling problems
4. Naturally occurring thiamine

Lifestyle changes
Please see the handout in the appendix on Adrenal restoration measures

NOTES:

232. Afternoon headache

An afternoon headache has many possible causes. It is important to rule out and correct any structural component and to assess how often this happens. Many times afternoon headaches occur only at work and are linked with poor ergonomics in the workplace and excess time at a computer screen without a break, which places tremendous strain on the eyes and upper body. If these are ruled out consider hypofunctioning adrenal glands, hypo-functioning thyroid and reactive hypoglycemia.

1° indication

Low adrenal function

Further assessment	1. Check for tenderness in the inguinal ligament bilaterally 2. Check for tenderness at the medial knee bilaterally, at the insertion of the sartorius muscle at the Pes Anserine. 3. Check for a paradoxical pupillary reflex by shining a light into a client's eye and grading the reaction of the pupil. A pupil that fails to constrict indicates adrenal exhaustion 4. Check for the presence of postural hypotension. A drop of more than 10 points is an indication of adrenal insufficiency 5. Check for a chronic short leg due to a posterior-inferior ilium. An adrenal indicator when confirmed with postural hypotension and a paradoxical pupillary response. 6. Check the cortisol/DHEA rhythm with a salivary adrenal stress profile e.g. ASI 7. Assess for adrenal insufficiency with the Acoustic Cardiogram (ACG), which will show static in both the systolic and diastolic rest phases. You will also see an elevated S2 sound.

2° Indication

Low thyroid function

Further assessment	1. Check for tenderness in the Chapman reflex for the thyroid located in the right 2nd intercostal space near the sternum right 2. Check for a delayed Achilles return reflex, which is a strong sign of a hypo-functioning thyroid 3. Check for general costochondral tenderness, which is a thyroid indicator 4. Check for pre-tibial edema, which is a sign of a hypo-functioning thyroid 5. Iodine test: Use a tincture of 2% iodine solution, and paint a 3" by 3" square on the client's abdomen. The client is to leave the patch unwashed until it disappears. The square should still be there in 24 hours. If it has disappeared, there is an indication of iodine need 6. Have client assess their basal metabolic temperature by taking their axillary temperature first thing in the morning for 5 straight days. An average temperature below 36.6°C is an indication of hypo-thyroidism

3° Indication
Reactive hypoglycemia

Further assessment	1. Check for tenderness in the Chapman reflex for the liver-gallbladder located over the 6th intercostal space on the right side 2. Check for tenderness in the Liver point located on the 3rd rib, 3 " to the right of the sternum, at the costochondral junction. 3. Check for tenderness underneath the right rib cage 4. Check for tenderness or nodularity in the right thenar pad, which is a pancreas indicator if tender 5. Check for tenderness in the Chapman reflex for the pancreas located in the 7th intercostal space on the left 6. Check for tenderness or guarding at the head of the pancreas located in the upper left quadrant of the abdominal region 1/2 to 2/3 of the way between the umbilicus and the angel of the ribs 7. Run a 6 hour glucose-insulin tolerance test

Supplemental Support

1. Adrenal tissue (neonatal bovine)
2. Adaptogenic herbs to support adrenal function
3. Multiple nutrients for blood sugar handling problems
4. Pyridoxal-5-phosphate
5. Multiple nutrients to support thyroid function with pituitary glandular
6. Potassium iodide

Lifestyle changes
Please see the handout in the appendix on Adrenal restoration measures

NOTES:

233. Asthma, wheezing or difficulty breathing

There are many causes of asthma including low adrenal function, dysbiosis, digestive dysfunction, allergies and increased intestinal hyperpermeability.

1° indication

Low adrenal function

Further assessment	1. Check for tenderness in the inguinal ligament bilaterally 2. Check for tenderness at the medial knee bilaterally, at the insertion of the sartorius muscle at the Pes Anserine. 3. Check for a paradoxical pupillary reflex by shining a light into a client's eye and grading the reaction of the pupil. A pupil that fails to constrict indicates adrenal exhaustion 4. Check for the presence of postural hypotension. A drop of more than 10 points is an indication of adrenal insufficiency 5. Check for a chronic short leg due to a posterior-inferior ilium. An adrenal indicator when confirmed with postural hypotension and a paradoxical pupillary response. 6. Check the cortisol/DHEA rhythm with an adrenal stress profile e.g. ASI 7. Assess for adrenal insufficiency with the Acoustic Cardiogram (ACG), which will show static in both the systolic and diastolic rest phases. You will also see an elevated S2 sound.

2° Indication

Toxic bowel with dysbiosis and /or increased intestinal hyperpermeability

Further assessment	1. Increased urinary indican 2. Stool analysis for candida and/or parasites 3. Check for tenderness in the Chapman reflex for the colon located bilaterally along the iliotibial band on the thighs. Palpate the colon for tenderness and tension. 4. Check for tenderness in the Chapman reflex for the small intestine located on the 8th, 9th and 10th intercostal spaces near the tip of the rib. Also palpate four quadrants in a 2" to 3" radius around the umbilicus for tenderness and tension. 5. Decreased secretory IgA on stool analysis.

Other indications

1. Allergies
2. Hypochlorhydria
3. Pancreatic insufficiency

Supplemental Support

1. Adrenal support: Adrenal tissue (neonatal bovine) and adrenal adaptogenic herbs
2. Multiple nutrients for blood sugar handling problems
3. Micro Emulsified Oregano
4. Digestive support: Nutrients to heal the intestines, Betaine HCL, Pepsin, & pancreatin
5. Colon support: Water soluble fiber & Lactobacillus acidophilus & Bifidobacterium bifidus

234. Pain on the medial or inner side of the knee

The medial or inner side of the knee is the insertion of the Sartorius muscle into the area known as the Pes Anserine. This area is one of the reflex areas for the adrenal glands. Tenderness in this area is an indication of adrenal insufficiency. Assessing the other reflex points and other adrenal tests will give a larger view of the adrenal system, and whether or not it needs support. It is obviously important to make sure that there are no structural problems in this area.

1° indication

Further adrenal assessment needed

Further assessment	1. Check for tenderness in the inguinal ligament bilaterally 2. Check for a paradoxical pupillary reflex by shining a light into a client's eye and grading the reaction of the pupil. A pupil that fails to constrict indicates adrenal exhaustion 3. Check for the presence of postural hypotension. A drop of more than 10 points is an indication of adrenal insufficiency 4. Check for a chronic short leg due to a posterior-inferior ilium. An adrenal indicator when confirmed with postural hypotension and a paradoxical pupillary response. 5. Check the cortisol/DHEA rhythm with a salivary adrenal stress profile 6. Assess for adrenal insufficiency with the Acoustic Cardiogram (ACG), which will show static in both the systolic and diastolic rest phases. You will also see an elevated S2 sound.

Supplemental Support

1. Adrenal tissue (neonatal bovine)
2. Adaptogenic herbs to support adrenal function
3. Multiple nutrients for blood sugar handling problems
4. Naturally occurring thiamine

Lifestyle changes

Please see the handout in the appendix on Adrenal restoration measures

NOTES:

235. Tendency to sprain ankles or "shin splints"

People with a tendency towards spraining ankles and shin splints are often suffering from poor adrenal function. Adrenal dysfunction causes increased weakness in the ligaments of the body. For some people the ankles are the area in the body that is most affected. For others it is the sacroiliac joint. It is important to not overlook other causes, especially the structural components. A thorough assessment of the ankle will determine if there is a structural cause.

1° indication

Low functioning adrenals

Further assessment	1. Check for tenderness in the inguinal ligament bilaterally 2. Check for a paradoxical pupillary reflex by shining a light into a client's eye and grading the reaction of the pupil. A pupil that fails to constrict indicates adrenal exhaustion 3. Check for the presence of postural hypotension. A drop of more than 10 points is an indication of adrenal insufficiency 4. Check for a chronic short leg due to a posterior-inferior ilium. An adrenal indicator when confirmed with postural hypotension and a paradoxical pupillary response. 5. Check the cortisol/DHEA rhythm with a salivary adrenal stress profile 6. Assess for adrenal insufficiency with the Acoustic Cardiogram (ACG), which will show static in both the systolic and diastolic rest phases. You will also see an elevated S2 sound.

Supplemental Support

1. Adrenal tissue (neonatal bovine)
2. Adaptogenic herbs to support adrenal function
3. Multiple nutrients for blood sugar handling problems
4. Naturally occurring thiamine

Lifestyle changes

Please see the handout in the appendix on Adrenal restoration measures

NOTES:

236. Tendency to need sunglasses

The ability of the pupil to adequately constrict in the presence of direct light is partly under the influence of the adrenal glands. Many people with poor adrenal health will display a paradoxical pupillary response to direct light. Instead of constriction, the pupil of the eye will first constrict a little and then dilate. This is an indication of adrenal fatigue. It is important to remember that contact lenses can increase a person's sensitivity to light. There may be neurological reasons for eyes that do not restrict or accommodate in the presence of direct light.

1° indication

Further adrenal assessment needed

Further assessment	1. Check for tenderness in the inguinal ligament bilaterally 2. Check for a paradoxical pupillary reflex by shining a light into a client's eye and grading the reaction of the pupil. A pupil that fails to constrict indicates adrenal insufficiency 3. Check for the presence of postural hypotension. A drop of more than 10 points is an indication of adrenal insufficiency 4. Check for a chronic short leg due to a posterior-inferior ilium. An adrenal indicator when confirmed with postural hypotension and a paradoxical pupillary response. 5. Check the cortisol/DHEA rhythm with a salivary adrenal stress profile e.g. ASI 6. Assess for adrenal insufficiency with the Acoustic Cardiogram (ACG), which will show static in both the systolic and diastolic rest phases. You will also see an elevated S2 sound.

Supplemental Support

1. Adrenal tissue (neonatal bovine)
2. Adaptogenic herbs to support adrenal function
3. Multiple nutrients for blood sugar handling problems
4. Naturally occurring thiamine

Lifestyle changes

Please see the handout in the appendix on Adrenal restoration measures

NOTES:

237. Allergies/Intolerances and / or hives

There are many causes of allergies and hives including low adrenal function, dysbiosis, digestive dysfunction, and increased intestinal hyperpermeability.

1° indication
Low adrenal function

Further assessment	1. Check for tenderness in the inguinal ligament bilaterally 2. Check for tenderness at the medial knee bilaterally, at the insertion of the sartorius muscle at the Pes Anserine. 3. Check for a paradoxical pupillary reflex by shining a light into a client's eye and grading the reaction of the pupil. A pupil that fails to constrict indicates adrenal exhaustion 4. Check for the presence of postural hypotension. A drop of more than 10 points is an indication of adrenal insufficiency 5. Check for a chronic short leg due to a posterior-inferior ilium. 6. Check the cortisol/DHEA rhythm with an adrenal stress profile 7. Assess for adrenal insufficiency with the Acoustic Cardiogram (ACG), which will show static in both the systolic and diastolic rest phases. You will also see an elevated S2 sound.

2° Indication
Toxic bowel with dysbiosis and /or increased intestinal hyperpermeability

Further assessment	1. Increased urinary indican 2. Stool analysis- either comprehensive digestive analysis or a parasite profile 3. Check for tenderness in the Chapman reflex for the colon located bilaterally along the iliotibial band on the thighs. Palpate the colon for tenderness and tension. 4. Check for tenderness in the Chapman reflex for the small intestine located on the 8th, 9th and 10th intercostal spaces near the tip of the rib. Also palpate four quadrants in a 2" to 3" radius around the umbilicus for tenderness and tension

Supplemental Support

1. Adrenal tissue (neonatal bovine)
2. Adaptogenic herbs to support adrenal function
3. Multiple nutrients for blood sugar handling problems
4. Micro Emulsified Oregano
5. Nutrients that heal the intestines
6. Multiple herbal anti-histamines
7. Betaine HCL, Pepsin, and pancreatin
8. Water soluble fiber and colon health nutrients
9. Multiple nutrients that support the immune system
10. Lactobacillus acidophilus and Bifidobacterium bifidus

Lifestyle changes
Please see the handout in the appendix on Adrenal restoration measures

238. Weakness, dizziness

Weakness and dizziness are classic signs of low functioning adrenal glands. The adrenal glands provide the initial control of blood pressure when you first stand up. If the adrenals are not functioning well, the client will complain of dizziness, especially when standing up. This client needs further adrenal assessment.

1° indication

Further adrenal assessment needed

Further assessment	1. Check for tenderness in the inguinal ligament bilaterally 2. Check for tenderness at the medial knee bilaterally, at the insertion of the sartorius muscle at the Pes Anserine. 3. Check for a paradoxical pupillary reflex by shining a light into a client's eye and grading the reaction of the pupil. A pupil that fails to constrict indicates adrenal exhaustion 4. Check for the presence of postural hypotension. A drop of more than 10 points is an indication of adrenal insufficiency 5. Check for a chronic short leg due to a posterior-inferior ilium. An adrenal indicator when confirmed with postural hypotension and a paradoxical pupillary response. 6. Check the cortisol/DHEA rhythm with a salivary adrenal stress profile 7. Assess for adrenal insufficiency with the Acoustic Cardiogram (ACG), which will show static in both the systolic and diastolic rest phases. You will also see an elevated S2 sound.

Supplemental Support

1. Adrenal tissue (neonatal bovine)
2. Adaptogenic herbs to support adrenal function
3. Multiple nutrients for blood sugar handling problems
4. Naturally occurring thiamine

Lifestyle changes

Please see the handout in the appendix on Adrenal restoration measures

NOTES:

PITUITARY

239. Over 6' 6" tall (Mature height) (1 = yes, 0 = no)
240. Early sexual development (before age 10) (1 = yes, 0 = no)
241. Increased libido
242. Splitting type headache
243. Memory failing
244. Tolerate sugar, feel fine when eating sugar (1 = yes, 0 = no)
245. Under 4' 10" (Mature height) (1 = yes, 0 = no)
246. Decreased libido
247. Excessive thirst
248. Weight gain around hips or waist
249. Menstrual disorders
250. Delayed sexual development (after age 13) (1 = yes, 0 = no)
251. Tendency to ulcers or colitis

239. Over 6' 6" tall (mature height)

Being over 6'6" tall can be a sign of hyper-pituitary function. Optimal pituitary function is essential for healthy hormonal regulation in the body. The hormonal hierarchy starts with the hypothalamus, which is linked to the central nervous system where, in many cases, the initial stimulus for a hormonal response begins. The pituitary gland acts as a sort of junction box and biological feedback gland between the hypothalamus and the end organs of hormone production. The pituitary can be separated into two distinct portions, the anterior pituitary and the posterior pituitary. The anterior pituitary hormones control peripheral endocrine glands from which an end hormone is released. "Releasing hormones" from the hypothalamus control the release of hormones from the anterior pituitary. Some of the anterior pituitary hormones include somatotropin or growth hormone (GH), follicular stimulating hormone (FSH), Lutenising hormone (LH), adrenocorticotropic hormone (ACTH), thyroid stimulating hormone (TSH) and prolactin. The influence of the anterior pituitary extends from the thyroid to the adrenal glands and the ovaries. In contrast, the hormones of the posterior pituitary are synthesized in the hypothalamus, transported to the posterior pituitary and released by nervous signals. The posterior pituitary produces only two hormones, oxytocin and anti-diuretic hormone, which act directly on the target cell.

Increased activity of the anterior pituitary can lead to an increased output of somatotropin or growth hormone. If this happens before puberty, one can get large increases in height. Hyper-pituitary activity in the anterior pituitary is uncommon. This question is referring to the possibility of a functional increase in anterior pituitary activity giving rise to an increased signal to the end organs of hormonal output: thyroid, adrenals, gonads etc. An overt increase in anterior pituitary output is suggestive of a tumor and should be investigated by a clinician trained in such diagnoses.

Supplemental Support

1. Pituitary/hypothalamus tissue (neonatal bovine)
2. Multi-gland (bovine neonatal)

Lifestyle changes

1. Eliminate all refined carbohydrates, alcohol and caffeine (fizzy drinks, coffee, tea and chocolate) from the diet
2. Increase fresh raw fruits and vegetables in the diet
3. Increase pure water (6-8 cups) daily
4. Get adequate rest and exercise

NOTES:

240. Early sexual development (before age 10) (1 = yes, 0 = no)

Early sexual development can be a sign of hyper-pituitary function. Optimal pituitary function is essential for healthy hormonal regulation in the body. The hormonal hierarchy starts with the hypothalamus, which is linked to the central nervous system where, in many cases, the initial stimulus for a hormonal response begins. The pituitary gland acts as a sort of junction box and biological feedback gland between the hypothalamus and the end organs of hormone production.

The pituitary can be separated into two distinct portions, the anterior pituitary and the posterior pituitary. The anterior pituitary hormones control peripheral endocrine glands from which an end hormone is released. "Releasing hormones" from the hypothalamus control the release of hormones from the anterior pituitary. Some of the anterior pituitary hormones include somatotropin or growth hormone (GH), follicular stimulating hormone (FSH), Lutenising hormone (LH), adrenocorticotropic hormone (ACTH), thyroid stimulating hormone (TSH) and prolactin. The influence of the anterior pituitary extends from the thyroid to the adrenal glands and the ovaries. In contrast, the hormones of the posterior pituitary are synthesized in the hypothalamus, transported to the posterior pituitary and released by nervous signals. The posterior pituitary produces only two hormones, oxytocin and anti-diuretic hormone, which act directly on the target cell.

Increased activity of the anterior pituitary before puberty can lead to an increased output of FSH and LH. This can cause the onset of early sexual development. Hyper-pituitary activity in the anterior pituitary is uncommon. This question is referring to the possibility of a functional increase in anterior pituitary activity giving rise to an increased signal to the end organs of hormonal output: thyroid, adrenals, gonads etc. An overt increase in anterior pituitary output is suggestive of a tumor and should be investigated by a clinician trained in such diagnoses.

Supplemental Support

1. Pituitary/hypothalamus tissue (neonatal bovine)
2. Multi-gland (bovine neonatal)

<u>Lifestyle changes</u>

- Eliminate all refined carbohydrates, alcohol and caffeine (fizzy drinks, coffee, tea and chocolate) from the diet
- Increase fresh raw fruits and vegetables in the diet
- Increase pure water (6-8 cups) daily
- Get adequate rest and exercise

NOTES:

241. Increased libido

An increased libido can be a sign of hyper-pituitary function. Optimal pituitary function is essential for healthy hormonal regulation in the body. The hormonal hierarchy starts with the hypothalamus, which is linked to the central nervous system where, in many cases, the initial stimulus for a hormonal response begins. The pituitary gland acts as a sort of junction box and biological feedback gland between the hypothalamus and the end organs of hormone production.

The pituitary can be separated into two distinct portions, the anterior pituitary and the posterior pituitary. The anterior pituitary hormones control peripheral endocrine glands from which an end hormone is released. "Releasing hormones" from the hypothalamus control the release of hormones from the anterior pituitary. Some of the anterior pituitary hormones include somatotropin or growth hormone (GH), follicular stimulating hormone (FSH), Lutenising hormone (LH), adrenocorticotropic hormone (ACTH), thyroid stimulating hormone (TSH) and prolactin. The influence of the anterior pituitary extends from the thyroid to the adrenal glands and the ovaries. In contrast, the hormones of the posterior pituitary are synthesized in the hypothalamus, transported to the posterior pituitary and released by nervous signals. The posterior pituitary produces only two hormones, oxytocin and anti-diuretic hormone, which act directly on the target cell.

Increased activity of the anterior pituitary can cause an increased output of the precursors of the sex hormones, leading to increased libido. Hyper-pituitary activity in the anterior pituitary is uncommon. This question is referring to the possibility of a functional increase in anterior pituitary activity giving rise to an increased signal to the end organs of hormonal output: thyroid, adrenals, gonads etc. An overt increase in anterior pituitary output is suggestive of a tumor and should be investigated by a clinician trained in such diagnoses.

Supplemental Support

1. Pituitary/hypothalamus tissue (neonatal bovine)
2. Multi-gland (bovine neonatal)

Lifestyle changes

- Eliminate all refined carbohydrates, alcohol and caffeine (fizzy drinks, coffee, tea and chocolate) from the diet
- Increase fresh raw fruits and vegetables in the diet
- Increase pure water (6-8 cups) daily
- Get adequate rest and exercise

NOTES:

242. Splitting type headache

There can be many causes of splitting type headaches. This should be assessed from a structural perspective. If all structural causes are ruled out, splitting type headaches may be due to biliary stasis or pituitary dysfunction, especially increased activity in the anterior pituitary.

Increased activity in the anterior pituitary is uncommon. This question is referring to the possibility of a functional increase in anterior pituitary activity giving rise to an increased signal to the end organs of hormonal output: thyroid, adrenals, gonads etc. An overt increase in anterior pituitary output is suggestive of a tumor and should be investigated by a clinician trained in such diagnoses.

1° Indication

Biliary stasis due to gallbladder dysfunction

Further assessment	1. Check for tenderness underneath the right rib cage 2. Check for tenderness and nodulation on the web between thumb and fore-finger of right hand 3. Check for tenderness in the Chapman reflex for the liver-gallbladder located over the 6th intercostal space on the right side 4. Blood chemistry and CBC testing for SGOT, SGPT, GGT 5. Assess for Hepato-biliary congestion with the Acoustic Cardiogram (ACG), which will show post-systolic rounding due to increased backpressure on the pulmonic and aortic valve. It may also show through to the tricuspid valve if chronic.

Supplemental Support

1. Beet juice, taurine, vitamin C and pancreolipase with or without bile salts
2. Phosphatidylcholine
3. Pancreatic enzymes
4. Pituitary/hypothalamus tissue (neonatal bovine)
5. Neonatal Multi Gland

Lifestyle changes

- Please see the handout in the appendix on Healthy lifestyle for a healthy gallbladder
- Eliminate all refined carbohydrates, alcohol and caffeine (fizzy drinks, coffee, tea and chocolate) from the diet
- Increase fresh raw fruits and vegetables in the diet
- Increase pure water (6-8 cups) daily
- Get adequate rest and exercise

NOTES:

243. Memory failing

There are many reasons for a memory loss including, but not limited to Alzheimer's disease, food allergy/sensitivity, carotid stenosis (atherosclerosis), heavy metal body burden, normal memory loss associated with aging, lack of exercise, thyroid hypo-function, reactive hypoglycemia, dysbiosis with an overgrowth of Candida, and amino acid imbalance. Obviously many of these conditions need to be thoroughly evaluated.

A hyper functioning pituitary can often cause failing memory, as can low thyroid function and poor cerebral blood flow to the brain from atherosclerosis. There may also be a need for supplemental RNA, which can be very helpful for failing memory especially in the elderly.

1° Indication
Hyperfunctioning of the pituitary gland

2° Indication
Low thyroid function

Further assessment	1. Check for tenderness in the Chapman reflex for the thyroid located in second intercostal space near the sternum on the right 2. Check for a delayed Achilles return reflex, which is a strong sign of a hypo-functioning thyroid 3. Check for general costochondral tenderness, a thyroid indicator 4. Check for pre-tibial edema, a sign of a hypo-functioning thyroid 5. Iodine test: Use a tincture of 2% iodine solution, and paint a 3" by 3" square on the client's abdomen. The client is to leave the patch unwashed until it disappears. The square should still be there in 24 hours. If it has disappeared iodine is indicated. 6. Have client assess their basal metabolic temperature by taking their axillary temperature first thing in the morning for 5 straight days. An average temperature below 36.6° is an indication of hypo-thyroidism

Other indications

1. Food allergy/sensitivity 2. Normal memory loss assoc. with aging 3. Heavy metal body burden	4. Reactive hypoglycemia 5. Dysbiosis with an overgrowth of Candida 6. Amino acid imbalance

Supplemental Support

1. Pituitary/hypothalamus tissue (neonatal bovine)
2. Multiple nutrients to support thyroid function with pituitary glandular
3. Gamma oryzanol (fortified)
4. Potassium iodide
5. Neonatal multi gland
6. Flax seed oil

Lifestyle changes: Eliminate all refined carbohydrates, alcohol and caffeine (fizzy drinks, coffee, tea and chocolate) from the diet, increase fresh raw fruits & vegetables in the diet, increase pure water (6-8 cups) daily.

244. Tolerate sugar, feel fine when eating sugar

A tolerance for sugar is a sign of hyper pituitary activity. Optimal pituitary function is essential for healthy hormonal regulation in the body. The hormonal hierarchy starts with the hypothalamus, which is linked to the central nervous system where, in many cases, the initial stimulus for a hormonal response begins. The pituitary gland acts as a sort of junction box and biological feedback gland between the hypothalamus and the end organs of hormone production. The pituitary can be separated into two distinct portions, the anterior pituitary and the posterior pituitary. The anterior pituitary hormones control peripheral endocrine glands from which an end hormone is released. “Releasing hormones” from the hypothalamus control the release of hormones from the anterior pituitary. Some of the anterior pituitary hormones include somatotropin or growth hormone (GH), follicular stimulating hormone (FSH), Lutenising hormone (LH), adrenocorticotropic hormone (ACTH), thyroid stimulating hormone (TSH) and prolactin. The influence of the anterior pituitary extends from the thyroid to the adrenal glands and the ovaries. In contrast, the hormones of the posterior pituitary are synthesized in the hypothalamus, transported to the posterior pituitary and released by nervous signals.
Increased activity of the anterior pituitary can lead to a reduced tolerance for sugar output. This is possibly due to increased amounts of somatotropin or growth hormone, which acts to increase blood sugar. It is important to remember that hyper-pituitary activity in the anterior pituitary is uncommon. This question is referring to the possibility of a functional increase in anterior pituitary activity giving rise to an increased signal to the end organs of hormonal output: thyroid, adrenals, gonads etc. An overt increase in anterior pituitary output is suggestive of a tumor and should be investigated by a clinician trained in such diagnoses.
With a decreased tolerance to sugar it is important to rule out diabetes and reactive hypoglycemia by assessing for blood sugar dysregulation.

1° Indication

Hyperfunctioning of the pituitary gland

2° Indication

Blood sugar dysregulation and hypoglycemia.

Further assessment	1. Check for tenderness in the Chapman reflex for the liver-gallbladder located over the 6th intercostal space on the right 2. Check for tenderness in the Liver point located on the 3rd rib, 3 “ to the right of the sternum, at the costochondral junction. 3. Check for tenderness underneath the right rib cage 4. Check for tenderness or nodularity in the right thenar pad, which is a pancreas indicator if tender 5. Check for tenderness in the Chapman reflex for the pancreas located in the 7th intercostal space on the left 6. Check for tenderness or guarding at the head of the pancreas located in the upper left quadrant of the abdominal region 1/2 to 2/3 of the way between the umbilicus and the angel of the ribs 7. Check fasting blood glucose 8. Run a six hour glucose-insulin tolerance test.

3° Indication

Low adrenal function

Further assessment	1. Check for tenderness in the inguinal ligament bilaterally 2. Check for tenderness at the medial knee bilaterally, at the insertion of the sartorius muscle at the Pes Anserine. 3. Check for a paradoxical pupillary reflex by shining a light into a client's eye and grading the reaction of the pupil. A pupil that fails to constrict indicates adrenal exhaustion 4. Check for the presence of postural hypotension. A drop of more than 10 points is an indication of adrenal insufficiency 5. Check for a chronic short leg due to a posterior-inferior ilium. 6. Assess for adrenal insufficiency with the Acoustic Cardiogram (ACG), which will show static in both the systolic and diastolic rest phases. You will also see an elevated S2 sound.

Supplemental Support

1. Pituitary/hypothalamus tissue (neonatal bovine)
2. Multi-gland (bovine neonatal)
3. Multiple nutrients for blood sugar handling problems
4. Adrenal tissue (neonatal bovine)
5. High potency multiple nutrients for sugar handling
6. Adaptogenic herbs to support adrenal function

Lifestyle changes

Please see the handout in the appendix on Recommendations for controlling blood sugar

NOTES:

245. Height under 4' 10"

Being less than 4' 10" can be a sign of hypo-pituitary function. Optimal pituitary function is essential for healthy hormonal regulation in the body. The hormonal hierarchy starts with the hypothalamus, which is linked to the central nervous system where, in many cases, the initial stimulus for a hormonal response begins. The pituitary gland acts as a sort of junction box and biological feedback gland between the hypothalamus and the end organs of hormone production. The pituitary can be separated into two distinct portions, the anterior pituitary and the posterior pituitary. The anterior pituitary hormones control peripheral endocrine glands from which an end hormone is released. "Releasing hormones" from the hypothalamus control the release of hormones from the anterior pituitary. Some of the anterior pituitary hormones include somatotropin or growth hormone (GH), follicular stimulating hormone (FSH), Lutenising hormone (LH), adrenocorticotropic hormone (ACTH), thyroid stimulating hormone (TSH) and prolactin. The influence of the anterior pituitary extends from the thyroid to the adrenal glands and the ovaries. In contrast, the hormones of the posterior pituitary are synthesized in the hypothalamus, transported to the posterior pituitary and released by nervous signals. The posterior pituitary produces only two hormones, oxytocin and anti-diuretic hormone, which act directly on the target cell.

Decreased activity of the anterior pituitary can cause a decreased output of somatotropin or growth hormone, leading to a decrease in height at puberty.

This question is referring to the possibility of a functional decrease in anterior pituitary activity giving rise to decreased signals to the end organs of hormonal output: thyroid, adrenals, gonads etc.

Supplemental Support

1. Pituitary/hypothalamus tissue (neonatal bovine)
2. Multi-gland (bovine neonatal)

Lifestyle changes

1. Eliminate all refined carbohydrates, alcohol and caffeine (fizzy drinks, coffee, tea and chocolate) from the diet
2. Increase fresh raw fruits and vegetables in the diet
3. Increase pure water (6-8 cups) daily
4. Get adequate rest and exercise

NOTES:

246. Decreased libido

A decreased libido is suggestive of low thyroid function. In men a decreased testosterone can cause a lower libido. In women, low androgens in general, may be the cause. In both of these cases there is probably a decrease in pituitary function. Optimal pituitary function is essential for healthy hormonal regulation in the body., and a low libido is suggestive of hormonal dysregulation. The hormonal hierarchy starts with the hypothalamus, which is linked to the central nervous system where, in many cases, the initial stimulus for a hormonal response begins. The pituitary gland acts as a sort of junction box and biological feedback gland between the hypothalamus and the end organs of hormone production. The pituitary can be separated into two distinct portions, the anterior pituitary and the posterior pituitary. The anterior pituitary hormones control peripheral endocrine glands from which an end hormone is released. "Releasing hormones" from the hypothalamus control the release of hormones from the anterior pituitary. Some of the anterior pituitary hormones include somatotropin or growth hormone (GH), follicular stimulating hormone (FSH), Lutenising hormone (LH), adrenocorticotropic hormone (ACTH), thyroid stimulating hormone (TSH) and prolactin. The influence of the anterior pituitary extends from the thyroid to the adrenal glands and the ovaries. In contrast, the hormones of the posterior pituitary are synthesized in the hypothalamus, transported to the posterior pituitary and released by nervous signals. The posterior pituitary produces only two hormones, oxytocin and anti-diuretic hormone, which act directly on the target cell.

Decreased activity in the anterior pituitary can lead to a decreased output of FSH and LH, which can impact on the production of androgen hormones such as androstenedione and testosterone, hormones responsible for libido.

<u>1° Indication</u>

Low thyroid function

Further assessment	1. Check for tenderness in the Chapman reflex for the thyroid located in the second intercostal space near the sternum on the right 2. Check for a delayed Achilles return reflex, which is a strong sign of a hypo-functioning thyroid 3. Check for general costochondral tenderness, which is a thyroid indicator 4. Check for pre-tibial edema, which is a sign of a hypo-functioning thyroid 5. Iodine test: Use a tincture of 2% iodine solution, and paint a 3" by 3" square on the client's abdomen. The client is to leave the patch unwashed until it disappears. The square should still be there in 24 hours. If it has disappeared, there is an indication of iodine need 6. Have client assess their basal metabolic temperature by taking their axillary temperature first thing in the morning for 5 straight days. An average temperature below 36.6°C is an indication of hypo-thyroidism

2° Indication

Dysregulation in the ovaries/testicles

Further assessment	1. Check for tenderness in the Chapman reflex for the ovaries/testes located lateral to the pubic symphisis on the rami attachment of the Rectus abdominus muscle.

Supplemental Support

1. Multiple nutrients to support thyroid function with pituitary glandular
2. Potassium iodide
3. Pituitary/hypothalamus tissue (neonatal bovine)
4. Multi-gland (bovine neonatal)
5. Ovary tissue (neonatal bovine)
6. Multi nutrients supporting female endocrine health
7. Orchic tissue (neonatal bovine)
8. Saw palmetto and other nutrients to support prostate health
9. Peruvian maca and deer antler velvet

Lifestyle changes

- Eliminate all refined carbohydrates, alcohol and caffeine (fizzy drinks, coffee, tea and chocolate) from the diet
- Increase fresh raw fruits and vegetables in the diet
- Increase pure water (6-8 cups) daily
- Get adequate rest and exercise

NOTES:

247. Excessive thirst

Excessive thirst is suggestive of a problem in the posterior pituitary gland. The posterior pituitary gland produces Anti diuretic hormone (ADH), which is responsible for regulating water in the body. Thirst is under the control of the thirst centre in the hypothalamus, which triggers the release of ADH to increase the resorption of water in the kidney. Excessive thirst can be due to a hypo functioning in the posterior pituitary and/or hypothalamus causing a decreased secretion of ADH.

Excessive thirst is also a hallmark sign of diabetes; therefore blood sugar control should be assessed.

1° Indication

Hypo functioning of the posterior pituitary in relation to decreased ADH secretion

Further assessment	1. Check for a decreased BUN/creatinine ratio on blood chemistry screen. When the ratio is decreased below 10, this frequently indicates inappropriate secretion of ADH due to posterior pituitary dysfunction.

2° Indication

Blood sugar dysregulation and hypoglycemia.

Further assessment	1. Check for tenderness in the Chapman reflex for the liver-gallbladder located over the 6th intercostal space on the right 2. Check for tenderness in the Liver point located on the 3rd rib, 3 " to the right of the sternum, at the costochondral junction. 3. Check for tenderness underneath the right rib cage 4. Check for tenderness or nodularity in the right thenar pad, which is a pancreas indicator if tender 5. Check for tenderness in the Chapman reflex for the pancreas located in the 7th intercostal space on the left 6. Check for tenderness or guarding at the head of the pancreas located in the upper left quadrant of the abdominal region 1/2 to 2/3 of the way between the umbilicus and the angel of the ribs 7. Check fasting blood glucose 8. Run a six hour glucose-insulin tolerance test.

3° Indication

Low adrenal function

Further assessment	1. Check for tenderness in the inguinal ligament bilaterally 2. Check for tenderness at the medial knee bilaterally, at the insertion of the sartorius muscle at the Pes Anserine. 3. Check for a paradoxical pupillary reflex by shining a light into a client's eye and grading the reaction of the pupil. A pupil that fails to constrict indicates adrenal exhaustion 4. Check for the presence of postural hypotension. A drop of more than 10 points is an indication of adrenal insufficiency 5. Check for a chronic short leg due to a posterior-inferior ilium. 6. Assess for adrenal insufficiency with the Acoustic Cardiogram (ACG), which will show static in both the systolic and diastolic rest phases. You will also see an elevated S2 sound.

Supplemental Support

1. Pituitary/hypothalamus tissue (neonatal bovine)
2. Multi-gland (bovine neonatal)
3. Multiple nutrients for blood sugar handling problems
4. Adrenal tissue (neonatal bovine)
5. High potency multiple nutrients for sugar handling
6. Adaptogenic herbs to support adrenal function

Lifestyle changes

Please see the handout in the appendix on Recommendations for controlling blood sugar

NOTES:

248. Weight gain around hips or waist

Weight gain around the hips or waist is suggestive of a dysfunction in the pituitary gland. Optimal pituitary function is essential for healthy hormonal regulation in the body. The hormonal hierarchy starts with the hypothalamus, which is linked to the central nervous system where, in many cases, the initial stimulus for a hormonal response begins. The pituitary gland acts as a sort of junction box and biological feedback gland between the hypothalamus and the end organs of hormone production. The pituitary can be separated into two distinct portions, the anterior pituitary and the posterior pituitary. The anterior pituitary hormones control peripheral endocrine glands from which an end hormone is released. "Releasing hormones" from the hypothalamus control the release of hormones from the anterior pituitary. Some of the anterior pituitary hormones include somatotropin or growth hormone (GH), follicular stimulating hormone (FSH), Lutenising hormone (LH), adrenocorticotropic hormone (ACTH), thyroid stimulating hormone (TSH) and prolactin. The influence of the anterior pituitary extends from the thyroid to the adrenal glands and the ovaries. In contrast, the hormones of the posterior pituitary are synthesized in the hypothalamus, transported to the posterior pituitary and released by nervous signals. The posterior pituitary produces only two hormones, oxytocin and anti-diuretic hormone, which act directly on the target cell.
Changes in the output of any of the hormones of the pituitary gland can have an impact anywhere in the body, including the metabolism and mobilization of fat around the body.

Supplemental Support

1. Pituitary/hypothalamus tissue (neonatal bovine)
2. Multi-gland (bovine neonatal)

Lifestyle changes

- Eliminate all refined carbohydrates, alcohol and caffeine (fizzy drinks, coffee, tea and chocolate) from the diet
- Increase fresh raw fruits and vegetables in the diet
- Increase pure water (6-8 cups) daily
- Get adequate rest and exercise

NOTES:

249. Menstrual disorders

Menstrual disorders have many possible causes, and should be evaluated by a clinician skilled in identifying the causes. However, many menstrual disorders have origins in the hormonal system and a hypo-functioning pituitary gland can have tremendous impact on menstruation. Optimal pituitary function is essential for healthy hormonal regulation in the body. The hormonal hierarchy starts with the hypothalamus, which is linked to the central nervous system where, in many cases, the initial stimulus for a hormonal response begins. The pituitary gland acts as a sort of junction box and biological feedback gland between the hypothalamus and the end organs of hormone production. The pituitary can be separated into two distinct portions, the anterior pituitary and the posterior pituitary. The anterior pituitary hormones control peripheral endocrine glands from which an end hormone is released. "Releasing hormones" from the hypothalamus control the release of hormones from the anterior pituitary. Some of the anterior pituitary hormones include somatotropin or growth hormone (GH), follicular stimulating hormone (FSH), Lutenising hormone (LH), adrenocorticotropic hormone (ACTH), thyroid stimulating hormone (TSH) and prolactin. The influence of the anterior pituitary extends from the thyroid to the adrenal glands and the ovaries. In contrast, the hormones of the posterior pituitary are synthesized in the hypothalamus, transported to the posterior pituitary and released by nervous signals. The posterior pituitary produces only two hormones, oxytocin and anti-diuretic hormone, which act directly on the target cell.
Decreased activity in the anterior pituitary can lead to decreased output of FSH and LH. This can cause a myriad of symptoms, including menstrual disorders. This question is referring to the possibility of a functional decrease in anterior pituitary activity giving rise to a decreased signal to the end organs of hormonal output: thyroid, adrenals, gonads etc.

1° Indication

Hypo-pituitary function with its impact on the ovaries

Further assessment	1. Check for tenderness in the Chapman reflex for the ovaries located lateral to the pubic symphisis on the rami attachment of the Rectus abdominus muscle.

Supplemental Support

1. Pituitary/hypothalamus tissue (neonatal bovine)
2. Multi-gland (bovine neonatal)
3. Ovary tissue (neonatal bovine)
4. Multi nutrients supporting female endocrine health

Lifestyle changes

- Eliminate all refined carbohydrates, alcohol and caffeine (fizzy drinks, coffee, tea and chocolate) from the diet
- Increase fresh raw fruits and vegetables in the diet
- Increase pure water (6-8 cups) daily
- Get adequate rest and exercise

250. Delayed sexual development (after age 13) (1 = yes, 0 = no)

Delayed sexual development can be a sign of hypo-pituitary function. Optimal pituitary function is essential for healthy hormonal regulation in the body. The hormonal hierarchy starts with the hypothalamus, which is linked to the central nervous system where, in many cases, the initial stimulus for a hormonal response begins. The pituitary gland acts as a sort of junction box and biological feedback gland between the hypothalamus and the end organs of hormone production. The pituitary can be separated into two distinct portions, the anterior pituitary and the posterior pituitary. The anterior pituitary hormones control peripheral endocrine glands from which an end hormone is released. "Releasing hormones" from the hypothalamus control the release of hormones from the anterior pituitary. Some of the anterior pituitary hormones include somatotropin or growth hormone (GH), follicular stimulating hormone (FSH), Lutenising hormone (LH), adrenocorticotropic hormone (ACTH), thyroid stimulating hormone (TSH) and prolactin. The influence of the anterior pituitary extends from the thyroid to the adrenal glands and the ovaries. In contrast, the hormones of the posterior pituitary are synthesized in the hypothalamus, transported to the posterior pituitary and released by nervous signals. The posterior pituitary produces only two hormones, oxytocin and anti-diuretic hormone, which act directly on the target cell.
Decreased activity of the anterior pituitary before puberty can lead to a decreased output of FSH and LH. This can cause a late onset of sexual development. This question is referring to the possibility of a functional decrease in anterior pituitary activity giving rise to decreased signals to the end organs of hormonal output: thyroid, adrenals, gonads etc.

Supplemental Support

1. Pituitary/hypothalamus tissue (neonatal bovine)
2. Multi-gland (bovine neonatal)

Lifestyle changes

- Eliminate all refined carbohydrates, alcohol and caffeine (fizzy drinks, coffee, tea and chocolate) from the diet
- Increase fresh raw fruits and vegetables in the diet
- Increase pure water (6-8 cups) daily
- Get adequate rest and exercise

NOTES:

251. Tendency to ulcers or colitis

This question, at first glance, appears to concern the digestive tract. The primary dysfunction with a tendency towards ulcers and colitis, are gastric hyperacidity and an imbalanced gastrointestinal environment or terrain, with a possible Helicobacter pylori infection. A secondary indication is hypo-pituitary function.

1° Indication

Gastric irritation with possible ulcer and/or H. pylori infection. May be an indication of gastric hyperacidity.

Further assessment	1. Check Ridler HCL reflex for tenderness 1 inch below xyphoid and over to the left edge of the rib cage 2. Check for tenderness in the Chapman reflex for the stomach and upper digestion located in 6th intercostal space on the left 3. Increased urinary indican levels 4. Test for H. pylori 5. Gastric assessment with Gastrotest to determine ambient stomach pH 6. Check for a positive zinc tally: A client holds a solution of aqueous zinc sulfate in their mouth and tells you if and when they can taste it. An almost immediate very bitter taste indicates the client does not need zinc. Clients who are zinc deficient will report no taste from the solution.

2° indication

Hypo-functioning pituitary gland

Supplemental Support

1. Gut healing nutrients and vitamin U 2. Chlorophyllins 3. Deglycerizzinated Licorice 4. Nutrients that heal the intestines	5. Beet juice, taurine, vitamin C and pancreolipase 6. Pancreatic Enzymes 7. Pituitary/hypothalamus tissue (neonatal bovine) 8. Multi-gland (bovine neonatal)

Lifestyle changes

Please see the handout in the appendix on the Diet to aid digestion

NOTES:

THYROID

252. Sensitive/allergic to iodine
253. Difficulty gaining weight, even with large appetite
254. Nervous, emotional, can't work under pressure
255. Inward trembling
256. Flush easily
257. Fast pulse at rest
258. Intolerance to high temperatures
259. Difficulty losing weight
260. Mentally sluggish, reduced initiative
261. Easily fatigued, sleepy during the day
262. Sensitive to cold, poor circulation (cold hands and feet)
263. Constipation, chronic
264. Excessive hair loss and / or coarse hair
265. Morning headaches, wear off during the day
266. Loss of lateral 1/3 of eyebrow
267. Seasonal sadness

252. Sensitive/allergic to iodine

An allergy to iodine is often confused with iodism, a condition of too much iodine in the body, which is marked by tachycardia, skin irritation, thinning of secretions (eyes, nose and saliva), nervousness, and headache. A client may say that they are allergic to iodine, but usually the symptoms they associate with allergy are symptoms of iodism. That is not to say that there are not individuals with allergies to iodine. Generally these are symptoms associated with an overactive thyroid. Iodine is an essential nutrient for optimal thyroid hormone production and activity. The body can become sensitized to iodine if there is too much thyroid hormone floating around the body. If you suspect an allergy to iodine do not perform the iodine skin test.

1° Indication

Increased thyroid function

Further assessment	1. Check for tenderness in the Chapman reflex for the thyroid located in the second intercostal space near the sternum on the right 2. Check for a delayed Achilles return reflex, which is a strong sign of a hypo-functioning thyroid 3. Check for general costochondral tenderness, which is a thyroid indicator 4. Check for pre-tibial edema, which is a sign of a hypo-functioning thyroid 5. Have client assess their basal metabolic temperature by taking their axillary temperature first thing in the morning for 5 straight days. An average temperature below 36.6° is an indication of hypo-thyroidism

Supplemental Support

1. Lithium
2. Thymus tissue (bovine neonatal)
3. Emulsified vitamin A drops
4. Flax Seed Oil

Lifestyle changes

Please see the handout in the appendix on recommendations for dealing with increased thyroid function.

NOTES:

253. Difficulty gaining weight, even with large appetite

Difficulty gaining weight, even with a large appetite, is a symptom of an overactive thyroid. The thyroid gland and the hormones that it produces, act as an accelerator for the metabolism. Increased thyroid hormone can be produced from a thyroid tumor, or by a diffuse goiter, as in Grave's disease, which is marked by increased levels of thyroid stimulating immunoglobulins.

This symptom is also seen in clients with intestinal parasites or extreme cases of dysbiosis. The increased levels of microorganisms will use the food consumed as their source of energy, thus depriving the "host" of the nutrients ingested from their meals.

1° Indication

Increased thyroid function

Further assessment	1. Check for tenderness in the Chapman reflex for the thyroid located in the second intercostal space near sternum on right. 2. Check for general costochondral tenderness, which is a thyroid indicator. 3. Check thyroid panel on Blood chemistry screen. Look for low TSH and high levels of T4. 4. If you suspect a hyperthyroid condition order thyroid antibody studies

2° Indication

Intestinal parasites

Further assessment	1. CBC- look for elevated eosinophils and basophils 2. Stool test for ova and parasite can help detect which parasite, if any, is present. Start with one random stool. If no parasite is found and the index of suspicion is high repeat the stool test, but this time do a purged sample with either a large bolus of vitamin C or magnesium sulfate. Collect the next two stools for testing. 3. Check for tenderness in the Chapman reflex for the colon located bilaterally along the iliotibial band on the thighs. Palpate the colon for tenderness and tension.

Supplemental Support

1. Lithium
2. Thymus tissue (bovine neonatal)
3. Emulsified vitamin A drops
4. Flax Seed Oil
5. Digestive support: Nutrients to heal the intestines, Betaine HCL, Pepsin, & pancreatin
6. Larch arabinogalactans
7. Micro Emulsified Oregano

Lifestyle changes

Please see the handout in the appendix on Recommendations for dealing with increased thyroid function.

254. Nervous, emotional, can't work under pressure
255. Inward trembling

Symptoms of being nervous, emotional, not being able to work under pressure and a sense of inner trembling are suggestive of an overactive thyroid. The thyroid gland and the hormones that it produces, act as an accelerator for the metabolism. Increased thyroid hormone can be produced from a thyroid tumor, or by a diffuse goiter, as in Grave's disease, which is marked by increased levels of thyroid stimulating immunoglobulins.

1° Indication

Increased thyroid function

Further assessment	1. Check for tenderness in the Chapman reflex for the thyroid located in the second intercostal space near the sternum on the right. 2. Check for general costochondral tenderness, which is a thyroid indicator. 3. Check thyroid panel on Blood chemistry screen. Look for low TSH and high levels of T4. 4. If you suspect a hyperthyroid condition order thyroid antibody studies

2° Indication

Vitamin B1 (Thiamine) deficiency

Further assessment	1. An excellent way to assess for Thiamine (vitamin B1) deficiency is with the Acoustic Cardiogram (ACG), which will show a depressed S1 heart sound reading. There will not be enough amplitude in the graph.

Other indications

Adrenal hyper-functioning

Supplemental Support

1. Lithium
2. Thymus tissue (bovine neonatal)
3. Emulsified Vitamin A drops
4. Naturally occurring thiamine

Lifestyle changes

Please see the handout in the appendix on recommendations for dealing with increased thyroid function.

NOTES:

256. Flush easily

Clients who indicate that they get flushed easily may be suffering from liver congestion. Women who are going through menopause may indicate that they experience their hot flashes in the face. Acne Rosacea can have symptoms of flushing. The primary cause of acne rosacea includes hypochlorhydria. An overactive thyroid may also contribute to this symptom.

1° Indication
Liver and gallbladder congestion

Further assessment	1. Check for tenderness in the Chapman reflex for the liver-gallbladder located over the 6th intercostal space on the right 2. Check for tenderness in the Liver point located on the 3rd rib, 3 " to the right of the sternum, at the costochondral junction. 3. Check for tenderness underneath the right rib cage 4. Check for tenderness and nodulation on the web between thumb and fore-finger of right hand

2° Indication
Hypochlorhydria

Further assessment	1. Check Ridler HCL reflex for tenderness 1 inch below xyphoid and over to the left edge of the rib cage 2. Check for tenderness in the Chapman reflex for the stomach and upper digestion located in 6th intercostal space on the left 3. Gastric acid assessment using Gastrotest 4. Check for a positive zinc tally: A client holds a solution of aqueous zinc sulfate in their mouth and tells you if and when they can taste it. An almost immediate very bitter taste indicates the client does not need zinc. Clients who are zinc deficient will report no taste from the solution. 5. Increased urinary indican levels

3° Indication
Increased thyroid function

Further assessment	1. Check for tenderness in the Chapman reflex for the thyroid located in the second intercostal space near the sternum on the right. 2. Check for general costochondral tenderness, which is a thyroid indicator. 3. Check thyroid panel on Blood chemistry screen. Look for low TSH and high levels of T4. 4. If you suspect a hyperthyroid condition order thyroid antibody studies

Supplemental Support

1. Phosphatidylcholine
2. Beet juice, taurine, vitamin C and pancreolipase
3. Beet juice and bile salts
4. Herbs that cleanse the liver
5. Betaine HCL, Pepsin, and pancreatin
6. Pancreatic Enzymes
7. Thymus tissue (bovine neonatal)
8. Lithium

Lifestyle changes

- Please see the handouts in the appendix on Healthy lifestyle for a healthy gallbladder

NOTES:

257. Fast pulse at rest

Dr. Arthur Coca discovered that a fast pulse at rest is a strong indication of allergies. Allergies are overreactions of the immune system and are often precipitated by a disturbance in the digestive system with a dysbiosis. Dysbiosis can be described as an abnormal intestinal flora and an abnormally permeable intestinal mucous membrane. Over time the villi, the large absorptive surface of mucous membranes in the intestines, becomes irritated and inflamed, which causes it to become less dense. Large, incompletely digested macromolecules, especially proteins, start to be able to penetrate the intestinal mucous membrane. Once in the bloodstream, the body's immune system recognizes the small protein or part of a protein as foreign, and produces antibodies against it. It is the reaction of the antibody/antigen complex that produces the classic allergy symptoms.

Another cause of a fast pulse at rest is an overactive thyroid gland. The thyroid gland and the hormones that it produces, act as an accelerator for the metabolism. Increased thyroid hormone can be produced from a thyroid tumor, or by a diffuse goiter, as in Grave's disease, which is marked by increased levels of thyroid stimulating immunoglobulins.

1° Indication

Dysbiosis- abnormal intestinal flora and increased intestinal hyperpermeability

Further assessment	1. Increased urinary indican and sediment levels 2. Stool analysis- either comprehensive digestive analysis or a parasite profile 3. Check for tenderness in the Chapman reflex for the colon located bilaterally along the iliotibial band on the thighs. Palpate the colon for tenderness and tension. 4. Check for tenderness in the Chapman reflex for the small intestine located on the 8th, 9th and 10th intercostal spaces near the tip of the rib. Also palpate four quadrants in a 2” to 3” radius around the umbilicus for tenderness and tension. 5. Decreased secretory IgA on stool analysis.

2° Indication

Increased thyroid function

Further assessment	1. Check for tenderness in the Chapman reflex for the thyroid located in the second intercostal space near the sternum on the right. 2. Check for general costochondral tenderness, which is a thyroid indicator. 3. Check thyroid panel on Blood chemistry screen. Look for low TSH and high levels of T4. 4. With a hyperthyroid condition order thyroid antibody studies

Supplemental Support

1. Micro Emulsified Oregano
2. Nutrients that heal the intestines
3. L-glutamine
4. Lactobacillus acidophilus and Bifidobacterium bifidus
5. Thymus tissue (bovine neonatal)
6. Lithium

NOTES:

258. Intolerance to high temperatures

Being intolerant of high temperatures is suggestive of an overactive thyroid. The thyroid gland and the hormones that it produces, act as an accelerator for the metabolism. Increased thyroid hormone can be produced from a thyroid tumor, or by a diffuse goiter, as in Grave's disease, which is marked by increased levels of thyroid stimulating immunoglobulins.

1° Indication

Increased thyroid function

Further assessment	1. Check for tenderness in the Chapman reflex for the thyroid located in the second intercostal space near the sternum on the right. 2. Check for general costochondral tenderness, which is a thyroid indicator. 3. Check thyroid panel on Blood chemistry screen. Look for low TSH and high levels of T4. 4. If you suspect a hyperthyroid condition order thyroid antibody studies

2° Indication

Vitamin B1 (Thiamine) deficiency

Further assessment	1. An excellent way to assess for Thiamine (vitamin B1) deficiency is with the Acoustic Cardiogram (ACG), which will show a depressed S1 heart sound reading. There will not be enough amplitude in the graph. 2. An increased Anion gap and a decreased CO_2 on a chem. screen is indicative of low thiamine levels.

Supplemental Support

1. Lithium
2. Thymus tissue (bovine neonatal)
3. Emulsified Vitamin A drops
4. Naturally occurring thiamine

Lifestyle changes

Please see the handout in the appendix on recommendations for dealing with increased thyroid function.

NOTES:

259. Difficulty losing weight

A difficulty losing weight is one of the many signs of low thyroid function. The thyroid gland produces thyroid hormone, which acts as an accelerator to the body's metabolism. Some of the common signs and symptoms of hypothyroidism include constipation, weight gain with diminished food intake, cold intolerance, poor circulation, fluid retention, ringing in the ears, poor memory, fatigue, dry skin and hair, hair loss, broken nails, and slow thinking.

Certain lab values may be altered with hypothyroidism. Complete blood counts may show anemia; chemistry screens may show elevated serum cholesterol; thyroid panels may show decreased T3 uptake, total T4 and free T4 with elevated TSH. Some clients may not exhibit any laboratory changes, but have low basal body temperature readings.

There may also be other metabolic issues that will need to be investigated, including liver congestion, poor digestion and blood sugar dysregulation. Body composition analysis is an excellent way to follow clients with difficulty losing weight. It will show lean body mass, % body fat, and metabolic index. It will also indicate the presence of cellular toxicity by showing the balance of intracellular versus extracellular water.

1° Indication

Low thyroid function

Further assessment	1. Check for tenderness in the Chapman reflex for the thyroid located in the right second intercostal space near the sternum 2. Check for a delayed Achilles return reflex, which is a strong sign of a hypo-functioning thyroid 3. Check for general costochondral tenderness, a thyroid indicator 4. Check for pre-tibial edema, a sign of a hypo-functioning thyroid 5. Iodine test: Use a tincture of 2% iodine solution, and paint a 3" by 3" square on the client's abdomen. The client is to leave the patch unwashed until it disappears. The square should still be there in 24 hours. If it has disappeared, there is an indication of iodine need 6. Have client assess their basal metabolic temperature by taking their axillary temperature first thing in the morning for 5 straight days. An average temperature below 36.6° is an indication of hypo-thyroidism. 7. Order a thyroid panel and check TSH, T4, T3, Free T4 and free T3 levels. 8. Any suspected case of hypothyroidism that shows abnormalities on a chem. Screen should have a thyroid antibody study performed.

2° Indication

Vitamin B1 (Thiamine) deficiency

Further assessment	1. An excellent way to assess for Thiamine (vitamin B1) deficiency is with the Acoustic Cardiogram (ACG), which will show a depressed S1 heart sound reading. There will not be enough amplitude in the graph. 2. An increased Anion gap and a decreased CO_2 on a chem. screen is indicative of low thiamine levels.

3° Indication

Assess metabolism

Further assessment	1. Body composition analysis will help determine the ratio of lean body mass to fat. It is very helpful to run on a routine basis to monitor dietary and exercise habits.

Supplemental support

1. Multiple nutrients to support thyroid function with pituitary glandular
2. Potassium iodide
3. Pituitary/hypothalamus tissue (neonatal bovine)
4. Thyroid glandular
5. Naturally occurring thiamine
6. Nutrients to support thyroid function
7. Flax seed oil

Lifestyle changes

Please see the handout in the appendix on recommendations for dealing with low thyroid function

NOTES:

260. Mentally sluggish, reduced initiative
261. Easily fatigued, sleepy during the day

Being mentally sluggish, with reduced initiative and easily fatigued are signs of low thyroid function. The thyroid gland produces thyroid hormone, which acts as an accelerator to the body's metabolism. Some of the common signs and symptoms of hypothyroidism include constipation, weight gain with diminished food intake, cold intolerance, poor circulation, fluid retention, ringing in the ears, poor memory, fatigue, dry skin and hair, hair loss, broken nails, and slow thinking.

Certain lab values may be altered with hypothyroidism. Complete blood counts may show anemia; chemistry screens may show elevated serum cholesterol; thyroid panels may show decreased T3 uptake, total T4 and free T4 with elevated TSH. Some clients may not exhibit any laboratory changes, but have low basal body temperature readings.
The above symptoms are also signs of low adrenal function, which should be thoroughly assessed.

<u>1° Indication</u>
Low thyroid function

Further assessment	1. Check for tenderness in the Chapman reflex for the thyroid located in the right second intercostal space near the sternum 2. Check for a delayed Achilles return reflex, which is a strong sign of a hypo-functioning thyroid 3. Check for general costochondral tenderness, a thyroid indicator 4. Check for pre-tibial edema, a sign of a hypo-functioning thyroid 5. Iodine test: Use a tincture of 2% iodine solution, and paint a 3" by 3" square on the client's abdomen. The client is to leave the patch unwashed until it disappears. The square should still be there in 24 hours. If it has disappeared, there is an indication of iodine need 6. Have client assess their basal metabolic temperature by taking their axillary temperature first thing in the morning for 5 straight days. An average temperature below 36.6° is an indication of hypo-thyroidism. 7. Order a thyroid panel and check TSH, T4, T3, Free T4 and free T3 levels. 8. Any suspected case of hypothyroidism that shows abnormalities on a chem. screen should have a thyroid antibody study performed.

2° indication

Low adrenal function

Further assessment	1. Check for tenderness in the inguinal ligament bilaterally 2. Check for tenderness at the medial knee bilaterally, at the insertion of the sartorius muscle at the Pes Anserine. 3. Check for a paradoxical pupillary reflex by shining a light into a client's eye and grading the reaction of the pupil. A pupil that fails to constrict indicates adrenal exhaustion 4. Check for the presence of postural hypotension. A drop of more than 10 points is an indication of adrenal insufficiency 5. Check for a chronic short leg due to a posterior-inferior ilium. An adrenal indicator when confirmed with postural hypotension and a paradoxical pupillary response. 6. Check the cortisol/DHEA rhythm with an adrenal stress profile 7. Assess for adrenal insufficiency with the Acoustic Cardiogram (ACG), which will show static in both the systolic and diastolic rest phases. You will also see an elevated S2 sound.

Supplemental support

1. Multiple nutrients to support thyroid function with pituitary glandular
2. Potassium iodide
3. Pituitary/hypothalamus tissue (neonatal bovine)
4. Thyroid glandular
5. Nutrients to support thyroid function
6. Flax seed oil
7. Adrenal tissue (bovine neonatal)
8. Adaptogenic herbs to support adrenal function

Lifestyle changes

Please see the handout in the appendix on recommendations for dealing with low thyroid function

NOTES:

262. Sensitive to cold, poor circulation (cold hands and feet)

An increased sensitivity to cold with poor circulation and cold hands and feet are classic signs of low thyroid function. The thyroid gland produces thyroid hormone, which acts as an accelerator to the body's metabolism. Some of the common signs and symptoms of hypothyroidism include constipation, weight gain with diminished food intake, cold intolerance, poor circulation, fluid retention, ringing in the ears, poor memory, fatigue, dry skin and hair, hair loss, broken nails, and slow thinking.

Certain lab values may be altered with hypothyroidism. Complete blood counts may show anemia; chemistry screens may show elevated serum cholesterol; thyroid panels may show decreased T3 uptake, total T4 and free T4 with elevated TSH. Some clients may not exhibit any laboratory changes, but have low basal body temperature readings
It is also important to rule out Raynaud's disease, Raynaud's syndrome and vascular insufficiency. Atherosclerosis of small vessels can contribute to a diminished blood flow to the extremities.

1° Indication
Low thyroid function

Further assessment	1. Check for tenderness in the Chapman reflex for the thyroid located in the right second intercostal space near the sternum 2. Check for a delayed Achilles return reflex, which is a strong sign of a hypo-functioning thyroid 3. Check for general costochondral tenderness, a thyroid indicator 4. Check for pre-tibial edema, a sign of a hypo-functioning thyroid 5. Iodine test: Use a tincture of 2% iodine solution, and paint a 3" by 3" square on the client's abdomen. The client is to leave the patch unwashed until it disappears. The square should still be there in 24 hours. If it has disappeared, there is an indication of iodine need 6. Have client assess their basal metabolic temperature by taking their axillary temperature first thing in the morning for 5 straight days. An average temperature below 36.6° is an indication of hypo-thyroidism. 7. Order a thyroid panel and check TSH, T4, T3, Free T4 and free T3 levels. 8. Any suspected case of hypothyroidism that shows abnormalities on a chem. screen should have a thyroid antibody study performed.

Other indications
Raynaud's disease and syndrome
Atherosclerosis (cold hands and feet)

Supplemental support

1. Multiple nutrients to support thyroid function with pituitary glandular
2. Potassium iodide
3. Pituitary/hypothalamus tissue (neonatal bovine)
4. Thyroid glandular
5. Naturally occurring thiamine
6. Nutrients to support thyroid function
7. Flax seed oil

Lifestyle changes

Please see the handout in the appendix on recommendations for dealing with low thyroid function

263. Constipation, chronic

Constipation is a subjective symptom where stools are too hard, too small, too infrequent, difficult to expel, or when the client has a feeling of incomplete evacuation after the bowel movement is over. Other objective signs are fewer than *3-5* stools per week, or more than 3 days without a stool. Average bowel transit time is 50-100 hours. The optimum bowel transit time is 17-30 hours. From a functional perspective a client should be considered constipated if a day passes without a bowel movement. Even if the client has a bowel movement every day, there still may be problems. Any significant, sudden change in bowel habits can be a sign of organic disease and must therefore be pursued.

The most common cause of constipation is a lack of dietary fiber and adequate hydration. Many people do not take their supplementary fiber with adequate amounts of water. This can make the constipation much worse, and cause the stool to be harder and more difficult to pass. Treating constipation is a process of trying one approach, seeing if it works and if it doesn't moving to the next step. Following. A low functioning thyroid can also be a cause for chronic constipation.

<u>1° Indication</u>

Assess the colon for lack of fiber and adequate hydration.

Further assessment	1. Have a client check their bowel transit time. Give 6 "00" caps of activated charcoal and ask them to record how long it takes for the black to appear and to go completely away. Various dyes, including beets, sweetcorn, and un-popped popcorn can also be used. 2. Assess the client's hydration status. Have client stand with hands by their side and check and palpate the veins in the right hand. Have them slowly raise their hand to heart level and see if the veins still stick out. Veins that are only just visible or not visible at all are a sign of dehydration 3. Check for tenderness in the Chapman reflex for the colon located bilaterally along the iliotibial band on the thighs. 4. Palpate the colon for tenderness and tension.

<u>2° Indication</u>

Low thyroid function

Further assessment	1. Check for tenderness in the Chapman reflex for the thyroid located in the right second intercostal space near the sternum 2. Check for a delayed Achilles return reflex, which is a strong sign of a hypo-functioning thyroid 3. Check for general costochondral tenderness, a thyroid indicator 4. Check for pre-tibial edema, a sign of a hypo-functioning thyroid 5. Iodine test: Use a tincture of 2% iodine solution, and paint a 3" by 3" square on the client's abdomen. The client is to leave the patch unwashed until it disappears. The square should still be there in 24 hours. If it has disappeared, there is an

	indication of iodine need 6. Have client assess their basal metabolic temperature by taking their axillary temperature first thing in the morning for 5 straight days. An average temperature below 36.6° is an indication of hypo-thyroidism. 7. Order a thyroid panel and check TSH, T4, T3, Free T4 and free T3 levels. 8. Any suspected case of hypothyroidism that shows abnormalities on a chem. screen should have a thyroid antibody study performed.

Supplemental support

1. Water soluble fiber and colon health nutrients
2. Betaine HCL, Pepsin, and pancreatin
3. Thyroid glandular
4. Multiple nutrients to support thyroid function with pituitary glandular
5. Potassium iodide

Lifestyle changes

Please see the handout in the appendix on recommendations for dealing with low thyroid function

NOTES:

264. Excessive hair loss and / or coarse hair

Excessive hair loss and/or coarse hair are classic symptoms of low thyroid function. The thyroid gland produces thyroid hormone, which acts as an accelerator to the body's metabolism. Some of the common signs and symptoms of hypothyroidism include constipation, weight gain with diminished food intake, cold intolerance, poor circulation, fluid retention, ringing in the ears, poor memory, fatigue, dry skin and hair, hair loss, broken nails, and slow thinking.

Certain lab values may be altered with hypothyroidism. Complete blood counts may show anemia; chemistry screens may show elevated serum cholesterol; thyroid panel's may show decreased T3 uptake, total T4 and free T4 with elevated TSH. Some clients may not exhibit any laboratory changes, but have low basal body temperature readings. Excessive hair loss and/or coarse hair are also signs of essential fatty acid deficiency and/or poor protein assimilation.

1° Indication

Low thyroid function

Further assessment	1. Check for tenderness in the Chapman reflex for the thyroid located in the right second intercostal space near the sternum 2. Check for a delayed Achilles return reflex, which is a strong sign of a hypo-functioning thyroid 3. Check for general costochondral tenderness, a thyroid indicator 4. Check for pre-tibial edema, a sign of a hypo-functioning thyroid 5. Iodine test: Use a tincture of 2% iodine solution, and paint a 3" by 3" square on the client's abdomen. The client is to leave the patch unwashed until it disappears. The square should still be there in 24 hours. If it has disappeared, there is an indication of iodine need 6. Have client assess their basal metabolic temperature by taking their axillary temperature first thing in the morning for 5 straight days. An average temperature below 36.6° is an indication of hypo-thyroidism. 7. Order a thyroid panel and check TSH, T4, T3, Free T4 and free T3 levels. 8. Any suspected case of hypothyroidism that shows abnormalities on a chem. screen should have a thyroid antibody study performed.

2° Indication

Essential fatty acid insufficiency.

Further assessment	1. Oral pH less that 7.2 indicates essential fatty acid deficiency 2. Repeated muscle challenge. This challenge involves a simple, normal muscle test repeated once per second, 20 times with regular intensity. As in a standard muscle test, the joint is positioned in such a way that the muscle to be tested is shortened. The practitioner applies pressure to the joint to lengthen the muscle, until a "locking" is noted. A positive result occurs when "locking" of the muscle and joint does not occur, indicating deficient free fatty acids. 3. Fatty acid profile via laboratory testing of blood

Supplemental support

1. Multiple nutrients to support thyroid function with pituitary glandular
2. Potassium iodide
3. Pituitary/hypothalamus tissue (neonatal bovine)
4. Nutrients to support thyroid function
5. Flax Seed Oil
6. Mixed fatty acids (walnut, hazelnut, sesame, and apricot)
7. EPA and DHA from fish oil
8. Black Currant Seed Oil

Lifestyle changes

Please see the handout in the appendix on recommendations for dealing with low thyroid function

NOTES:

265. Morning headaches, wear off during the day

Morning headaches that wear off during the day are a sign of a low functioning thyroid gland and/or hypoglycemia. It is important to rule out and correct any structural component and to assess how often these headaches happen.

The thyroid gland produces thyroid hormone, which acts as an accelerator to the body's metabolism. Some of the common signs and symptoms of hypothyroidism include constipation, weight gain with diminished food intake, cold intolerance, poor circulation, fluid retention, ringing in the ears, poor memory, fatigue, dry skin and hair, hair loss, broken nails, and slow thinking.

Certain lab values may be altered with hypothyroidism. Complete blood counts may show anemia; chemistry screens may show elevated serum cholesterol; thyroid panel's may show decreased T3 uptake, total T4 and free T4 with elevated TSH. Some clients may not exhibit any laboratory changes, but have low basal body temperature readings.

1° Indication

Low thyroid function

Further assessment	1. Check for tenderness in the Chapman reflex for the thyroid located in the right second intercostal space near the sternum 2. Check for a delayed Achilles return reflex, which is a strong sign of a hypo-functioning thyroid 3. Check for general costochondral tenderness, a thyroid indicator 4. Check for pre-tibial edema, a sign of a hypo-functioning thyroid 5. Iodine test: Use a tincture of 2% iodine solution, and paint a 3" by 3" square on the client's abdomen. The client is to leave the patch unwashed until it disappears. The square should still be there in 24 hours. If it has disappeared, there is an indication of iodine need 6. Have client assess their basal metabolic temperature by taking their axillary temperature first thing in the morning for 5 straight days. An average temperature below 36.6° is an indication of hypo-thyroidism. 7. Order a thyroid panel and check TSH, T4, T3, Free T4 and free T3 levels. 8. Any suspected case of hypothyroidism that shows abnormalities on a chem. screen should have a thyroid antibody study performed.

2° Indication

Blood sugar dysregulation and hypoglycemia.

Further assessment	1. Check for tenderness in the Chapman reflex for the liver-gallbladder located over the 6th intercostal space on the right 2. Check for tenderness in the Liver point located on the 3rd rib, 3 " to the right of the sternum, at the costochondral junction.

	3. Check for tenderness underneath the right rib cage 4. Check for tenderness or nodularity in the right thenar pad, which is a pancreas indicator if tender 5. Check for tenderness in the Chapman reflex for the pancreas located in the 7th intercostal space on the left 6. Check for tenderness or guarding at the head of the pancreas located in the upper left quadrant of the abdominal region 1/2 to 2/3 of the way between the umbilicus and the angel of the ribs 7. Check fasting blood glucose 8. Run a six hour glucose-insulin tolerance test.

Supplemental support

1. Multiple nutrients to support thyroid function with pituitary glandular
2. Potassium iodide
3. Pituitary/hypothalamus tissue (neonatal bovine)
4. Thyroid glandular
5. Multiple nutrients for blood sugar handling problems
6. Nutrients to support thyroid function
7. Flax Seed Oil
8. Adrenal tissue (bovine neonatal)

Lifestyle changes

Please see the handout in the appendix on recommendations for dealing with low thyroid function

NOTES:

266. Loss of lateral 1/3 of eyebrow

The loss of lateral 1/3 of the eyebrows is a sign of a low functioning thyroid gland. It is hard to find a reason why this is so except that it is! Clinical observation has shown that a person with a hypofunctioning thyroid gland is more susceptible to losing hair from their eyebrows. It may have something to do with the way low thyroid hormone levels affect the hair. In hypothyroidism the hair is typically sparse, coarse and falls out easily. The hair follicles of the eyebrows may be particularly sensitive.

The thyroid gland produces thyroid hormone, which acts as an accelerator to the body's metabolism. Some of the common signs and symptoms of hypothyroidism include constipation, weight gain with diminished food intake, cold intolerance, poor circulation, fluid retention, ringing in the ears, poor memory, fatigue, dry skin and hair, hair loss, broken nails, and slow thinking.

Certain lab values may be altered with hypothyroidism. Complete blood counts may show anemia; chemistry screens may show elevated serum cholesterol; thyroid panel's may show decreased T3 uptake, total T4 and free T4 with elevated TSH. Some clients may not exhibit any laboratory changes, but have low basal body temperature readings.

<u>1° Indication</u>
Low thyroid function

Further assessment	1. Check for tenderness in the Chapman reflex for the thyroid located in the right second intercostal space near the sternum 2. Check for a delayed Achilles return reflex, which is a strong sign of a hypo-functioning thyroid 3. Check for general costochondral tenderness, a thyroid indicator 4. Check for pre-tibial edema, a sign of a hypo-functioning thyroid 5. Iodine test: Use a tincture of 2% iodine solution, and paint a 3" by 3" square on the client's abdomen. The client is to leave the patch unwashed until it disappears. The square should still be there in 24 hours. If it has disappeared, there is an indication of iodine need 6. Have client assess their basal metabolic temperature by taking their axillary temperature first thing in the morning for 5 straight days. An average temperature below 36.6° is an indication of hypo-thyroidism. 7. Order a thyroid panel and check TSH, T4, T3, Free T4 and free T3 levels. 8. Any suspected case of hypothyroidism that shows abnormalities on a chem. screen should have a thyroid antibody study performed.

Supplemental support

1. Multiple nutrients to support thyroid function with pituitary glandular
2. Potassium iodide
3. Pituitary/hypothalamus tissue (neonatal bovine)
4. Nutrients to support thyroid function
5. Flax Seed Oil
6. Thyroid glandular

Lifestyle changes

Please see the handout in the appendix on recommendations for dealing with low thyroid function.

NOTES:

267. Seasonal sadness

Seasonal sadness is a sign of a low functioning thyroid gland and low adrenal function. It is often due to interruptions in the diurnal rhythms of the body, which will alter adrenal hormone output. This is especially true during the winter months in the northern latitudes. The pituitary gland is especially sensitive to shifts in daylight and this will affect the output of both TSH (which stimulates the thyroid gland) and ACTH (which stimulates the adrenal glands to produce cortisol). Therefore, an assessment of the adrenal glands is called for.

The thyroid gland produces thyroid hormone, which acts as an accelerator to the body's metabolism. Some of the common signs and symptoms of hypothyroidism include constipation, weight gain with diminished food intake, cold intolerance, poor circulation, fluid retention, ringing in the ears, poor memory, fatigue, dry skin and hair, hair loss, broken nails, and slow thinking.

Certain lab values may be altered with hypothyroidism. Complete blood counts may show anemia; chemistry screens may show elevated serum cholesterol; thyroid panel's may show decreased T3 uptake, total T4 and free T4 with elevated TSH. Some clients may not exhibit any laboratory changes, but have low basal body temperature readings.

<u>1° indication</u>

Low thyroid function

Further assessment	1. Check for tenderness in the Chapman reflex for the thyroid located in the right second intercostal space near the sternum 2. Check for a delayed Achilles return reflex, which is a strong sign of a hypo-functioning thyroid 3. Check for general costochondral tenderness, a thyroid indicator 4. Check for pre-tibial edema, a sign of a hypo-functioning thyroid 5. Iodine test: Use a tincture of 2% iodine solution, and paint a 3" by 3" square on the client's abdomen. The client is to leave the patch unwashed until it disappears. The square should still be there in 24 hours. If it has disappeared, there is an indication of iodine need 6. Have client assess their basal metabolic temperature by taking their axillary temperature first thing in the morning for 5 straight days. An average temperature below 36.6° is an indication of hypo-thyroidism. 7. Order a thyroid panel and check TSH, T4, T3, Free T4 and free T3 levels. 8. Any suspected case of hypothyroidism that shows abnormalities on a chem. screen should have a thyroid antibody study performed.

Supplemental support

1. Multiple nutrients to support thyroid function with pituitary glandular
2. Potassium iodide
3. Pituitary/hypothalamus tissue (neonatal bovine)
4. Nutrients to support thyroid function
5. Flax seed oil
6. Thyroid glandular

Lifestyle changes

Please see the handout in the appendix on recommendations for dealing with low thyroid function.

NOTES:

MALE ONLY

268. Prostate problems
269. Difficulty with urination, dribbling
270. Difficult to start and stop urine stream
271. Pain or burning with urination
272. Waking to urinate at night
273. Interruption of stream during urination
274. Pain on inside of legs or heels
275. Feeling of incomplete bowel evacuation
276. Decreased sexual function

268. Prostate problems
269. Urination difficult or dribbling
270. Difficult to start and stop urine stream

The above symptoms are highly suggestive of prostatic problems. The prostate is a small gland that surrounds the urethra. Symptoms of urinary frequency, urgency, nocturia, hesitancy and intermittency with decreased size and force of the urinary stream with sensations of incomplete emptying, terminal dribbling, continuous overflow incontinence, or complete urinary retention, are indicative of Benign Prostatic Hypertrophy or BPH. 50-60% of males between the ages of 40-59 years have BPH and by age 80 90% of all males have BPH with 75% having prostate cancer according to biopsy.

Pain in the prostate is not necessarily related to infection of the prostate; only 5% of all prostatitis is bacterial, usually E. coli. Any swelling or inflammation of the prostate causes constriction to the urethra, hence all the urinary symptoms.

BPH may be due to increased levels of di-hydrotestosterone (DHT), which stimulates prostate growth. There are also prostaglandins, nutrient deficiencies and altered sex hormones as possible causes.

It is important to run appropriate lab work on these clients to assess creatinine, PSA and Prostatic Acid Phosphatase (PAP) levels. It is also essential to either perform or refer out for a digital rectal examination. This is to be considered an annual screening exam for men over 45, because prostate cancer is becoming an epidemic in this country.
With Prostatic problems make sure you rule out the following: sensitivity to dairy products, obesity, infrequent sexual activity, hereditary factors and lack of exercise.

1° Indication
Prostatic dysfunction with a likelihood of Benign Prostatic hypertrophy (BPH)

Further assessment	1. Check for tenderness in the Chapman's reflex for the prostate located lateral to the pubic symphisis on the rami 2. Check for tenderness in the middle portion of the illio-tibial band, an indicator for the prostate 3. Check creatinine levels on a blood chemistry screen. If the client has a creatinine 1.2 or > they have a developing prostate problem e.g. BPH. PSA will only show prostatic problem when it's too late. 4. Check client's PSA and PAP levels to follow course of therapy 5. Check client's zinc levels with a zinc test

Supplemental Support

1. Saw palmetto and other nutrients to support prostate health
2. Essential fatty acids: EPA and DHA from fish oil and/or flax seed oil
3. Nutritional zinc
4. Potassium iodide

Lifestyle changes: Please see handout in appendix on recommendations for the prostate

271. Pain or burning with urination

Pain or burning with urination is a sign of a urinary tract infection (UTI). UTIs are fairly uncommon in men and should be investigated with the appropriate urinalysis and lab work. This may be a more common symptom in older men, who are at an increased risk of Benign Prostatic Hypertrophy, which can lead to prostatitis. It is important to remember that pain with urination may not necessarily be related to infection of the prostate; only 5% of all prostatitis is bacterial, usually E. coli. Any swelling or inflammation of the prostate causes constriction to the urethra, hence all the urinary symptoms. A thorough evaluation should be performed to rule out the possibility of kidney involvement.

1° Indication

Possible UTI and BPH

Further assessment	1. Check for nitrites, lymphocytes and RBCs in the urine. If necessary order or perform urine culture and microscopy. 2. Check for tenderness in the Chapman's reflex for the prostate located lateral to the pubic symphisis on the rami 3. Check for tenderness in the middle portion of the illio-tibial band, an indicator for the prostate 4. Check creatinine levels on a blood chemistry screen. If the client has a creatinine 1.2 or > they have a developing prostate problem e.g. BPH. PSA will only show prostatic problem when it's too late. 5. Check client's PSA and PAP levels to follow course of therapy 6. Check client's zinc levels with a zinc tally test

Supplemental Support

1. Saw palmetto and other nutrients to support prostate health
2. Essential fatty acids: EPA and DHA from fish oil and/or flax seed oil
3. Nutritional zinc
4. Potassium iodide

Lifestyle changes

Please see the handout in the appendix on recommendations for the prostate

NOTES:

272. Waking to urinate at night
273. Interruption of stream during urination
274. Pain on inside of legs or heels

The above symptoms are highly suggestive of prostatic problems. The prostate is a small gland that surrounds the urethra. Symptoms of urinary frequency, urgency, nocturia, hesitancy and intermittency with decreased size and force of the urinary stream with sensations of incomplete emptying, terminal dribbling, continuous overflow incontinence, or complete urinary retention, are indicative of Benign Prostatic Hypertrophy or BPH. 50-60% of males between the ages of 40-59 years have BPH and by age 80 90% of all males have BPH with 75% having prostate cancer according to biopsy.

BPH may be due to increased levels of di-hydrotestosterone (DHT), which stimulates prostate growth. There are also prostaglandins, nutrient deficiencies and altered sex hormones as possible causes.

It is important to run appropriate lab work on these clients to assess creatinine, PSA and Prostatic Acid Phosphatase (PAP) levels. It is also essential to either perform or refer out for a digital rectal examination. This is to be considered an annual screening exam for men over 45, because prostate cancer is becoming an epidemic in this country.

With Prostatic problems make sure you rule out the following: sensitivity to dairy products, obesity, infrequent sexual activity, hereditary factors and lack of exercise.

1° Indication

Prostatic dysfunction with a likelihood of Benign Prostatic hypertrophy (BPH)

Further assessment	1. Check for tenderness in the Chapman's reflex for the prostate located lateral to the pubic symphisis on the rami 2. Check for tenderness in the middle portion of the illio-tibial band, an indicator for the prostate 3. Check creatinine levels on a blood chemistry screen. If the client has a creatinine 1.2 or > they have a developing prostate problem e.g. BPH. PSA will only show prostatic problem when it's too late. 4. Check client's PSA and PAP levels to follow course of therapy 5. Check client's zinc levels with a zinc tally test

Supplemental Support

5. Saw palmetto and other nutrients to support prostate health 6. Essential fatty acids: EPA and DHA from fish oil and/or flax seed oil 7. Nutritional zinc 8. Potassium iodide

Lifestyle changes

Please see the handout in the appendix on recommendations for the prostate

275. Feeling of incomplete bowel evacuation

A feeling of incomplete bowel evacuation is a symptom of either Prostatic difficulty or liver congestion. Some of the other symptoms of BPH include: urinary frequency, urgency, nocturia, hesitancy and intermittency with decreased size and force of the urinary stream with sensations of incomplete emptying, terminal dribbling, continuous overflow incontinence, or complete urinary retention. The prostate is a small gland that surrounds the urethra. Any swelling or inflammation of the prostate causes constriction to the urethra, hence all of the above urinary symptoms.

It is important to run appropriate lab work on these clients to assess creatinine, PSA and Prostatic Acid Phosphatase (PAP) levels. It is also essential to either perform or refer out for a digital rectal examination. This is to be considered an annual screening exam for men over 45, because prostate cancer is becoming an epidemic in this country.

With Prostatic problems make sure you rule out the following: sensitivity to dairy products, obesity, infrequent sexual activity, hereditary factors and lack of exercise.

<u>1° Indication</u>

Prostatic dysfunction with a likelihood of Benign Prostatic hypertrophy (BPH)

Further assessment	1. Check for tenderness in the Chapman's reflex for the prostate located lateral to the pubic symphisis on the rami 2. Check for tenderness in the middle portion of the illio-tibial band, an indicator for the prostate 3. Check creatinine levels on a blood chemistry screen. If the client has a creatinine 1.2 or > they have a developing prostate problem e.g. BPH. PSA will only show prostatic problem when it's too late. 4. Check client's PSA and PAP levels to follow course of therapy 5. Check client's zinc levels with a zinc tally test

<u>2° indication</u>

Liver congestion

Further assessment	1. Check for tenderness in the Chapman reflex for the liver-gallbladder located over the 6th intercostal space on the right 2. Check for tenderness in the Liver point located on the 3rd rib, 3 " to the right of the sternum, at the costochondral junction. 3. Check for tenderness underneath the right rib cage 4. Check for tenderness and nodulation on the web between thumb and fore-finger of right hand 5. Assess for Hepato-biliary congestion with the Acoustic Cardiogram (ACG), which will show post-systolic rounding due to increased backpressure on the pulmonic and aortic valve. It may also show through to the tricuspid valve if chronic.

Supplemental Support

1. Saw palmetto and other nutrients to support prostate health
2. EPA and DHA from fish oil
3. Nutritional Zinc
4. Flax Seed Oil
5. Potassium iodide
6. Beet juice and bile salts
7. Herbs that cleanse the liver
8. Glutathione, cysteine, and Glycine
9. Powdered detoxification support formula

Lifestyle changes

Please see the handout in the appendix on recommendations for the prostate

NOTES:

276. Decreased sexual function

Decreased sexual function may be due to some kind of prostate difficulty or Benign Prostatic Hypertrophy (swelling of the prostate gland).

The prostate is a small gland that surrounds the urethra. Symptoms of urinary frequency, urgency, nocturia, hesitancy and intermittency with decreased size and force of the urinary stream with sensations of incomplete emptying, terminal dribbling, continuous overflow incontinence, or complete urinary retention, are indicative of Benign Prostatic Hypertrophy or BPH. 50-60% of males between the ages of 40-59 years have BPH and by age 80 90% of all males have BPH with 75% having prostate cancer according to biopsy. Pain in the prostate is not necessarily related to infection of the prostate; only 5% of all prostatitis is bacterial, usually E. coli. Any swelling or inflammation of the prostate causes constriction to the urethra, hence all the urinary symptoms.

BPH may be due to increased levels of di-hydrotestosterone (DHT), which stimulates prostate growth. There are also prostaglandins, nutrient deficiencies and altered sex hormones as possible causes.

It is important to run appropriate lab work on these clients to assess creatinine, PSA and Prostatic Acid Phosphatase (PAP) levels. It is also essential to either perform or refer out for a digital rectal examination. This is to be considered an annual screening exam for men over 45, because prostate cancer is becoming an epidemic in this country.
With Prostatic problems make sure you rule out the following: sensitivity to dairy products, obesity, infrequent sexual activity, hereditary factors and lack of exercise.

1° Indication

Prostatic dysfunction with a likelihood of Benign Prostatic hypertrophy (BPH)

Further assessment	1. Check for tenderness in the Chapman's reflex for the prostate located lateral to the pubic symphisis on the rami 2. Check for tenderness in the middle portion of the illio-tibial band, an indicator for the prostate 3. Check creatinine levels on a blood chemistry screen. If the client has a creatinine 1.2 or > they have a developing prostate problem e.g. BPH. PSA will only show prostatic problem when it's too late. 4. Check client's PSA and PAP levels to follow course of therapy 5. Check client's zinc levels with a zinc tally test

Supplemental Support

9. Saw palmetto and other nutrients to support prostate health
10. Essential fatty acids: EPA and DHA from fish oil and/or flax seed oil
11. Nutritional zinc
12. Potassium iodide

Lifestyle changes

Please see the handout in the appendix on recommendations for the prostate

FEMALE ONLY

277. Depression during periods
278. Mood swings associated with periods (PMS)
279. Crave chocolate around periods
280. Breast tenderness associated with cycle
281. Excessive menstrual flow
282. Scanty blood flow during periods
283. Occasional skipped periods
284. Variations in menstrual cycles
285. Endometriosis
286. Uterine fibroids
287. Breast fibroids, benign masses
288. Painful intercourse (dyspareunia)
289. Vaginal discharge
290. Vaginal dryness
291. Vaginal itchiness
292. Gain weight around hips, thighs and buttocks
293. Excess facial or body hair
294. Hot flashes
295. Night sweats (in menopausal females)
296. Thinning skin

277. Depression during periods

Depression during the period is often a sign of magnesium deficiency or low thyroid function. There has been some interesting work done that postulates low serotonin levels in some women after ovulation and into menstruation. Low serotonin levels are linked to depression. There is evidence that estrogen levels have some impact on serotonin levels in the body.

1° Indication
Magnesium deficiency

Further assessment	1. Assess for mineral deficiency using Tissue mineral assessment test. Place a standard blood pressure cuff around the largest portion of the client's calf muscle (sitting). Instruct the client to let you know when they feel the onset of cramping pain and gradually inflate the cuff. Stop and deflate immediately when threshold has been reached. Less than 200 mmHg is considered deficient in minerals. Use the neurolingual testing to challenge the body with several different types of minerals and other co-factors to see which combination of minerals and co-factors increases the threshold above 200mmHg. 2. Assess for mineral insufficiency by using Dr. Kane's mineral assessment tests. 3. Assess the impact of mineral deficiencies on the body's acid buffering capacities by using Dr. Bieler's salivary pH acid challenge.

2° Indication
Thyroid dysfunction

Further assessment	1. Check for tenderness in the Chapman reflex for the thyroid located in the right second intercostal space near the sternum 2. Check for a delayed Achilles return reflex, which is a strong sign of a hypo-functioning thyroid 3. Check for general costochondral tenderness, a thyroid indicator 4. Check for pre-tibial edema, a sign of a hypo-functioning thyroid 5. Iodine test: Use a tincture of 2% iodine solution, and paint a 3" by 3" square on the client's abdomen. The client is to leave the patch unwashed until it disappears. The square should still be there in 24 hours. If it has disappeared, there is an indication of iodine need 6. Have client assess their basal metabolic temperature by taking their axillary temperature first thing in the morning for 5 straight days. An average temperature below 36.6° is an indication of hypo-thyroidism. 7. Order a thyroid panel and check TSH, T4, T3, Free T4 and free T3 levels. 8. Any suspected case of hypothyroidism that shows abnormalities on a chem. screen should have a thyroid antibody study performed.

Other indications

1. B6 deficiency
2. Increased refined carbohydrates in diet
3. Hypoglycemia
4. Essential fatty acid need

Supplemental support

1. Magnesium
2. Calcium and magnesium formula with or without parathyroid tissue
3. Multiple nutrients to support thyroid function with pituitary glandular
4. Potassium iodide
5. Flax Seed Oil

Lifestyle changes

Please see the handout in the appendix on recommendations for a healthy menstrual cycle

NOTES:

278. Mood swings associated with periods (PMS)

PMS seems to be most common in women in their 30's and 40's, but may occur at puberty or later in life. It is believed that as many as one third to one half of women between the ages of twenty and fifty are affected. PMS may run in families or may start as a result of pregnancy, hysterectomy, birth control pills, or tubal ligation.

PMS symptoms usually begin ten to fourteen days prior to the onset of the menstrual period, and become progressively worse until the onset of menstruation or, for some women, several days after the onset. More than 150 symptoms have been documented and can affect almost every organ system of the body.

There are a number of theories that attempt to explain why PMS occurs. No one theory is universally accepted. Though, one of the most widely accepted theories for PMS is an imbalance between the ovarian hormones estrogen and progesterone. Estrogen is the principle hormone in the early part of the cycle, the follicular phase, joined by progesterone at mid-cycle, ovulation. Both estrogen and progesterone decrease about 5 days before the next menstrual period. It is felt that PMS may be due to an imbalance in the normal ratio of progesterone to estrogen. Some PMS sufferers have higher levels of estrogen or lower levels of progesterone; others have lower levels of estrogen and higher levels of progesterone.

There are other factors in the body that have an impact on the hormonal regulation. The liver helps convert estrogen to its proper metabolites for circulation. Thyroid hormone has effects that regulate estrogen levels. The pineal gland secretes a hormone that also regulates estrogen production. Another hormone, prolactin, is secreted in response to stress, estrogen, oral contraceptives, and lactation, and inhibits progesterone production, and thereby aggravates the problem.

Nutritional supplementation has been shown to be effective for the treatment of PMS. The most important nutrients to consider are the B vitamins, especially B6, vitamins A and E, and the minerals calcium and magnesium.

Vitamin B6: Supplementation with vitamin B6 improves hepatic clearance of estrogen. In studies with rats, B6 blocks estrogen metabolism. Although PMS is of multifactorial origin, B6 supplementation alone appears to benefit most clients.

Vitamin A: Vitamin A deficiency has been associated with increased estrogen levels. New research suggests that vitamin A is needed to synthesize progesterone; therefore a deficiency can disrupt the balance of estrogen to progesterone. PMS symptoms have been reduced with supplemental vitamin A, though beta-carotene may be a better choice, as it is less toxic than Vitamin A.

Vitamin E: In studies on vitamin E, the PMS symptoms of anxiety, headache, fatigue, depression and insomnia were all significantly reduced despite a lack of deficiency of vitamin E.

Magnesium: Magnesium deficiency can cause hyperirritability to the muscular and nervous systems. Hyperirritable nerves can result in emotional irritability and nervousness. Magnesium has been shown to cause a major reduction in water retention, behavioral changes, and mood swings.

Calcium: A diet that averages 500-1300 mg a day in calcium shows a marked reduction in the symptoms of PMS across the board. The exact mechanism is not understood.

1° Indication

Need for increased liver function

Further assessment	1. Check for tenderness in the Chapman reflex for the liver-gallbladder located over the 6th intercostal space on the right 2. Check for tenderness in the Liver point located on the 3rd rib, 3 " to the right of the sternum, at the costochondral junction. 3. Check for tenderness underneath the right rib cage 4. Increased SGOT, SGPT on a blood chemistry panel 5. Various labs do liver detoxification panels 6. Assess for Hepato-biliary congestion with the Acoustic Cardiogram (ACG), which will show post-systolic rounding due to increased backpressure on the pulmonic and aortic valve. It may also show through to the tricuspid valve if chronic.

2° Indication

Low Thyroid function

Further assessment	1. Check for tenderness in the Chapman reflex for the thyroid located in the right second intercostal space near the sternum 2. Check for a delayed Achilles return reflex, which is a strong sign of a hypo-functioning thyroid 3. Check for general costochondral tenderness, a thyroid indicator 4. Check for pre-tibial edema, a sign of a hypo-functioning thyroid 5. Iodine test: Use a tincture of 2% iodine solution, and paint a 3" by 3" square on the client's abdomen. The client is to leave the patch unwashed until it disappears. The square should still be there in 24 hours. If it has disappeared, there is an indication of iodine need 6. Have client assess their basal metabolic temperature by taking their axillary temperature first thing in the morning for 5 straight days. An average temperature below 36.6° is an indication of hypo-thyroidism. 7. Order a thyroid panel and check TSH, T4, T3, Free T4 and free T3 levels. 8. Any suspected case of hypothyroidism that shows abnormalities on a chem. screen should have a thyroid antibody study performed.

3° Indication

Imbalanced progesterone to estrogen ratio

Further assessment	1. Assess client's hormonal status across the menstrual cycle with a cycling female salivary hormone assessment.

Other indications

1. B vitamin need
2. Magnesium need
3. Imbalance in pituitary output
4. Essential fatty acid need
5. Blood sugar dysregulation

Supplemental support

1. Multi nutrients supporting female endocrine health
2. Nutrients to support Phase II liver detoxification
3. Beet juice, taurine, vitamin C and pancreolipase
4. Magnesium
5. Black Currant Seed Oil
6. Herbs that cleanse the liver
7. Ovarian tissue (bovine neonatal)
8. Pituitary/hypothalamus tissue (neonatal bovine)

Lifestyle changes

Please see the handout in the appendix on Recommendations for a healthy menstrual cycle

NOTES:

279. Crave chocolate around periods

Craving chocolate around the time of the period is a sign of magnesium deficiency. It may also be a sign of blood sugar abnormalities and a need for adrenal support. The period is a time of hormonal upheaval and the body may be having a more difficult time controlling blood sugar.

1° Indication

Magnesium deficiency

Further assessment	1. Assess for mineral deficiency using Tissue mineral assessment test. Place a standard blood pressure cuff around the largest portion of the client's calf muscle (sitting). Instruct the client to let you know when they feel the onset of cramping pain and gradually inflate the cuff. Stop and deflate immediately when threshold has been reached. Less than 200 mmHg is considered deficient in minerals. Use the neurolingual testing to challenge the body with several different types of minerals and other co-factors to see which combination of minerals and co-factors increases the threshold above 200mmHg. 2. Assess for mineral insufficiency by using Dr. Kane's mineral assessment tests. 3. Assess the impact of mineral deficiencies on the body's acid buffering capacities by using Dr. Bieler's salivary pH acid challenge.

2° Indication

Blood sugar dysregulation and hypoglycemia.

Further assessment	1. Check for tenderness in the Chapman reflex for the liver-gallbladder located over the 6th intercostal space on the right 2. Check for tenderness in the Liver point located on the 3rd rib, 3 " to the right of the sternum, at the costochondral junction. 3. Check for tenderness underneath the right rib cage 4. Check for tenderness or nodularity in the right thenar pad, which is a pancreas indicator if tender 5. Check for tenderness in the Chapman reflex for the pancreas located in the 7th intercostal space on the left 6. Check for tenderness or guarding at the head of the pancreas located in the upper left quadrant of the abdominal region 1/2 to 2/3 of the way between the umbilicus and the angel of the ribs 7. Check for tenderness in the inguinal ligament bilaterally, an adrenal indicator 8. Check for tenderness at the medial knee bilaterally, at the insertion of the sartorius muscle at the Pes Anserine. This is an adrenal indicator. 9. Check for a paradoxical pupillary reflex by shining a light into

	a client's eye and grading the reaction of the pupil. A pupil that fails to constrict indicates adrenal exhaustion 10. Check for the presence of postural hypotension. A drop of more than 10 points is an indication of adrenal insufficiency 11. Check for a chronic short leg due to a posterior-inferior ilium. An adrenal indicator when confirmed with postural hypotension and a paradoxical pupillary response. 12. Check fasting blood glucose 13. Run a six hour glucose-insulin tolerance test.

Supplemental Support

1. Magnesium
2. Calcium and magnesium formula with or without parathyroid tissue
3. Multiple nutrients for blood sugar handling problems
4. Adaptogenic herbs to support adrenal function
5. Adrenal tissue (neonatal bovine)
6. Beet juice, taurine, vitamin C and pancreolipase
7. Pancreatic tissue (neonatal bovine)
8. Herbs that cleanse the liver

Lifestyle changes

Please see the handout in the appendix on recommendations for a healthy menstrual cycle

NOTES:

280. Breast tenderness associated with cycle

A woman's health throughout her menstrual cycle is like a barometer for her overall health. Many disorders in the body can be mirrored in the menstrual cycle. Breast tenderness associated with the menstrual cycle is one such symptom, which indicates a need for liver support. Symptoms associated with the menstrual cycle can also indicate dysbiosis, thyroid or adrenal problems and colon support.

1° Indication

Liver dysfunction

Further assessment	1. Check for tenderness in the Chapman reflex for the liver-gallbladder located over the 6th intercostal space on the right side 2. Check for tenderness in the Liver point located on the 3rd rib, 3 " to the right of the sternum, at the costochondral junction. 3. Check for tenderness underneath the right rib cage 4. Increased SGOT, SGPT on a blood chemistry panel 5. Various labs do liver detoxification panels 6. Assess for Hepato-biliary congestion with the Acoustic Cardiogram (ACG), which will show post-systolic rounding due to increased backpressure on the pulmonic and aortic valve. It may also show through to the tricuspid valve if chronic.

Other indications

1. Dysbiosis
2. Low thyroid function
3. Adrenal insufficiency
4. Need for colon support

Supplemental Support

1. Multi nutrients supporting female endocrine health
2. Nutrients to support Phase II liver detoxification
3. Ovarian tissue (neonatal bovine)
4. Beet juice, taurine, vitamin C and pancreolipase
5. Magnesium
6. Black currant seed oil

Lifestyle changes

Please see the handout in the appendix on Recommendations for a healthy menstrual cycle

NOTES:

281. Excessive menstrual flow

An average blood loss during a period is 60 - 250 ml or 20 menstrual pads. It is important to determine just what excessive menstrual flow means to your client. Excessive menstrual flow or menorrhagia can be an indication of something serious: pregnancy, endometriosis, cervical cancer, polyps and endometrial hyperplasic to name but a few. Therefore it is essential to rule out serious pathology. One of the problems with excessive menstrual flow is the likelihood of developing iron deficiency anemia. Doing a CBC to monitor red blood cell indices is indicated to make sure any anemia is being treated. Another important screening test is to run a pregnancy test.

In the absence of any serious pathology excessive menstrual flow can be a sign of general health disturbances in the body.

1° Indication

Need for increased liver function

Further assessment	1. Check for tenderness in the Chapman reflex for the liver-gallbladder located over the 6th intercostal space on the right side 2. Check for tenderness in the Liver point located on the 3rd rib, 3 " to the right of the sternum, at the costochondral junction. 3. Check for tenderness underneath the right rib cage 4. Increased SGOT, SGPT on a blood chemistry panel 5. Assess for Hepato-biliary congestion with the Acoustic Cardiogram (ACG), which will show post-systolic rounding due to increased backpressure on the pulmonic and aortic valve. It may also show through to the tricuspid valve if chronic.

Other indications

1. Dysbiosis
2. Low thyroid function
3. Adrenal insufficiency
4. Need for colon support

Supplemental Support

1. Multi nutrients supporting female endocrine health
2. Nutrients to support Phase II liver detoxification
3. Ovarian tissue (neonatal bovine)
4. Beet juice, taurine, vitamin C and pancreolipase
5. Magnesium
6. Black Currant Seed Oil

Lifestyle changes

Please see the handout in the appendix on Recommendations for a healthy menstrual cycle

282. Scanty blood flow during periods

A scanty flow during menstruation can be an indication of anemia. Deficient iron in the body can trigger the body to conserve blood during the period. Another strong possibility is a generalized hormonal deficit in this client that is causing a reduced flow during the menses. There are other factors in the body that have an impact on the hormonal regulation. The liver helps convert estrogen to its proper metabolites for excretion. Thyroid hormone has effects that regulate estrogen levels. The pineal gland secretes a hormone that also regulates estrogen production. Another hormone, prolactin, is secreted in response to stress, estrogen, oral contraceptives, and lactation, and inhibits progesterone production, and thereby aggravates the problem.

1° Indication

Need for increased liver function

Further assessment	1. Check for tenderness in the Chapman reflex for the liver-gallbladder located over the 6th intercostal space on the right side 2. Check for tenderness in the Liver point located on the 3rd rib, 3 " to the right of the sternum, at the costochondral junction. 3. Check for tenderness underneath the right rib cage 4. Increased SGOT, SGPT on a blood chemistry panel 5. Various labs do liver detoxification panels 6. Assess for Hepato-biliary congestion with the Acoustic Cardiogram (ACG), which will show post-systolic rounding due to increased backpressure on the pulmonic and aortic valve. It may also show through to the tricuspid valve if chronic.

2° Indication

Low Thyroid function

Further assessment	1. Check for tenderness in the Chapman reflex for the thyroid located in the second intercostal space near the sternum on the right 2. Check for a delayed Achilles return reflex, which is a strong sign of a hypo-functioning thyroid 3. Check for general costochondral tenderness, which is a thyroid indicator 4. Check for pre-tibial edema, which is a sign of a hypo-functioning thyroid 5. Iodine test: Use a tincture of 2% iodine solution, and paint a 3" by 3" square on the client's abdomen. The client is to leave the patch unwashed until it disappears. The square should still be there in 24 hours. If it has disappeared, there is an indication of iodine need 6. Have client assess their basal metabolic temperature by taking their axillary temperature first thing in the morning for 5 straight days. An average temperature below 36.6° is an indication of hypo-thyroidism

3° Indication

Monitor for anemia

Further assessment	1. Assess anemia from blood chemistry and CBC for possible nutritional causes

Supplemental support

1. Multi nutrients supporting female endocrine health
2. Nutrients to support Phase II liver detoxification
3. Beet juice, taurine, vitamin C and pancreolipase
4. Magnesium
5. Black Currant Seed Oil
6. Herbs that cleanse the liver
7. Ovarian tissue (neonatal bovine)
8. Pituitary/hypothalamus tissue (neonatal bovine)

Lifestyle changes

Please see the handout in the appendix on recommendations for a healthy menstrual cycle

NOTES:

283. Occasional skipped periods

Occasional skipped periods indicate a condition called amenorrhea. To evaluate amenorrhea it is necessary to know what would be considered normal menstruation. The duration of a menstrual cycle is 28 ± 3 days for about 65% of women, with a possible range of 18 to 40 days; once a menstrual pattern has been established it tends not to fluctuate by more than 5 days. The average duration of flow is 5 ± 2 days with a blood loss averaging 130 ml, usually heavier on the second day.

There are three main categories of amenorrhea:

1. Primary amenorrhea where menstruation has never happened.
2. Secondary amenorrhea when menstruation stops after at least one period. This is a common occurrence with causes including pregnancy, stress, loss or gain of weight, adrenal and/or thyroid dysfunction, menopause, breast-feeding, anemia, excessive exercise, stopping contraceptive pill intake, some drugs, ovarian cysts or tumors, problems in the hypothalamus and/or pituitary etc.
3. Erratic or irregular menstruation. There may be 3 or 4 periods in a year, or 3 close together followed by none for a few months. A similar range of cause is possible.

Doing a cycling female salivary hormone panel will give some very useful information, as would looking at FSH and LH levels. Any sexually active woman who presents with problems with the menstrual cycle should have a screening pregnancy test performed. An unknown pregnancy will cause many of the problems seen in the menstrual cycle.

1° indication

Need for adrenal support

Further assessment	1. Check for tenderness in the inguinal ligament bilaterally 2. Check for tenderness at the medial knee bilaterally, at the insertion of the sartorius muscle at the Pes Anserine. 3. Check for a paradoxical pupillary reflex by shining a light into a client's eye and grading the reaction of the pupil. A pupil that fails to constrict indicates adrenal exhaustion 4. Check for the presence of postural hypotension. A drop of more than 10 points is an indication of adrenal insufficiency 5. Check for a chronic short leg due to a posterior-inferior ilium. An adrenal indicator when confirmed with postural hypotension and a paradoxical pupillary response. 6. Check the cortisol/DHEA rhythm with a salivary adrenal stress index 7. Increased chloride in the urine is a sign of low adrenal function 8. Assess for adrenal insufficiency with the Acoustic Cardiogram (ACG), which will show static in both the systolic and diastolic rest phases. You will also see an elevated S2 sound.

2° Indication

Thyroid dysfunction

Further assessment	1. Check for tenderness in the Chapman reflex for the thyroid located in the second intercostal space near the sternum on the right 2. Check for a delayed Achilles return reflex, which is a strong sign of a hypo-functioning thyroid 3. Check for general costochondral tenderness, which is a thyroid indicator 4. Check for pre-tibial edema, which is a sign of a hypo-functioning thyroid 5. Iodine test: Use a tincture of 2% iodine solution, and paint a 3" by 3" square on the client's abdomen. The client is to leave the patch unwashed until it disappears. The square should still be there in 24 hours. If it has disappeared, there is an indication of iodine need 6. Have client assess their basal metabolic temperature by taking their axillary temperature first thing in the morning for 5 straight days. An average temperature below 36.6° is an indication of hypo-thyroidism

Supplemental Support

1. Multi nutrients supporting female endocrine health
2. Adrenal tissue (neonatal bovine)
3. Adaptogenic herbs to support adrenal function
4. Pituitary/hypothalamus tissue (neonatal bovine)
5. Ovarian tissue (neonatal bovine)
6. Beet juice, taurine, vitamin C and pancreolipase
7. Magnesium
8. Black Currant Seed Oil

Lifestyle changes

Please see the handout in the appendix on recommendations for a healthy menstrual cycle

NOTES:

284. Variations in menstrual cycles

Depending on a woman's age, variations in the menstrual cycle can indicate a peri-menopausal state. The year or so before the onset of menopause a woman should expect to see her periods beginning to fluctuate. If the client is in her teens, 20s or 30s any variation of the menstrual cycle can be problematic, and should be assessed for secondary amenorrhea. Secondary amenorrhea occurs when menstruation stops after at least one period. This is a common occurrence with causes including pregnancy, stress, loss or gain of weight, adrenal and/or thyroid dysfunction, menopause, breast-feeding, anemia, excessive exercise, stopping contraceptive pill intake, some drugs, ovarian cysts or tumors, problems in the hypothalamus and/or pituitary etc.

1° indication

Need for adrenal support

Further assessment	1. Check for tenderness in the inguinal ligament bilaterally 2. Check for tenderness at the medial knee bilaterally, at the insertion of the sartorius muscle at the Pes Anserine. 3. Check for a paradoxical pupillary reflex by shining a light into a client's eye and grading the reaction of the pupil. A pupil that fails to constrict indicates adrenal exhaustion 4. Check for the presence of postural hypotension. A drop of more than 10 points is an indication of adrenal insufficiency 5. Check for a chronic short leg due to a posterior-inferior ilium. An adrenal indicator when confirmed with postural hypotension and a paradoxical pupillary response. 6. Check the cortisol/DHEA rhythm with a salivary adrenal stress index e.g. ASI

2° Indication

Thyroid dysfunction

Further assessment	1. Check for tenderness in the Chapman reflex for the thyroid located in the right second intercostal space near the sternum 2. Check for a delayed Achilles return reflex, which is a strong sign of a hypo-functioning thyroid 3. Check for general costochondral tenderness, a thyroid indicator 4. Check for pre-tibial edema, a sign of a hypo-functioning thyroid 5. Iodine test: Use a tincture of 2% iodine solution, and paint a 3" by 3" square on the client's abdomen. The client is to leave the patch unwashed until it disappears. The square should still be there in 24 hours. If it has disappeared, there is an indication of iodine need 6. Have client assess their basal metabolic temperature by taking their axillary temperature first thing in the morning for 5 straight days. An average temperature below 36.6° is an indication of hypo-thyroidism.

	7. Order a thyroid panel and check TSH, T4, T3, Free T4 and free T3 levels. 8. Any suspected case of hypothyroidism that shows abnormalities on a chem. screen should have a thyroid antibody study performed.

3° Indication

Assess female hormones

Further assessment	1. Assess female hormones by running a cycling female salivary hormone panel 2. Assess pituitary hormonal influences by running serum FSH and LH levels

Supplemental Support

1. Multi nutrients supporting female endocrine health
2. Adrenal tissue (neonatal bovine)
3. Adaptogenic herbs to support adrenal function
4. Pituitary/hypothalamus tissue (neonatal bovine)
5. Ovarian tissue (neonatal bovine)
6. Beet juice, taurine, vitamin C and pancreolipase
7. Magnesium
8. Black Currant Seed Oil

Lifestyle changes

Please see the handout in the appendix on recommendations for a healthy menstrual cycle

NOTES:

285. Endometriosis

Endometriosis is a condition marked by retrograde movement of uterine tissue through the fallopian tubes. Ectopic endometrial tissue migrates out of the uterus and can implant anywhere in the pelvic or abdominal cavity. This tissue then goes through the menstrual cycle just as if it were normal endometrium, and responds to ovarian hormones like estrogen. It can be extremely painful and cause many compilations.

There is no known cause of this disease but general hormone dysfunction can play a large part, as can liver detoxification problems, dysbiosis and the general build up of toxicity in the body.

It is a difficult disorder to diagnose without the aid of laparoscopic surgery, as many of the routine lab tests are negative. It may be useful to assess the liver as well. General treatment and balancing of the body can be very helpful for people with endometriosis.

1° Indication
Assess uterus and ovaries

Further assessment	1. Check for tenderness in the Chapman reflex for the ovaries and uterus located lateral to the pubic symphisis on the rami attachment of the Rectus abdominus muscle. 2. Check for tenderness in the Chapman reflex for the uterus located in the middle portion of the iliotibial band bilaterally

2° Indication
Need for increased liver function

Further assessment	1. Check for tenderness in the Chapman reflex for the liver-gallbladder located over the 6th intercostal space on the right side 2. Check for tenderness in the Liver point located on the 3rd rib, 3 " to the right of the sternum, at the costochondral junction. 3. Check for tenderness underneath the right rib cage 4. Increased SGOT, SGPT on a blood chemistry panel 5. Various labs do liver detoxification panels 6. Assess for Hepato-biliary congestion with the Acoustic Cardiogram (ACG), which will show post-systolic rounding due to increased backpressure on the pulmonic and aortic valve. It may also show through to the tricuspid valve if chronic.

Supplemental support

1. Multi nutrients supporting female endocrine health
2. Nutrients to support Phase II liver detoxification
3. Beet juice, taurine, vitamin C and pancreolipase
4. Herbs that cleanse the liver
5. Black Currant Seed Oil
6. Herbs that cleanse the liver
7. Adrenal tissue (bovine neonatal)
8. Pituitary/hypothalamus tissue (neonatal bovine)

Lifestyle changes

FOODS TO INCLUDE

a. **Foods high in fiber:** whole grain breads, brown rice, raw vegetables, ground flax seeds
b. **High protein vegetarian diet**
   i. Animal fats, especially red meat, increase inflammatory prostaglandins and thus inflammation and pain
   ii. **Vegetable proteins** include: almond and other nut butters, salmon and other fatty fish, beans
c. **Increase intake of vegetables** especially liver-friendly vegetables
   i. Liver-friendly foods include carrots, kale, cabbage family vegetables: broccoli, Brussels sprouts, cabbage and cauliflower, beet root, artichokes, lemons, dandelion greens, watercress, onions, garlic and leeks.
d. **Use seasonings** such as turmeric, ginger
e. Grind a tablespoon of ground flax seeds and put in cereals and salads

FOODS TO AVOID

a. **Sugar**
b. **Caffeine**- endometriosis is found to be associated with caffeine consumption especially coffee
c. **Dairy**- Milk, cottage cheese and cheese will tip the balance in favor of prostaglandins that cause inflammation, smooth muscle contraction and vascular constriction
d. **Alcohol**- depletes B vitamins in the liver and has an estrogenic effects on the body
e. **All sources of hydrogenated oils**

NOTES:

286. Uterine fibroids

Uterine fibroids are the most common benign tumor in women. They tend to be estrogen dependent and their growth corresponds with rises and falls in estrogen levels. Their growth tends to increase during pregnancy and estrogen therapy, and tends to shrink during menopause. They can be an indication of a need for extra liver support, as the liver is responsible for clearing up estrogen in the body. They may also be an indication of dysbiosis in the body.

<u>1° Indication</u>

Need for increased liver function

Further assessment	1. Check for tenderness in the Chapman reflex for the liver-gallbladder located over the 6th intercostal space on the right side 2. Check for tenderness in the Liver point located on the 3rd rib, 3 " to the right of the sternum, at the costochondral junction. 3. Check for tenderness underneath the right rib cage 4. Increased SGOT, SGPT on a blood chemistry panel 5. Various labs do liver detoxification panels 6. Assess for Hepato-biliary congestion with the Acoustic Cardiogram (ACG), which will show post-systolic rounding due to increased backpressure on the pulmonic and aortic valve. It may also show through to the tricuspid valve if chronic.

<u>2° Indication</u>

Dysbiosis

Further assessment	1. Increased urinary indican 2. Stool analysis- either comprehensive digestive analysis or a parasite profile 3. Check for tenderness in the Chapman reflex for the colon located bilaterally along the iliotibial band on the thighs. Palpate the colon for tenderness and tension. 4. Check for tenderness in the Chapman reflex for the small intestine located on the 8th, 9th and 10th intercostal spaces near the tip of the rib. Also palpate four quadrants in a 2" to 3" radius around the umbilicus for tenderness and tension. 5. Decreased secretory IgA on stool analysis.

<u>Other indications</u>

1. Essential fatty acid deficiency
2. Allergies

Supplemental support

1. Multi nutrients supporting female endocrine health
2. Nutrients to support Phase II liver detoxification
3. Beet juice, taurine, vitamin C and pancreolipase
4. Herbs that cleanse the liver
5. Black Currant Seed Oil
6. Herbs that cleanse the liver
7. Micro Emulsified Oregano
8. Nutrients that heal the intestines

Lifestyle changes

FOODS TO INCLUDE

a. **Foods high in fiber:** whole grain breads, brown rice, raw vegetables, ground flax seeds
b. **High protein vegetarian diet**
    i. Animal fats, especially red meat, increase inflammatory prostaglandins and thus inflammation and pain
    ii. **Vegetable proteins** include: almond and other nut butters, salmon and other fatty fish, beans
c. **Increase intake of vegetables** especially liver-friendly vegetables
    i. Liver-friendly foods include carrots, kale, cabbage family vegetables: broccoli, Brussels sprouts, cabbage and cauliflower, beet root, artichokes, lemons, dandelion greens, watercress, onions, garlic and leeks.
d. **Use seasonings** such as turmeric, ginger
e. Grind a tablespoon of ground flax seeds and put in cereals and salads

FOODS TO AVOID

a. **Sugar**
b. **Caffeine**- endometriosis is found to be associated with caffeine consumption especially coffee
c. **Dairy**- Milk, cottage cheese and cheese will tip the balance in favor of prostaglandins that cause inflammation, smooth muscle contraction and vascular constriction
d. **Alcohol**- depletes B vitamins in the liver and has an estrogenic effects on the body
e. **All sources of hydrogenated oils**

NOTES:

287. Breast fibroids, benign masses

Breast fibroids, fibrocystic breast disease and benign masses in the breast are characterized by a growth of fibrous tissues that most frequently appears in the 30s and 40s but disappears with menopause. Whilst uncomfortable they are not dangerous, with up to 20% of women developing them to some degree during their lives.

These masses are largely influenced by hormonal fluctuations, becoming larger and more painful just prior to the onset of menstrual bleeding. The key to successful treatment lies in normalizing hormonal fluctuations and treating the liver, as these masses are a strong indication of a need for additional liver support. These conditions have been associated with an abnormal estrogen to progesterone ratio and the liver plays an important role in clearing the body of excess hormones. If the liver is not working well, and is congested, the hormones can increase and cause these types of problems.

There has been a strong association with the consumption of caffeine and other methylxanthines and breast fibroids. It is important for clients with this complaint to stop all forms of caffeine at once.

Dr. Jonathan Wright and Dr Alan Gaby have taught that fibrocystic breast disease is related to thyroid deficient and iodine deficiency. Using supplemental iodine can be very helpful for this condition, but you must monitor thyroid hormone levels with a thyroid panel.

1° Indication

Need for increased liver function

Further assessment	1. Check for tenderness in the Chapman reflex for the liver-gallbladder located over the 6th intercostal space on the right side 2. Check for tenderness in the Liver point located on the 3rd rib, 3 " to the right of the sternum, at the costochondral junction. 3. Check for tenderness underneath the right rib cage 4. Increased SGOT, SGPT on a blood chemistry panel 5. Various labs do liver detoxification panels 6. Assess for Hepato-biliary congestion with the Acoustic Cardiogram (ACG), which will show post-systolic rounding due to increased backpressure on the pulmonic and aortic valve. It may also show through to the tricuspid valve if chronic.

2° Indication

Assess female hormones

Further assessment	1. Assess female hormones by running a cycling female salivary hormone panel 2. Assess pituitary hormonal influences by running serum FSH and LH levels

3° Indication

Assess thyroid and iodine insufficiency

Further assessment	1. Check for tenderness in the Chapman reflex for the thyroid located in the right second intercostal space near the sternum 2. Check for a delayed Achilles return reflex, which is a strong sign of a hypo-functioning thyroid 3. Check for general costochondral tenderness, a thyroid indicator 4. Check for pre-tibial edema, a sign of a hypo-functioning thyroid 5. Iodine test: Use a tincture of 2% iodine solution, and paint a 3" by 3" square on the client's abdomen. The client is to leave the patch unwashed until it disappears. The square should still be there in 24 hours. If it has disappeared, there is an indication of iodine need 6. Have client assess their basal metabolic temperature by taking their axillary temperature first thing in the morning for 5 straight days. An average temperature below 36.6° is an indication of hypo-thyroidism. 7. Order a thyroid panel and check TSH, T4, T3, Free T4 and free T3 levels. 8. Any suspected case of hypothyroidism that shows abnormalities on a chem. screen should have a thyroid antibody study performed.

Supplemental Support

1. Multi nutrients supporting female endocrine health
2. Nutrients to support Phase II liver detoxification
3. Herbs that cleanse the liver
4. Potassium iodide
5. Powdered detoxification formula
6. Glutathione, cysteine, and Glycine

Lifestyle changes

Please see the handout in the appendix on recommendations for a healthy menstrual cycle and also the handout for dealing with low thyroid function.

NOTES:

288. Painful intercourse (dyspareunia)

Dyspareunia is associated with menopausal changes in the vaginal tissue. As the hormones begin to change in menopause, the tissue of the vagina begins to atrophy and thin causing painful intercourse. In a woman prior to menopause, painful intercourse can be associated with candidiasis.

1° Indication

Assess female hormones

Further assessment	1. Assess female hormones by running a post-menopause female salivary hormone panel 2. Assess pituitary hormonal influences by running serum FSH and LH levels

2° Indication

Dysbiosis with Candida overgrowth

Further assessment	1. Increased urinary indican 2. Stool analysis- either comprehensive digestive analysis or a Candida profile 3. Check for tenderness in the Chapman reflex for the colon located bilaterally along the iliotibial band on the thighs. Palpate the colon for tenderness and tension. 4. Check for tenderness in the Chapman reflex for the small intestine located on the 8th, 9th and 10th intercostal spaces near the tip of the rib. Also palpate four quadrants in a 2" to 3" radius around the umbilicus for tenderness and tension. 5. Decreased secretory IgA on stool analysis.

Other indications

Need for Vitamin A, Vitamin E and Zinc

Supplemental support

1. Multi nutrients supporting female endocrine health
2. Emulsified vitamin A drops
3. Emulsified vitamin E
4. Micro Emulsified Oregano
5. Nutrients that heal the intestines
6. Water soluble fiber and nutrients to support healthy colon
7. Lactobacillus acidophilus and Bifidobacterium bifidus

NOTES:

289. Vaginal discharge
290. Vaginal dryness
291. Vaginal itchiness

Vaginal discharge and/or itching are indications of candidiasis or dysbiosis. Perform a smear for testing in the office, or refer out to another clinician. It is important to know what it is you are dealing with.

Vaginal dryness is a problem associated with peri-menopause or menopause.

1° Indication

Dysbiosis with Candida overgrowth

Further assessment	1. Increased urinary indican 2. Stool analysis- either comprehensive digestive analysis or a Candida profile 3. Check for tenderness in the Chapman reflex for the colon located bilaterally along the iliotibial band on the thighs. Palpate the colon for tenderness and tension. 4. Check for tenderness in the Chapman reflex for the small intestine located on the 8th, 9th and 10th intercostal spaces near the tip of the rib. Also palpate four quadrants in a 2" to 3" radius around the umbilicus for tenderness and tension. 5. Decreased secretory IgA on stool analysis.

2° Indication

Assess female hormones

Further assessment	1. Assess female hormones by running a cycling female or a post menopausal salivary hormone panel

Supplemental Support

1. Micro Emulsified Oregano
2. Nutrients that heal the intestines
3. Betaine HCL, Pepsin, and pancreatin
4. Multi nutrients supporting female endocrine health
5. Water soluble fiber and colon health nutrients
6. Multiple nutrients that support the immune system
7. Lactobacillus acidophilus and Bifidobacterium bifidus

Lifestyle changes

Please see the handout in the appendix on the dysbiosis diet

NOTES:

292. Gain weight around hips, thighs and buttocks

Gaining weight around the hips thighs and buttocks is an indication of either female hormone imbalance or blood sugar dysregulation.

1° Indication
Assess female hormones

Further assessment	2. Assess female hormones by running a cycling female or a post menopausal salivary hormone panel

2° Indication
Blood sugar dysregulation

Further assessment	1. Check for tenderness in the Chapman reflex for the liver-gallbladder located over the 6th intercostal space on the right side 2. Check for tenderness in the Liver point located on the 3rd rib, 3 " to the right of the sternum, at the costochondral junction. 3. Check for tenderness underneath the right rib cage 4. Check for tenderness in the Chapman reflex for the pancreas located in the 7th intercostal space on the left 5. Check for tenderness or guarding at the head of the pancreas located in the upper left quadrant of the abdominal region 1/2 to 2/3 of the way between the umbilicus and the angel of the ribs 6. Check for tenderness or nodularity in the right thenar pad, which is a pancreas indicator if tender 7. Run a fasting glucose and/or a six hour glucose insulin tolerance test

Supplemental support

1. Multi nutrients supporting female endocrine health
2. Multiple nutrients for blood sugar handling problems
3. Adrenal tissue (neonatal bovine)
4. Beet juice, taurine, vitamin C and pancreolipase

NOTES:

293. Excess facial or body hair

Excess facial hair is called hirsuitism and is often associated with androgen hormone excess. It can also be an indication of a pituitary dysfunction. Optimal pituitary function is essential for healthy hormonal regulation in the body. The hormonal hierarchy starts with the hypothalamus, which is linked to the central nervous system where, in many cases, the initial stimulus for a hormonal response begins. The pituitary gland acts as a sort of junction box and biological feedback gland between the hypothalamus and the end organs of hormone production.

The pituitary can be separated into two distinct portions, the anterior pituitary and the posterior pituitary. The anterior pituitary hormones control peripheral endocrine glands from which an end hormone is released. "Releasing hormones" from the hypothalamus control the release of hormones from the anterior pituitary. Some of the anterior pituitary hormones include somatotropin or growth hormone (GH), follicular stimulating hormone (FSH), Lutenising hormone (LH), adrenocorticotropic hormone (ACTH), thyroid stimulating hormone (TSH) and prolactin. The influence of the anterior pituitary extends from the thyroid to the adrenal glands and the ovaries. In contrast, the hormones of the posterior pituitary are synthesized in the hypothalamus, transported to the posterior pituitary and released by nervous signals. The posterior pituitary produces only two hormones, oxytocin and anti-diuretic hormone, which act directly on the target cell.

Increased facial hair may be due to too much stimulation for the production of testosterone and other androgen hormones.

1° Indication

Assess female hormones

Further assessment	1. Assess female hormones by running a cycling female salivary hormone panel 2. Assess pituitary hormonal influences by running serum FSH and LH levels

2° Indication

Assess ovaries

Further assessment	1. Check for tenderness in the Chapman reflex for the ovaries located lateral to the pubic symphisis on the rami attachment of the Rectus abdominus muscle.

Supplemental support

1. Multi nutrients supporting female endocrine health
2. Pituitary/hypothalamus tissue (neonatal bovine)

NOTES:

294. Hot flashes
295. Night sweats (in menopausal females)
296. Thinning skin

These are all symptoms associated with menopause, a time of dramatic hormonal changes in a woman's body. Menopause is defined as the cessation of menses (periods), which is caused by the body's decreased production of sex hormones (estrogen and progesterone). Most women will experience the beginning of menopause between ages 50 and 55, although some women may note changes earlier. Surgical menopause is caused by removal of the ovaries and uterus.

There are three phases of menopause:

1. The climacteric phase in which the periods become irregular;
2. Actual menopause which is the last menstrual cycle, diagnosed only in retrospect and
3. Post-menopause which begins one year after the cessation of the menses. In this last phase, there may be signs of declining estrogen.

The most common symptoms resulting from the menopausal decline in estrogen secretion are hot flashes or flushing, feelings of warmth and sweating. About 85 % of women over age 50 are affected. The onset is sudden, and when associated with palpitation, dizziness or faintness, they can be a frightening experience. Emotional stress, exercise, alcohol and certain foods can bring them on in some individuals. Typically they occur several times a day and last a few minutes at a time.

As the hormones begin to change in menopause, the tissue of the vagina begins to atrophy and thin causing painful intercourse. Doing a general assessment of function in the body and assessing the levels of female hormones is an important place to start.

1° Indication

Assess female hormones

Further assessment	1. Assess female hormones by running a cycling female salivary hormone panel 2. Assess pituitary hormonal influences by running serum FSH and LH levels

Supplemental support

1. Multi nutrients supporting female endocrine health
2. Flax Seed Oil
3. Beet juice, taurine, vitamin C and pancreolipase
4. Adrenal tissue (neonatal bovine)
5. Black Currant Seed Oil

Lifestyle changes

Diet:

1. A vegetarian diet with occasional chicken and fish
2. Avoid all caffeine (tea, coffee, chocolate, cola) and sugars. Alcohol consumption adds a burden to the liver.
3. Avoid all sources of hydrogenated oils
4. Include in your diet: whole grains (wheat, spelt, oat, barley, millet, rye, quinoa), fresh fruit and vegetables at least 5 servings each day (raw or steamed is best).
5. Liver cleansing foods are beets, artichokes, and carrots (raw or puree)
6. Licorice root extract 20-30 drops in ½ cup of water up to 3 times a day will help support the adrenal glands which will continue to produce estrogen (in small amounts) when the ovaries stop.

Exercise: Regular daily exercise that you *enjoy* is most important to enhance circulation and help bones keep their strength and prevent osteoporosis. Walking/running, T'ai Chi, dance/movement, etc. are a few examples.

Relaxation: A balance between exercise and our work is essential, so relaxation needs to be part of our daily routine. Meditation, Yoga, relaxation tapes, and massage are some suggestions.

NOTES:

CARDIOVASCULAR

297. Aware of heavy and / or irregular breathing
298. Discomfort at high altitudes
299. "Air hunger" and / or yawn frequently
300. Compelled to open windows in a closed room
301. Shortness of breath with moderate exertion
302. Ankles swell, especially at end of day
303. Cough at night
304. Blush or face turns red for no reason
305. Dull pain or tightness in chest and / or radiate into right arm, worse with exertion
306. Muscle cramps with exertion

297. Aware of heavy and / or irregular breathing
298. Discomfort at high altitudes
299. "Air hunger" and / or sigh frequently
300. Compelled to open windows in a closed room
301. Shortness of breath with moderate exertion
302. Ankles swell, especially at end of day

The heart is one area to do both a thorough traditional cardiac workup in addition to a nutritional assessment. If you do not these assessments in your office, refer out to a local cardiologist. It is important to protect the life of the client, and any of the above symptoms could be symptoms of an impending cardiovascular incident. An acute condition such as a myocardial infarct is best left up to the traditional doctors, who treat acute things well. Long-term conditions respond well to nutritional and dietary therapies.

Heart disease can be split up into two different categories, each with a different presentation:

Congestive type
Characterized by low blood pressure and a craving for sugar. They often feel bad or run down and get sick often. They need Vitamin B1 (thiamine) and are generally thyroid types.

Myocardial type
Characterized by hypertension, a craving for alcohol, a need for vitamin B2 (riboflavin), not getting sick easily, and lots of adrenal energy.

The above symptoms are all indications for the congestive type of cardiovascular stress Each of these types will require slightly different supplementation, especially in their B vitamin needs.

MI types need riboflavin and the associated B vitamins.

Congestive types need naturally occurring thiamine.

Cardiovascular stress results from, among other things, an over consumption of refined and processed foods. The heart is often a mirror for the rest of the body.

1° Indication
Assess cardiovascular system

Further assessment	1. Check for tenderness in the Chapman reflex for the heart located in the left second intercostal space near the sternum Check for tenderness in the Chapman reflex for the kidney located 1" lateral and 1" superior from the umbilicus on the medial margin of the Rectus abdominus muscle (have client tighten stomach muscle to palpate.

	2. Assess for tenderness over the transverse processes at T1 for the MI type, and T2 for the myocardium and the congestive type, 3. Assess blood pressure 4. An excellent way to assess the heart from a functional perspective is with the Acoustic Cardiogram (ACG). By analyzing the graphical output of the heart sounds one can determine many functional disturbances that can be assessed and corrected using nutrition.

2° Indication

Vitamin B1 (Thiamine) deficiency

Further assessment	1. An excellent way to assess for Thiamine (vitamin B1) deficiency is with the Acoustic Cardiogram (ACG), which will show a depressed S1 heart sound reading. There will not be enough amplitude in the graph. 2. An increased Anion gap and a decreased CO_2 on a chem. screen is indicative of low thiamine levels.

Supplemental Support

1. Nutrients to support cardiovascular health
2. Heart tissue (neonatal bovine)
3. CoQ10
4. EPA and DHA from fish oil
5. Naturally occurring thiamine
6. Bio-Cardio Packs

Lifestyle changes

See the handout in the appendix on recommendations for a healthy heart

NOTES:

303. Cough at night

A cough at night is a sign of congestive heart failure. Backpressure on the aorta will increase the pressure on the pulmonary arteries and veins leading from the heart to the lungs. This is especially true when the client is lying down at night. The lungs are in danger of filling with fluid, which causes the client to cough. Obviously a client should also be assessed for other conditions more closely associated with the lungs.

1° Indication
Assess cardiovascular system

Further assessment	1. Check for tenderness in the Chapman reflex for the heart located in the second intercostal space near the sternum on the left 2. Check for tenderness in the Chapman reflex for the kidney located 1" lateral and 1" superior from the umbilicus on the medial margin of the Rectus abdominus muscle (have client tighten stomach muscle to palpate. 3. Assess for tenderness over the transverse processes at T1 for the MI type, and T2 for the myocardium and the congestive type, 4. Assess blood pressure 5. An excellent way to assess the heart from a functional perspective is with the Acoustic Cardiogram (ACG). By analyzing the graphical output of the heart sounds one can determine many functional disturbances that can be assessed and corrected using nutrition.

2° Indication
Vitamin B1 (Thiamine) deficiency

Further assessment	1. An excellent way to assess for Thiamine (vitamin B1) deficiency is with the Acoustic Cardiogram (ACG), which will show a depressed S1 heart sound reading. There will not be enough amplitude in the graph. 2. An increased Anion gap and a decreased CO_2 on a chem. screen is indicative of low thiamine levels.

Supplemental Support

1. Nutrients to support cardiovascular health
2. Heart tissue (neonatal bovine)
3. CoQ10
4. EPA and DHA from fish oil
5. Naturally occurring thiamine

Lifestyle changes
See the handout in the appendix on recommendations for a healthy heart

NOTES:

304. Blush or face turns red for no reason

This is a sign of cardiovascular dysfunction and/or blood pressure issues. Some of the underlying causes of high blood pressure are kidney dysfunction, liver and gallbladder stasis, adrenal dysfunction, circulatory stress, mineral imbalances, sugar handling problems and thyroid dysfunction. Obviously the cardiovascular system needs to be adequately assessed and any pathology ruled out. Nutrition is an essential part of treating the cardiovascular system. It is important to remember that the health of the heart reflects the health of the body. One of the main causes of cardiovascular stress is the over consumption of processed foods. Working with the diet will be an important treatment.

1° Indication

Assess cardiovascular system

Further assessment	1. Check for tenderness in the Chapman reflex for the heart located in the second intercostal space near the sternum on the left 2. Check for tenderness in the Chapman reflex for the kidney located 1" lateral and 1" superior from the umbilicus on the medial margin of the Rectus abdominus muscle (have client tighten stomach muscle to palpate. 3. Assess for tenderness over the transverse processes at T1 for the heart, T2 for the myocardium and T11/12 for the kidney 4. Assess blood pressure 5. An excellent way to assess the heart from a functional perspective is with the Acoustic Cardiogram (ACG). By analyzing the graphical output of the heart sounds one can determine many functional disturbances that can be assessed and corrected using nutrition.

Other indications

1. Liver biliary stasis
2. Mineral imbalances
3. Sugar handling problems
4. Adrenal or thyroid dysfunction

Supplemental Support

1. Nutrients to support cardiovascular health
2. Heart tissue (neonatal bovine)
3. CoQ10
4. EPA and DHA from fish oil
5. Naturally occurring thiamine
6. Riboflavin and the associated B vitamins
7. Multiple nutrients for supporting renal function

Lifestyle changes

See the handout in the appendix on recommendations for a healthy heart

305. Dull pain or tightness in chest and / or radiate into right arm, worse with exertion
306. Muscle cramps with exertion

The heart is one area to do both a thorough traditional cardiac workup in addition to a nutritional assessment. If you do not do such assessments in your office, refer out to a local cardiologist. It is important to protect the life of the client, and any of the above symptoms could be symptoms of an impending cardiovascular incident. An acute condition such as a myocardial infarct is best left up to the traditional doctors, who treat acute things well. Long-term conditions respond well to nutritional and dietary therapies.

Heart disease can be split up into two different categories, each with a different presentation:

Myocardial type
Characterized by hypertension, a craving for alcohol, a need for vitamin B2 (riboflavin), not getting sick easily, and lots of adrenal energy.

Congestive type
Characterized by low blood pressure and a craving for sugar. They often feel bad or run down and get sick often. They need Vitamin B1 (thiamine) and are generally thyroid types.

The above symptoms are all indications for the myocardial type of cardiovascular stress Each of these types will require slightly different supplementation, especially in their B vitamin needs.

MI types need Riboflavin and the associated B vitamins.

Congestive types need naturally occurring thiamine.

Cardiovascular stress results from, among other things, an over consumption of refined and processed foods. The heart is often a mirror for the rest of the body.

1° Indication
Assess cardiovascular system

Further assessment	1. Check for tenderness in the Chapman reflex for the heart located in the left second intercostal space near the sternum 2. Check for tenderness in the Chapman reflex for the kidney located 1” lateral and 1” superior from the umbilicus on the medial margin of the Rectus abdominus muscle (have client tighten stomach muscle to palpate. 3. Assess for tenderness over the transverse processes at T1 for the MI type, and T2 for the myocardium and the congestive type, 4. Assess blood pressure 5. An excellent way to assess the heart from a functional perspective is with the Acoustic Cardiogram (ACG). By analyzing the graphical output of the heart sounds one can determine many functional disturbances that can be assessed and corrected using nutrition.

2° Indication

Vitamin B2 (Riboflavin) deficiency

Further assessment	1. An excellent way to assess for Riboflavin (vitamin B2) deficiency is with the Acoustic Cardiogram (ACG), which will show an elongated S1 heart sound reading due to weak aortic and pulmonic valve closure.

Supplemental Support

1. Nutrients to support cardiovascular health
2. Heart tissue (neonatal bovine)
3. CoQ10
4. EPA and DHA from fish oil
5. Naturally occurring thiamine

Lifestyle changes

See the handout in the appendix on recommendations for a healthy heart

NOTES:

KIDNEY AND BLADDER

307. Pain in mid back region
308. Puffy around the eyes, dark circles under eyes
309. History of kidney stones (1 = yes, 0 = no)
310. Cloudy, bloody or darkened urine
311. Urine has a strong odor

307. Pain in mid back region

Pain in the mid back region is a classic sign of kidney problems, especially infection. A kidney infection is a serious problem, and should be managed by a clinician experienced in dealing with them. If possible pathology has been ruled out; pain in the mid back region can be an indication of kidney stress.

1° Indication

Need to support kidney function to promote adequate elimination

Further assessment	1. Check for tenderness in the Chapman reflex for the kidneys located 1” lateral and 1” superior from the umbilicus on the medial margin of the Rectus abdominus muscle. Have clients tighten stomach muscles to palpate. 2. Check for an increase in blood pressure when the client goes from standing to supine 3. Check for tenderness with Murphy’s punch to the kidneys on the lower back 4. Routine and functional urinalysis 5. Blood chemistry renal function panel

Supplemental Support

1. Multiple nutrients for supporting renal function
2. Kidney tissue (neonatal bovine)
3. Culture of Beet Juice containing Arginase

Lifestyle changes

Please see the handout in the appendix on recommendations on how to strengthen the kidneys

NOTES:

308. Puffy around the eyes, dark circles under eyes

Dark circles under the eyes and/or puffy eyes are a classic sign of allergies, liver detoxification problems and kidney dysfunction. Allergies are overreactions of the immune system and are often precipitated by a disturbance in the digestive system with a dysbiosis. Dysbiosis can be described as an abnormal intestinal flora and an abnormally permeable intestinal mucous membrane. Over time the villi, the large absorptive surface of mucous membranes in the intestines, becomes irritated and inflamed, which causes it to become less dense. Large, incompletely digested macromolecules, especially proteins, start to be able to penetrate the intestinal mucous membrane. Once in the bloodstream, the body's immune system recognizes the small protein or part of a protein as foreign, and produces antibodies against it. It is the reaction of the antibody/antigen complex that produces the classic allergy symptoms.

The body's second layer of defense lies in the liver. The liver normally screens the blood for antigens. On each pass through the body, the blood must pass through the liver for cleaning and detoxification. The liver will normally take these foreign substances and destroy them or get them out of the body. Unfortunately liver dysfunction is a very common occurrence in our society. The destruction of foreign substances will not occur if the liver is not functioning as it should, if there is too much of the substance to get rid of easily or the liver's phase I and II detoxification pathways cannot destroy it.

The kidney is responsible for selecting what gets excreted and what gets resorbed. If it is exposed to allergenic material or is having to excrete large amounts of toxic waste, it can become congested

1° Indication

Dysbiosis- abnormal intestinal flora and increased intestinal hyperpermeability

Further assessment	1. Increased urinary indican and sediment levels 2. Stool analysis- either comprehensive digestive analysis or a parasite profile 3. Check for tenderness in the Chapman reflex for the colon located bilaterally along the iliotibial band on the thighs. Palpate the colon for tenderness and tension. 4. Check for tenderness in the Chapman reflex for the small intestine located on the 8th, 9th and 10th intercostal spaces near the tip of the rib. Also palpate four quadrants in a 2" to 3" radius around the umbilicus for tenderness and tension. 5. Decreased secretory IgA on stool analysis.

2° Indication

Liver congestion with detoxification problems, especially phase I and II detoxification

Further assessment	1. Check for tenderness in the Chapman reflex for the liver-gallbladder located over the 6th intercostal space on the right 2. Check for tenderness in the Liver point located on the 3rd rib, 3 " to the right of the sternum, at the costochondral junction. 3. Check for tenderness underneath the right rib cage

	4. Increased SGOT, SGPT on a blood chemistry panel 5. Assess for Hepato-biliary congestion with the Acoustic Cardiogram (ACG), which will show post-systolic rounding due to increased backpressure on the pulmonic and aortic valve.

3° Indication

Need to support kidney function to promote adequate elimination

Further assessment	1. Check for tenderness in the Chapman reflex for the kidneys located 1" lateral and 1" superior from the umbilicus on the medial margin of the Rectus abdominus muscle. Have clients tighten stomach muscles to palpate. 2. Check for tenderness with Murphy's punch to the kidneys on the lower back 3. Check for an increase in blood pressure when the client goes from standing to supine 4. Routine and functional urinalysis 5. Blood chemistry renal function panel

Other indications
1. Hypochlorhydria
2. Pancreatic insufficiency
3. Adrenal hypofunction
4. Mineral deficiency

Supplemental Support

1. Micro Emulsified Oregano 2. Nutrients that heal the intestines 3. L-glutamine 4. Lactobacillus acidophilus and Bifidobacterium bifidus 5. Water soluble fiber and colon health nutrients 6. Nutrients to support Phase II liver detoxification 7. Herbs that cleanse the liver 8. Glutathione, cysteine, and Glycine 9. Powdered detoxification support formula 10. Multiple nutrients for supporting renal function 11. Kidney tissue (neonatal bovine) 12. Culture of Beet Juice containing Arginase

Lifestyle changes

Please refer to the handouts in the appendix on the Dysbiosis diet, Recommendations on keeping the liver healthy

NOTES:

309. History of kidney stones (1 = yes, 0 = no)

The kidney is a filter for small amounts of solid waste in the blood stream, but not stones. Kidney stones can be a sign of serious pathology. In the past most stone formation occurred in the bladder while today most stone formation occurs in the upper urinary tract. The incidence has been steadily increasing, paralleling the rise of other diseases associated with the "western diet" i.e. ischemic heart disease, cholelithiasis, hypertension and diabetes. In the western hemisphere, kidney stones are usually composed of calcium salts (oxalates and/or phosphates) (75-85%), uric acid (5-8%) or struvite(10-15%). The incidence varies geographically, reflecting differences in environmental factors, diet, and components of drinking water.

Kidney stones can cause an infection of the kidneys, which should be adequately assessed and treated appropriately. A routine urinalysis will show if there is kidney damage and whether or not there are leukocytes, nitrites, sugar or protein in the urine. Occasionally the individual treated for repeated kidney infections will have a large kidney stone creating the symptoms of infection. An x-ray or intravenous pyelogram is often necessary.

Diagnosing the type of stone is critical to determining the appropriate therapy. Clinical evaluation, such as functional urinalysis, can usually determine the composition of the stone if one is not available for chemical evaluation. A person with a history of kidney stones may need to make some important changes to ensure the health of the urinary tract.

<u>1° Indication</u>

Need to support kidney function to promote adequate elimination

Further assessment	1. Check for tenderness in the Chapman reflex for the kidneys located 1" lateral and 1" superior from the umbilicus on the medial margin of the Rectus abdominus muscle. Have clients tighten stomach muscles to palpate. 2. Check for an increase in blood pressure when the client goes from standing to supine 3. Check for tenderness with Murphy's punch to the kidneys on the lower back 4. Routine and functional urinalysis 5. Check urine pH. Extremes of pH on the acid and alkaline side can determine whether or not certain stones will form 6. Blood chemistry renal function panel 7. X-ray or intravenous pyelogram may be necessary

Supplemental Support

1. Multiple nutrients for supporting renal function
2. Flax Seed Oil
3. Pyridoxal-5-phosphate
4. Magnesium
5. Emulsified vitamin A drops
6. Buffered vitamin C plus bioflavanoids
7. Larch arabinogalactans

Lifestyle changes

Please see the handout in the appendix on Recommendations on how to strengthen the kidneys.

NOTES:

310. Cloudy, bloody or darkened urine

This is a sign of hematuria. Hematuria can give rise to a red or brown color in the urine. If the amount of blood is small it might not show visually but can be detected by a dipstick urinalysis, which can detect both hemolized and non-hemolized blood. This symptom may be associated with a wide range of conditions, some minor and others quite severe. Competent diagnosis is crucial. The bleeding may occur at a site of physical trauma, such as a stone cutting the tissue or may bleed from foci of infection. Generalized kidney support is indicated for this client, but the cause of the symptom must be addressed. If blood is found on a dipstick, send the urine out for a culture and microscopic examination.

1° Indication

Need to support kidney function to promote adequate elimination

Further assessment	1. Check for blood on a urine diptick 2. Urine culture and microscopy may be indicated 3. Check for tenderness in the Chapman reflex for the kidneys located 1" lateral and 1" superior from the umbilicus on the medial margin of the Rectus abdominus muscle. Have clients tighten stomach muscles to palpate. 4. Check for an increase in blood pressure when the client goes from standing to supine 5. Blood chemistry renal function panel 6. Check for tenderness with Murphy's punch to the kidneys on the lower back 7. X-ray or intravenous pyelogram may be necessary

Supplemental Support

1. Multiple nutrients for supporting renal function
2. Flax Seed Oil
3. Pyridoxal-5-phosphate
4. Magnesium
5. Emulsified vitamin A drops
6. Buffered vitamin C plus bioflavanoids
7. Larch arabinogalactans

Lifestyle changes

Please see the handout in the appendix on Recommendations on how to strengthen the kidneys

NOTES:

311. Urine has a strong odor

A strong odor to the urine is an indication of a need for liver and/or kidney support. It is important to assess the urine for possible signs of infection. A client that is drinking inadequate amounts of water will have unusually concentrated urine, which can have a strong smell.

1° Indication
Liver congestion with detoxification problems, especially phase I and II detoxification

Further assessment	1. Check for tenderness in the Chapman reflex for the liver-gallbladder located over the 6th intercostal space on the right 2. Check for tenderness in the Liver point located on the 3rd rib, 3 " to the right of the sternum, at the costochondral junction. 3. Check for tenderness underneath the right rib cage 4. Increased SGOT, SGPT on a blood chemistry panel 5. Various labs do liver detoxification panels 6. Assess for Hepato-biliary congestion with the Acoustic Cardiogram (ACG), which will show post-systolic rounding due to increased backpressure on the pulmonic and aortic valve. It may also show through to the tricuspid valve if chronic.

2° Indication
Need to support kidney function to promote adequate elimination

Further assessment	1. Check for tenderness in the Chapman reflex for the kidneys located 1" lateral and 1" superior from the umbilicus on the medial margin of the Rectus abdominus muscle. Have clients tighten stomach muscles to palpate. 2. Check for an increase in blood pressure when the client goes from standing to supine 3. Routine and functional urinalysis 4. Check for tenderness with Murphy's punch to the kidneys 5. Blood chemistry renal function panel

3° Indication
Assess for adequate hydration

Further assessment	1. Assess the client's hydration status. Have client stand with hands by their side and check and palpate the veins in the right hand. Have them slowly raise their hand to heart level and see if the veins still stick out. Veins that are only just visible or not visible at all are a sign of dehydration

Supplement support

1. Nutrients to support Phase II liver detoxification
2. Herbs that cleanse the liver
3. Glutathione, cysteine, and Glycine
4. Powdered detoxification support formula
5. Multiple nutrients for supporting renal function

6. Kidney tissue (neonatal bovine)
7. Culture of Beet Juice containing Arginase
8. Flax Seed Oil

Lifestyle changes

Please see the handout in on how to strengthen the kidneys

IMMUNE SYSTEM

312. Runny or drippy nose
313. Catch colds at the beginning of winter
314. Mucus producing cough
315. Frequent colds or flu (0 = 1 or less per year, 1 = 2 to 3 times per year, 2 = 4 to 5 times per year, 3 = 6 or more times per year)
316. Other infections (ear, sinus, lung, skin, bladder, kidney, etc.) (0 = 1 or less per year, 1 = 2 to 3 times per year, 2 = 4 to 5 times per year, 3 = 6 or more times per year)
317. Never get sick (0 = sick only 1 or 2 times in last 2 years, 1 = not sick in last 2 years, 2 = not sick in last 4 years, 3 = not sick in last 7 years) Acne (adult)
318. Acne (adult)
319. Itchy skin (dermatitis)
320. Cysts, boils, rashes
321. History of Epstein Bar, Mono, Herpes, Shingles, Chronic Fatigue, Hepatitis or other chronic viral condition (0 = no, 1 = yes in the past, 2 = currently mild condition, 3 = severe)

312. Runny or drippy nose

A runny or drippy nose may be a sign of chronic sinusitis. Sinusitis can be traced to the digestive system and a series of events that trigger an increased susceptibility to infection: functional hypochlorhydria and pancreatic enzyme deficiency, which causes a maldigestion of carbohydrates, fats and proteins. The maldigestion of food leaves large macromolecules undigested, which form the substrate for dysbiosis formation. Dysbiosis can be described as an abnormal intestinal flora. When the intestinal flora is not intact, the absorptive ability of the intestinal mucous membranes becomes impaired and you get an abnormally permeable intestinal mucous membrane.

Over time the villi, the large absorptive surface of the intestines, becomes irritated and inflamed by the large macromolecules and the dysbiosis, which causes it to become less dense. The large, incompletely digested macromolecules, especially proteins, start to be able to penetrate the intestinal mucous membrane. With the destruction of the villi comes the reduction of the Gut Associated Lymphoid Tissue (GALT) and the secretory IgA, the body's first line defense against "foreign" invaders. Once in the bloodstream, the body's immune system recognizes the small protein or part of a protein as foreign, and produces antibodies against it. It is the reaction of the antibody/antigen complex that produces the symptoms of allergies that can cause asthma and a stuffy nose.

Sinus infections are a reflection of the dysbiosis in both the small intestine and more importantly in the sinuses themselves. New research has linked a chronic fungal infection with chronic sinus infections. Many people with chronic sinus infections have had numerous courses of antibiotics to treat the infection, with no success. This can also contribute the dysbiosis in the small intestine.

Treatment, therefore, needs to address the underlying cause by thoroughly assessing the digestive system and beginning therapy to restore a healthy gut function.

Additionally the dysbiosis can cause the client to need more bile salts. This is most often seen in the client with a chronically runny, nose, not stuffed up. Yeast and other unfriendly bacteria in the digestive system can degrade the bile salts, which cause gastrointestinal irritation and increased intestinal permeability. This may also lead to a decrease in fat-soluble nutrients.

A runny or drippy nose may also be the early stages of on upper respiratory infection.

<u>1° Indication</u>

Dysbiosis

Further assessment	1. Increased urinary indican and sediment levels 2. Stool analysis- either comprehensive digestive analysis or a parasite profile 3. Check for tenderness in the Chapman reflex for the colon located bilaterally along the iliotibial band on the thighs. Palpate the colon for tenderness and tension. 4. Check for tenderness in the Chapman reflex for the small intestine located on the 8th, 9th and 10th intercostal spaces

	near the tip of the rib. Also palpate four quadrants in a 2" to 3" radius around the umbilicus for tenderness and tension. 5. Decreased secretory IgA on stool analysis.

2° Indication

Need for supplementary bile salts

Further assessment	1. Check for tenderness underneath the right rib cage 2. Check for tenderness and nodulation on the web between thumb and fore-finger of right hand 3. Check for tenderness in the Chapman reflex for the liver-gallbladder located over the 6th intercostal space on the right side 4. Blood chemistry and CBC testing for SGOT, SGPT, GGT 5. Assess for Hepato-biliary congestion with the Acoustic Cardiogram (ACG), which will show post-systolic rounding due to increased backpressure on the pulmonic and aortic valve. It may also show through to the tricuspid valve if chronic.

Other indications

Hypochlorhydria and pancreatic insufficiency with a need for supplemental HCL and pancreatic enzymes

Supplemental Support

1. Micro Emulsified Oregano
2. Nutrients that heal the intestines
3. Betaine HCL, Pepsin, and pancreatin
4. Water soluble fiber and nutrients to support healthy colon
5. L-Glutamine
6. Multiple nutrients that support the immune system
7. Lactobacillus acidophilus and Bifidobacterium bifidus
8. Beet juice and bile salts

Lifestyle changes

Please see the handout in the appendix on the Dysbiosis diet

NOTES:

313. Catch colds at the beginning of winter

The beginning of the winter is a time when many people turn their heating on. For those with forced air heat, and a network of heating ducts, this may be a time of increased susceptibility to yeasts and moulds that are blown around the house. In the summer moist air, from the air conditioning, travels through the ductwork. In the winter heated air blows the mould and spores around. It is advisable to ask people what kind of heating they have and to recommend that they get the ductwork and furnace cleaned every fall.

This pattern can also be traced to the digestive system and a series of events that trigger an increased susceptibility to infection: functional hypochlorhydria and pancreatic enzyme deficiency leading to maldigestion, maldigestion leading to gastrointestinal irritation and dysbiosis, and dysbiosis leading to increased intestinal hyperpermeability. Foreign proteins in the form of antigenic material enter the bloodstream and interface with the antibodies of the immune system. It is the reaction of the antibody/antigen complex that produces the symptoms of allergies that can cause the stuffy nose and cold like symptoms, even causing decreased immune function and an increased susceptibility to catching colds.

A low functioning thyroid can lead to a symptom of catching colds at the beginning of winter. Low thyroid function can cause a diminished immune function.

1° Indication

Dysbiosis

Further assessment	1. Increased urinary indican and sediment levels 2. Stool analysis- either comprehensive digestive analysis or a parasite profile 3. Check for tenderness in the Chapman reflex for the colon located bilaterally along the iliotibial band on the thighs. Palpate the colon for tenderness and tension. 4. Check for tenderness in the Chapman reflex for the small intestine located on the 8th, 9th and 10th intercostal spaces near the tip of the rib. Also palpate four quadrants in a 2" to 3" radius around the umbilicus for tenderness and tension. 5. Decreased secretory IgA on stool analysis.

2° Indication

Low thyroid function

Further assessment	1. Check for tenderness in the Chapman reflex for the thyroid located in the right second intercostal space near the sternum 2. Check for a delayed Achilles return reflex, which is a strong sign of a hypo-functioning thyroid 3. Check for general costochondral tenderness, a thyroid indicator 4. Check for pre-tibial edema, a sign of a hypo-functioning thyroid 5. Iodine test: Use a tincture of 2% iodine solution, and paint a

	3" by 3" square on the client's abdomen. The client is to leave the patch unwashed until it disappears. The square should still be there in 24 hours. If it has disappeared, there is an indication of iodine need 6. Have client assess their basal metabolic temperature by taking their axillary temperature first thing in the morning for 5 straight days. An average temperature below 36.6° is an indication of hypo-thyroidism. 7. Order a thyroid panel and check TSH, T4, T3, Free T4 and free T3 levels. 8. Any suspected case of hypothyroidism that shows abnormalities on a chem. screen should have a thyroid antibody study performed.

Supplemental Support

1. Multiple nutrients that support the immune system
2. Herbal support against viruses
3. Micro Emulsified Oregano
4. Nutrients that heal the intestines
5. Betaine HCL, Pepsin, and pancreatin
6. Water soluble fiber and nutrients to support healthy colon
7. L-Glutamine
8. Lactobacillus acidophilus and Bifidobacterium bifidus
9. Multiple nutrients to support thyroid function with pituitary glandular
10. Potassium iodide
11. Thymus tissue (neonatal bovine)
12. Larch arabinogalactans

Lifestyle changes

Please see the handout in the appendix on recommendations for dealing with low thyroid function

NOTES:

314. Mucus producing cough

A mucous producing cough suggests a need for immune support. It may also be a sign of iodine need, especially if the mucous is very thick and the client is having a hard time coughing it up. Iodine has the ability to thin secretions.

Making sure that the bowels and kidneys are functioning properly to eliminate wastes from the body is important in keeping the immune system healthy. It is also important that the body not be inundated with toxins from the environment, and the diet that the liver needs to process. Improving diet, decreasing stress, and increasing bowel function will help improve immune function. Remember that the body uses the mucous producing function as a way to clean and discharge.

1° Indication

Need for immune support

Further assessment	1. Check for tenderness in the Chapman reflex for the thymus located in the 5th intercostal space on the right near the sternum 2. Check for tenderness in the Chapman reflex for the lungs located bilaterally in the 3rd and 4th intercostal space near the sternum 3. Check for tenderness in the histamine point located at five o'clock on the pectoralis muscle in the intercostal space between the 5th and 6th rib on the right side only 4. Assess the client for allergic tension. Take a full one-minute pulse sitting, then stand, wait 15 seconds and take another full minute pulse. If the standing pulse goes up by more than six beats, this is an indication of "allergic tension" 5. Assess the client's vitamin C status with the lingual and urinary ascorbic acid tests

Supplemental Support

1. Multiple nutrients that support the immune system
2. Thymus tissue (neonatal bovine)
3. Herbal support against viruses
4. Nutrients that support against bacteria
5. Lung tissue (neonatal bovine) and other nutrients to support lung function
6. Multiple herbal anti-histamines

Lifestyle changes

Please see the handout in the appendix on recommendations for decreasing coughs, colds and flus

NOTES:

315. Frequent colds or flu

Frequent colds and flus indicate a need for immune support, and are also associated with a low functioning thyroid. It is important to assess what the client means by frequent colds or flu. A cold once or twice a year is a sign of a healthy immune system, and is often used by the body to detoxify itself.

Insuring the bowels and kidneys are functioning properly to eliminate wastes from the body is important in keeping the immune system healthy. Make sure that the body is not inundated with toxins from the environment or diet that the liver needs to process. Improving diet, stress, and bowel function will help improve immune function.

1° Indication

Need for immune support

Further assessment	1. Check for tenderness in the Chapman reflex for the thymus located in the 5th intercostal space on the right near the sternum 2. Check for tenderness in the Chapman reflex for the lungs located bilaterally in the 3rd and 4th intercostal space near the sternum 3. Check for tenderness in the histamine point located at five o'clock on the pectoralis muscle in the intercostal space between the 5th and 6th rib on the right side only 4. Assess the client for allergic tension. Take a full one-minute pulse sitting, then stand, wait 15 seconds and take another full minute pulse. If the standing pulse goes up by more than six beats, this is an indication of "allergic tension" 5. Assess the client's tissue ascorbic acid status with the lingual and ascorbic acid test

2° Indication

Low thyroid function

Further assessment	1. Check for tenderness in the Chapman reflex for the thyroid located in the right second intercostal space near the sternum 2. Check for a delayed Achilles return reflex, which is a strong sign of a hypo-functioning thyroid 3. Check for general costochondral tenderness, a thyroid indicator 4. Check for pre-tibial edema, a sign of a hypo-functioning thyroid 5. Iodine test: Use a tincture of 2% iodine solution, and paint a 3"

	by 3" square on the client's abdomen. The client is to leave the patch unwashed until it disappears. The square should still be there in 24 hours. If it has disappeared, there is an indication of iodine need 6. Have client assess their basal metabolic temperature by taking their axillary temperature first thing in the morning for 5 straight days. An average temperature below 36.6° is an indication of hypo-thyroidism. 7. Order a thyroid panel and check TSH, T4, T3, Free T4 and free T3 levels. 8. Any suspected case of hypothyroidism that shows abnormalities on a chem. screen should have a thyroid antibody study performed.

Supplemental Support

1. Multiple nutrients that support the immune system
2. Thymus tissue (neonatal bovine)
3. Herbal support against viruses
4. Nutrients that support against bacteria
5. Lung tissue (neonatal bovine) and other nutrients to support lung function
6. Multiple herbal anti-histamines

Lifestyle changes

Please see the handout in the appendix on recommendations for decreasing coughs, colds and flus

NOTES:

316. Other infections (sinus, ear, lung, skin, bladder, kidney, etc.)

Other infections, such as sinus, ear, lung, bladder, kidney, suggest a need for immune support. They are a symptom of an imbalanced internal terrain or environment that can be traced to the digestive system and a series of events that trigger an increased susceptibility to infection: functional hypochlorhydria and pancreatic enzyme deficiency leading to maldigestion, maldigestion leading to gastrointestinal irritation and dysbiosis, and dysbiosis leading to increased intestinal hyperpermeability. Foreign proteins in the form of antigenic material enter the bloodstream and interface with the antibodies of the immune system. It is the reaction of the antibody/antigen complex that produces the symptoms of allergies that can cause the stuffy nose and cold like symptoms, even causing decreased immune function and an increased susceptibility to frequent infections. It is essential to assess and treat imbalances in the internal terrain or environment of the body, in order to prevent frequent infections.

Insuring the bowels and kidneys are functioning properly to eliminate wastes from the body is important in keeping the immune system healthy. Insuring that the body is not inundated with toxins that the liver needs to process such as from the environment, the occupation, or from the diet, and improving diet, stress, and bowel function will help improve immune function.

<u>1° Indication</u>
Dysbiosis

Further assessment	1. Stool analysis- either comprehensive digestive analysis or a parasite profile 2. Check for tenderness in the Chapman reflex for the colon located bilaterally along the iliotibial band on the thighs. Palpate the colon for tenderness and tension. 3. Check for tenderness in the Chapman reflex for the small intestine located on the 8th, 9th and 10th intercostal spaces near the tip of the rib. Also palpate four quadrants in a 2" to 3" radius around the umbilicus for tenderness and tension. 4. Decreased secretory IgA on stool analysis.

<u>2° Indication</u>
Need for immune support

Further assessment	1. Check for tenderness in the Chapman reflex for the thymus located in the 5th intercostal space on the right near the sternum 2. Check for tenderness in the Chapman reflex for the lungs located bilaterally in the 3rd and 4th intercostal space near the sternum 3. Check for tenderness in the histamine point located at five o'clock on the pectoralis muscle in the intercostal space between the 5th and 6th rib on the right side only 4. Assess the client for allergic tension. Take a full one-minute

	pulse sitting, then stand, wait 15 seconds and take another full minute pulse. If the standing pulse goes up by more than six beats, this is an indication of "allergic tension" 5. Assess the client's vitamin C status with the lingual ascorbic acid tests

Supplemental Support

6. Multiple nutrients that support the immune system
7. Thymus tissue (neonatal bovine)
8. Herbal support against viruses
9. Nutrients that support against bacteria
10. Lung tissue (neonatal bovine) and other nutrients to support lung function
11. Multiple herbal anti-histamines
12. Multiple nutrients to support thyroid function with pituitary glandular
13. Potassium iodide

Lifestyle changes

Please see the handout in the appendix on recommendations for decreasing coughs, colds and flus, and also the handout on the dysbiosis diet.

NOTES:

317. Never get sick (3 = not in last 7 yrs., 2 = not in last 4 yrs., 1 = not in last 2 yrs, 0 = sick only 1 or 2 times in last 2 years)

Despite what most people think, never getting sick is a bad thing. In fact getting a cold or flu once in a while is a good exercise for the immune system. The longer a person goes without getting sick the less active the immune system might be. This needs to be evaluated and supported nutritionally.

1° Indication

Need for immune support

Further assessment	1. Check for tenderness in the Chapman reflex for the thymus located in the 5th intercostal space on the right near the sternum 2. Check for tenderness in the Chapman reflex for the lungs located bilaterally in the 3rd and 4th intercostal space near the sternum 3. Check for tenderness in the histamine point located at five o'clock on the pectoralis muscle in the intercostal space between the 5th and 6th rib on the right side only 4. Assess the client for allergic tension. Take a full one-minute pulse sitting, then stand, wait 15 seconds and take another full minute pulse. If the standing pulse goes up by more than six beats, this is an indication of "allergic tension" 5. Assess the client's vitamin C status with the lingual and urinary ascorbic acid tests

Supplemental Support

1. Multiple nutrients that support the immune system
2. Thymus tissue (neonatal bovine)
3. Herbal support against viruses
4. Nutrients that support against bacteria
5. Lung tissue (neonatal bovine) and other nutrients to support lung function
6. Multiple herbal anti-histamines

NOTES:

318. Acne (adult)

Adult acne is most often due to allergies. There is also a connection to the liver, a need for calcium and/or essential fatty acids and an increased intake of sweets, candy and refined sugar. Allergies have a strong connection to imbalance in the digestive system and a series of events that trigger the susceptibility to allergies: functional hypochlorhydria and pancreatic enzyme deficiency leading to maldigestion, maldigestion leading to gastrointestinal irritation and dysbiosis, and dysbiosis leading to increased intestinal hyperpermeability. Foreign proteins in the form of antigenic material enter the bloodstream and interface with the antibodies of the immune system. It is the reaction of the antibody/antigen complex that produces the symptoms of allergies that can cause the acne and a decreased immune function.

Also look at blood sugar dysregulation. Acne in the adult has been called "diabetes of the face".

1° Indication

Dysbiosis

Further assessment	1. Increased urinary indican and sediment levels 2. Stool analysis- either comprehensive digestive analysis or a parasite profile 3. Check for tenderness in the Chapman reflex for the colon located bilaterally along the iliotibial band on the thighs. Palpate the colon for tenderness and tension. 4. Check for tenderness in the Chapman reflex for the small intestine located on the 8th, 9th and 10th intercostal spaces near the tip of the rib. Also palpate four quadrants in a 2" to 3" radius around the umbilicus for tenderness and tension. 5. Decreased secretory IgA on stool analysis.

2° Indication

Liver detoxification problems, especially phase I detoxification

Further assessment	7. Check for tenderness in the Chapman reflex for the liver-gallbladder located over the 6th intercostal space on the right 8. Check for tenderness in the Liver point located on the 3rd rib, 3 " to the right of the sternum, at the costochondral junction. 9. Check for tenderness underneath the right rib cage Increased SGOT, SGPT on a blood chemistry panel 10. Various labs do liver detoxification panels

Other indications

1. Blood sugar dysregulation
2. Calcium deficiency
3. Essential fatty acid deficiency

Supplemental Support

1. Multiple nutrients that support the immune system
2. Thymus tissue (neonatal bovine)
3. Herbal support against viruses
4. Nutrients that support against bacteria
5. Lung tissue (neonatal bovine) and other nutrients to support lung function
6. Multiple herbal anti-histamines

Lifestyle changes

Please see the handout in the appendix on the Dysbiosis diet and recommendations for controlling blood sugar.

NOTES:

319. Itchy skin / dermatitis
320. Cysts, boils, rashes

Skin symptoms often have a root cause in allergies and immune deficiency. There are many different kinds of dermatitis and in general the integrity of the digestive system plays a big role in the development of skin symptoms. Another cause of skin symptoms is a diet that is deficient in nutrients and is full of processed ingredients.

It is also important to remember that the integument plays a large role in detoxification, especially when the usual routes of elimination (liver, kidneys and digestive system) are not functioning well. Therefore, skin reactions such as itchy skin, rashes and dermatitis, should be seen as the body trying to eliminate. Supporting the liver, kidneys and digestive system will help. Cysts and boils are evidence of the body trying to wall something off.

1° Indication

Need for immune support

Further assessment	1. Check for tenderness in the Chapman reflex for the thymus located in the 5th intercostal space on the right near the sternum 2. Check for tenderness in the Chapman reflex for the lungs located bilaterally in the 3rd and 4th intercostal space near the sternum 3. Check for tenderness in the histamine point located at five o'clock on the pectoralis muscle in the intercostal space between the 5th and 6th rib on the right side only 4. Assess the client for allergic tension. Take a full one-minute pulse sitting, then stand, wait 15 seconds and take another full minute pulse. If the standing pulse goes up by more than six beats, this is an indication of "allergic tension" 5. Assess the client's vitamin C status with the lingual and urinary ascorbic acid tests

2° Indication

Digestive dysfunction with hydrochloric acid need

Further assessment	1. Check Ridler HCL reflex for tenderness 1 inch below xyphoid and over to the left edge of the rib cage 2. Check for tenderness in the Chapman reflex for the stomach and upper digestion located in 6th intercostal space on the left 3. Check for a positive zinc tally: A client holds a solution of aqueous zinc sulfate in their mouth and tells you if and when they can taste it. An almost immediate very bitter taste indicates the client does not need zinc. Clients who are zinc deficient will report no taste from the solution. 4. Gastric acid assessment using Gastrotest 5. Increased urinary indican levels

3° Indication

Pancreatic insufficiency with pancreatic enzyme need

Further assessment	1. Check Ridler enzyme point for tenderness 1 inch below xyphoid and over to the right edge of the rib cage 2. Check for tenderness in the Chapman reflex for the pancreas located in the 7th intercostal space 3. Increased urinary sediment levels

Other indications

1. Toxic bowel
2. General nutrient deficiency

Supplemental Support

1. Multiple nutrients that support the immune system
2. Thymus tissue (neonatal bovine)
3. Herbal support against viruses
4. Nutrients that support against bacteria
5. Lung tissue (neonatal bovine) and other nutrients to support lung function
6. Betaine HCL, Pepsin, and pancreatin
7. Pancreatic enzymes
8. Beet juice, taurine, vitamin C and pancreolipase
9. Multiple herbal anti-histamines

NOTES:

321. History of Epstein Bar, Mono, Herpes, Shingles, Chronic Fatigue, Hepatitis or other chronic viral condition

A history of the above infections is an indication that the immune system in the past has been compromised. Many of these diseases are latent in the body and require a vigilant immune system to keep them under control. This puts extra stress on an already compromised immune system. Decreasing the stress in this person's life will help keep these infections inactive.

1° Indication

Need for immune support

Further assessment	1. Check for tenderness in the Chapman reflex for the thymus located in the 5th intercostal space on the right near the sternum 2. Check for tenderness in the Chapman reflex for the lungs located bilaterally in the 3rd and 4th intercostal space near the sternum 3. Check for tenderness in the histamine point located at five o'clock on the pectoralis muscle in the intercostal space between the 5th and 6th rib on the right side only 4. Assess the client for allergic tension. Take a full one-minute pulse sitting, then stand, wait 15 seconds and take another full minute pulse. If the standing pulse goes up by more than six beats, this is an indication of "allergic tension" 5. Assess the client's vitamin C status with the lingual and urinary ascorbic acid tests

Supplemental Support

1. Multiple nutrients that support the immune system
2. Thymus tissue (neonatal bovine)
3. Herbal support against viruses
4. Nutrients that support against bacteria
5. Lung tissue (neonatal bovine) and other nutrients to support lung function
6. Multiple herbal anti-histamines

NOTES:

APPENDIX

DIET AND LIFESTYLE HANDOUTS

1. Adrenal restoration measures
2. Diabetes dietary recommendation
3. Diet to aid digestion
4. Diet and lifestyle recommendations for healthy bones
5. Dysbiosis diet: for control of Candida, bacteria, viruses and parasites
6. Food sources of calcium
7. Food sources of magnesium
8. Food sources of potassium
9. Food sources of zinc
10. Foods containing milk or dairy
11. Foods to be avoided on a gluten-free diet
12. Healthy lifestyle for a healthy gallbladder
13. Herpes diet
14. Life in the fast lane
15. Recommendations for a healthy heart
16. Recommendations for a healthy menstrual cycle
17. Recommendations for controlling blood sugar
18. Recommendations for dealing with increased thyroid activity
19. Recommendations for dealing with low thyroid function
20. Recommendations for decreasing clods, flus and infections
21. Recommendations for Diarrhea
22. Recommendations for keeping your liver healthy
23. Recommendations for the prostate
24. Recommendations for strengthening your kidneys

ADRENAL RESTORATION MEASURES

Diet

- Whole foods
- Avoid refined sugar
- No caffeine
- Avoid alcohol
- Adequate protein
-
- Avoid all food allergens, which can weaken the system and can be an adrenal stressor
- Fasting and detoxification/cleansing diets should be avoided, at least initially

Botanical support

- **Ginseng:** Has steroid-like activities, can increase resistance to a whole load of stressors, can prevent shrinking of the thymus gland and can prevent adrenal hyperplasia. Can prevent adrenal atrophy in cortisone treatment.
  Dose: 100mg capsule twice/day.
- **Licorice:** It can increase cortisol half-life and is extremely useful in correcting low cortisol states, giving the adrenal glands a "rest" and chance to restore. Can help prevent shrinking of the thymus and immunosupression from the administration of cortisone. May lessen the amount of cortisone needed to achieve a therapeutic effect.
  Dose: ¼ teaspoon of 5:1 solid extract three times/day or strong licorice tea or capsulated licorice 2 caps 3X/day

Stress management

- **Get adequate sleep**. 8 hours of sleep beginning at 10:00 p.m. is much more restoring to the adrenals than 8 hours beginning at 1:00 a.m. Nap if needed but not enough to interfere with night sleep.
- **Relaxation:** Breathing or skilled relaxation exercises, listen to relaxation tapes, meditate, biofeedback.
- **Accept nurturing and affection**
- **Laugh**

Exercise

- **Light to moderate exercise**. Do not push yourself and begin at a level that you can handle.

Natural light

- **Get outdoors into natural light** as much as possible. Direct sunlight is not necessary. Natural light is essential for healthy adrenal function
- **Use full spectrum lights in the home and work area**
- **Green light:** some research has come out about the benefits of green light. Obtain a Par 38 dichromatic 150-watt spot or flood green light to have as an ambient light somewhere in the home.

DIABETES DIETARY RECOMMENDATIONS

1. **MAINTENANCE DIET**
    a. A whole food diet that is moderate in protein, moderate in complex carbohydrates, moderate in fat, low in refined and concentrated sugars.
    b. **Macronutrient proportions**:
        - Complex carbohydrates consists of 40% of caloric intake
        - Proteins consist of 30% of caloric intake
        - Fats consist of 30% of caloric intake
        - Total fiber content is ideally 100 grams/day

        The benefits of a diet in these ratios are:
        1. Reduced after-mealtime hyperglycemia and delayed hypoglycemia
        2. Reduced cholesterol and triglyceride levels with ↑ HDL
        3. Progressive weight reduction
        4. Prevention of diabetic complications

    c. **Complex carbohydrates**:
        - Legumes--beans, peas, lentils, kidney beans
        - Whole grains--buckwheat, millet, oats, brown rice
        - Nuts--almonds, cashews, nut butters, seeds

    d. **Vegetables:**
    Eat vegetables with a low carbohydrate content, avoid starchy vegetables like potatoes and corn
    e. **Fruits:**
        - Small to moderate amounts of fruit with frequent blood sugar monitoring to see the response
        - Eliminate dried fruits

    f. **Fiber:**
        - Legumes
        - Whole grains
        - Vegetables and fruit
        - Nuts and seeds

    g. **Fat:**
        - Follow a moderate animal protein diet
        - Avoid hydrogenated and partially-hydrogenated oils
        - Eat healthy oils: Olive oil, flax oil, sesame, walnut

    h. **Protein:**
        - Lean red meat, chicken without the skin, fish

DIET TO AID DIGESTION

LIFESTYLE CHANGES

1. Chew food thoroughly. Most people eat too fast and swallow air with their food; this causes digestive stress leading to poor absorption of nutrients, digestive problems like gas and bloating, and possible growth of harmful yeast and bacteria in the digestive tract (toxic bowel).
2. Drink warm liquid before meals. Drinking warm water with lemon, broth, miso soup or soup before a meal will prepare digestive tract for digestion.
3. Avoid smoking, alcohol, coffee, refined sugars and flours and other irritants. These will all cause digestive stress depleting vitamins and minerals vital for enzyme activity, and deplete stomach acid.
4. Increase consumption of fresh vegetables. Increasing intake of fruits and vegetables with high water content, especially raw, will help digestion and increase bowel transit time.

DIETARY AND LIFESTYLE RECOMMENDATIONS FOR HEALTHY BONES

FOODS TO FOCUS ON

Foods High in Calcium

Canned sardines and canned salmon (with bones)

Non-fat yogurt	Kale
Mustard, collard and turnip greens	Celery
Dates, figs, raisins	Rutabagas
Broccoli	Sesame seeds
Carob flour	Sea vegetables
Blackstrap molasses	

Foods High in Vitamin K

Broccoli	Alfalfa
Green leafy vegetables, like spinach	Oats
Tomatoes	Rye
Wheat	Cauliflower

Foods High in Zinc

Wheat germ	Seafood
Pumpkin seeds	Nutritional yeast
Sunflower seeds	
Foods grown in organically enriched soils	

Foods High in Magnesium

Whole wheat	Nuts
Bran	Seeds
Green leafy vegetables	Asparagus
Celery	Cabbage
Bananas	Prunes
Oranges	Cashews
Legumes	Almonds

Foods High in Manganese

Celery	Bananas
Beets	Egg yolks
Bran	Legumes
Pineapple	Asparagus
Green leafy vegetables	Whole grains

Foods High in Potassium

Fruit (Bananas)	Raisins
Potatoes	Halibut
Salmon	Almonds
Carrots	

FOODS TO AVOID

- **Alcohol** - Decreases intestinal calcium absorption and vitamin D levels. It is also associated with hip fractures due to an increased number of falls.
- **Coffee or Black Tea** - Coffee and tea increase urinary and fecal calcium excretion. Heavy caffeine drinkers (> 2 cups of coffee/tea per day) are twice as likely to suffer hip fractures.
- **Damaged/Bad Fats** – A diet high in highly refined processed vegetable oils and particularly hydrogenated abd partially hydrogenated oils (a major source of trans fatty acids) should be strictly avoided because thay are so damaging to the body and will decrease calcium absorption. Fried foods of all kinds should be avoided also.
- **High Protein Foods/Meats** - A high protein diet increases calcium excretion.
- **Salt** - Increases calcium excretion.
- **Sugar** - Increases peaks in urinary calcium excretion.
- **Smoking** - The bone mineral content of smokers is 15-30% lower in women. Smokers are twice as likely to have osteoporosis as non-smokers.

EXERCISE

Weight-bearing exercise such as walking protects against bone loss. To be effective, exercise at least three times per week for an hour. Studies show that exercise can actually increase bone mass in postmenopausal women.

DYSBIOSIS DIET:
For control of Candida, Bacteria, Viruses & Parasites

DIRECTIONS: Eliminate the following foods from your diet, which have been shown to exacerbate dysbiosis, candidiasis and intestinal parasites due to their sugar, yeast and fermented food content. Okay fruits and Nuts/Butters are acceptable foods that will not exacerbate dysbiosis.

SUGARS
Beet sugar
Cane sugar (turbinado)
Corn sugar ("Cerelose," dextrose, "Dyno")
Corn syrup ("Cartose," glucose, "Sweetose")
Fructose
Honey and related products
Honeycomb
Maple syrup, sugar
Molasses

FRUITS
Apricot
Banana
Cantaloupe
Cherry (sour, sweet)
Coconut (oil, meal, milk, meat)
Currant (red, black, white)
Date
Date plum
Fig (all varieties)
Grape (all varieties)
Grapefruit (all varieties)
Kiwi fruit
Loganberry
Mango
Mulberry
Nectarine
Orange (all varieties)
Pear
Persimmon (American, Japanese)
Plum
Pomelo
Prune
Raisin (all varieties)
Raspberries

OKAY FRUIT
Casaba melon
Watermelon
Apples
Blackberries
Lemons, limes
Blueberries
Papaya
Pineapple
Pomegranate
Strawberries
Peaches

VEGETABLES
Chinese yam (potato)
Morel Mushroom
Plantain
Poi
Tapioca
Taro (root)
Yam (sweet Potato)

NUTS/NUT BUTTERS
Brazil nut
Butternut
Cashew
Cola nut (cola, Kola)
Hickory nut
Macadamia nut
Pecan
Pistachio
Walnut (black, English)

OKAY NUTS/NUT BUTTERS
Almond
Chestnut
Hazelnut
Filberts
Pine nuts

MISCELLANEOUS
Apple cider vinegar
Baker's yeast
Black tea
Brewer's yeast (nutritional yeast)
Buckthorn (tea)
Chocolate (cacao)
Cocoa
Cocoa butter
Cream of tartar
Hops (alcohol)
Pickles (cucumber, gherkin)
Vinegar (cider, wine)

ANIMAL PRODUCTS
Cheese (bacteria-, mould- or yeast ripened)
Asiago
Bel Paese
Bleu/blue
Brick
Brie
Camembert
Emmental
Gorgonzola
Gruyere
Muenster
Port de salut
Roquefort
Stilton
Swiss
Pork

Other suggestions for dealing with dysbiosis:

- **Eat two Large chopped salads each day:** Normal flora feed on vegetable fiber. Eating the chopped salads will help normal, beneficial bacteria to thrive.
- **Chew your food thoroughly:** This improves digestion, breaking down food particles and mixing them with salivary enzymes. The better your digestion, the easier it is to treat dysbiosis.
- **Don't eat a lot of meat:** You don't have to avoid it completely (unless allergies are an issue). Eating too much meat can feed certain species of undesirable bacteria. Your doctor will make specific dietary recommendations.
- **Avoid dairy products.**
- **Eat plenty of raw vegetables:** Raw foods contain enzymes and aid digestion.
- **Find and eliminate any allergens:** Avoiding hidden allergies will reduce the burden on the immune system.

FOOD SOURCES OF CALCIUM

FOOD SOURCES HIGH IN CALCIUM

Dairy products
Salmon, sardines, oysters, herring
Seaweed
Dark green leafy vegetables
Broccoli
Dried beans and peas
Nuts and seeds
Sprouts
Brewer's yeast
Blackstrap molasses
Whole grains
Herbs: Borage, lambs quarters, wild lettuce, amaranth, nettles, campion, burdock, and yellow dock leaves

RDA FOR CALCIUM

800 mg/day

1200 mg/day Pregnant/Lactating

Optimal levels:
1000-1500 mg Therapeutic

CALCIUM CONTENT OF FOODS

Dairy (1 cup)	**(Milligrams)**
Goat milk	315
Skim milk	300
Buttermilk	300
Whole milk	290
Breast milk (average)	80
Yogurt	270
Cottage cheese	230
Ice cream	200
Butter (1 Tbsp=3)	45
Swiss cheese (1 oz)	260
Edam cheese (1 oz)	220
Cheddar cheese (1 oz)	215
Parmesan (1 Tbsp grated)	70

Miscellaneous	**(Milligrams)**
Blackstrap molasses	280

Seafood (3 oz)	**(Milligrams)**
Sardines with bones	370
Salmon, red (4 oz)	285
Oysters	90
Smoked Salmon	15

Dark Green Leafy Vegetables (1 cup cooked)	**(Milligrams)**
Collard	360
Shepard's Purse*	300
Bok choy	250
Kale	210
Parsley*	200
Mustard greens	190
Broccoli (1 stalk)	160
Spinach*	230
Dandelion greens	150
Chard	125
Rutabaga	100
Leaf or Romaine lettuce	40
Head lettuce	10

*Contain oxalic acid and other phytic acids that binds calcium. Steam these vegetables to keep this from happening.

Seaweed (25 grams)	**(Milligrams)**
Hijiki	350
Wakame	325
Arame	290
Kombu	200

Beans and Peas	**(Milligrams)**
(1 cup cooked)	
Navy beans	140
Pinto	100
Garbanzo beans	95
Limas/black beans	60
Lentils and kidneys	50
Peanuts (1/4 cup)	25
Split peas	20

Grains	**(Milligrams)**
(1 cup dry)	
Masa Harina	140
Tortillas (2)	120
Cornmeal	24
Cornmeal (degermed)	8
Whole wheat flour	50
White enriched flour	20
Oats	40
Rice	25

Sprouts	**(Milligrams)**
(1 cup raw)	
Mung	35
Alfalfa	25

Nuts and Seeds	**(Milligrams)**
(1 Tbsp)	
Sesame seeds	70
Tahini-sesame butter	20
Pumpkin seeds	20
Sunflower seeds	10
Peanuts	7

FOOD SOURCES OF MAGNESIUM

Food	*Amount*	*Magnesium Content (mg)*
Black-Eyed Peas	1/2 cup	200
Millet	1/2 cup	185
White Beans	1/2 cup	175
Lima Beans	1/2 cup	160
Red Beans	1/2 cup	150
Wheat bran/germ	1/2 cup	140
Barley	1/2 cup	140
Beet Greens	1/4 pound	120
Spinach	1/4 pound	100
Lentils	1/2 cup	75
Cashews	14	75
Swiss Chard	1/4 pound	75
Cornmeal	1/2 cup	65
Collard Greens	1/4 pound	65
Brown Rice	1/2 cup	60
Oats	1 cup	50
Potato/Sweet Potato	1 large	50
Peas	1 cup	50
Brussels Sprouts	1/4 pound	45
Almonds	15	40
Beets	2 medium	30
Peanut Butter	1 tbs.	30
Milk	1 cup	30
Sesame Seeds	2 tbs.	30
Broccoli	1 stalk	25
Cauliflower	1 cup	25
Corn	1 ear	25
Peanuts	1 tbs.	20
Carrot or Onion	1 medium	20
Asparagus	5 spears	20
Mushrooms	4 large	15
Tomato or Green Pepper	1 medium	15

FOOD SOURCES OF POTASSIUM

POTASSIUM IS FOUND IN THE FOLLOWING FOODS:

Vegetable skins and peels
Fruit, especially skins
Nuts
Fish
Meat

POTASSIUM CONTENT OF FOOD (mg)

Protein Foods (4 oz)

915 Almonds
525 Halibut
420 Cashews
470 Salmon
420 White Beans
400 Hamburger
335 Beef
300 Lamb

Fruit

800 Raisins- 4 oz
600 1/2 Avocado
370 Banana
250 1/4 Cantaloupe
245 Pineapple- 1 cup
225 Orange Juice- 4 oz
200 Orange
135 1/2 Grapefruit

Vegetables

500 Potato
340 Carrot
250 Spinach- 1 cup
195 Lettuce or Cabbage- 1 cup
160 Cucumber
150 Beets- 1/2 cup
120 Onion- 1/2

FOOD SOURCES OF ZINC

MAJOR ZINC CONTAINING FOODS

- Oysters
- Vegetables
- Legumes
- Meat
- Dairy
- Seeds (esp. pumpkin seeds)
- Eggs
- Fruits
- Seafood
- Grains

RDA FOR ZINC

- Maintenance-15 mg
- Preventive-25 mg
- Pregnancy-30 mg
- Therapeutic-40-50 mg
- Breastfeeding -25 mg

ZINC CONTENT OF VARIOUS FOODS

Grains (1 cup dry)	Milligrams
Hard wheat berries	6.9
Soft wheat berries	5.4
Wheat bran	5.7
Buckwheat groats	3.9
Millet	3.6
Rice bran	3.1
Whole wheat flour	2.9
White flour	0.8
Brown rice	2.4
Oatmeal	2.4
White rice	1.2
Corn meal	2.1

Dairy	
Milk (1 cup)	0.9
Ice cream (1 cup)	0.6
Cheddar cheese (1 slice)	0.5

Legumes (1 cup cooked)	Milligrams
Black-eyed peas	3.0
Green peas	2.1
Garbanzo beans	2.1
Lentils	2.1
Lima beans	1.7
Peanut butter (1 tbs.)	0.5
Peanuts (1 tbs.)	0.3

Vegetables (1 cup)	
Spinach (cooked)	1.3
Sweet corn	0.7
Spinach (chopped/raw)	0.5
Onion	0.5

Eggs/Brewers Yeast	
Egg (1 egg, Zn mostly in yolk)	0.5
Brewer's yeast (1 tbs.)	0.4

FOODS CONTAINING MILK OR DAIRY

FOODS CONTAINING MILK

Cheese
Cottage cheese
Yogurt
Ice cream
Butter
Most margarines
Creamed soups and sauces
Chocolate
Pudding
Custard
Baked goods
Mashed potatoes
Some "non-dairy" products
Baked goods
Pancakes & waffles
Doughnuts
Meatloaf
Gravies
Many breads have whey
Calcium supplements may have casein
Protein powders
Check vitamins

MILK FREE

Almond milk
Hazlenut milk
Rice milk
Rice Dream (brown nut milks)
coconut milk
Rice Dream (ice cream substitute)
Try cereals with dilute fruit juice instead of milk e.g. Apple
Oat milk
Great Harvest Bread

MAY BE LISTED ON LABEL AS THE FOLLOWING INGREDIENTS:

Casein
Caseinate
Whey
Lactalbumin sodium caseinate lactose
Cream
Non-fat milk solids calcium caseinate

FOODS TO BE AVOIDED ON A GLUTEN-FREE DIET

The following foods may contain wheat, and should be avoided on a wheat- free diet.

Beverages:
- Beer
- Cocomalt
- Gin (any drink containing grain neutral spirits)
- Malted milk
- Ovaltine
- Postum
- Whiskeys

Breads:
- Biscuits
- Cornbread
- Crackers
- Gluten bread
- Graham bread
- Muffins
- Popovers
- Pretzels
- Pumpernickel bread
- Rolls
- Rye bread
- Soy bread
- Triscuits
- White bread

Cereals:
- Bran flakes
- Cornflakes
- Crackers
- Cream of wheat
- Farina
- Grapenuts
- Krumbles
- Muffets

Cereals cont.
- Pettijohn's
- Puffed wheat
- Ralston's wheat cereal
- Pep
- Rice Krispies
- Shredded wheat
- Wheatena & other malted cereals

Flours:
- Buckwheat flour*
- Corn flour*
- Gluten flour
- Graham flour
- Flour
- Lima bean flour*
- Paten flour
- Rice flour*
- Rye flour/White flour
- Whole-wheat flour
- One should not overlook mixtures with flour in them

Miscellaneous:
- Bologna
- Bouillon cubes
- Chocolate candy
- Chocolate, except bitter chocolate and bitter cocoa
- Cooked mixed meat dishes
- Fats used for frying foods rolled in flour
- Wieners
- Fish rolled in flour
- Fowl rolled in flour
- Gravies and sauces
- Griddle cakes
- Hamburger, etc.
- Hotcakes
- Ice cream cones
- Liverwurst
- Lunch ham
- Malt products or foods containing malt
- Matzos
- Mayonnaise*

Miscellaneous cont.
- Meat rolled in flour (do not overlook meat fried in frying fats, which has been used to fry meats rolled in flour, particularly in restaurants)
- Pancake mixtures
- Some yeasts
- Synthetic pepper

Pastries and Desserts:

- Cakes
- Candy bars
- Chocolate candy
- Frozen pies
- Cookies*
- Waffles
- Doughnuts
- Wheat cakes

Wheat Products:

- Bread and cracker crumbs
- Dumplings
- Hamburger mix
- Macaroni
- Noodles
- Rusk
- Spaghetti
- Vermicelli
- Zweiback
- Wheat germ
- Wheat starch
- Durum
- Farina
- Semolina
- Wheat bran
- Modified food starch
- Couscous

*** Can be homemade without wheat**

HEALTHY LIFESTYLE FOR A HEALTHY GALLBLADDER

DIET

1. Increase healthy fats and oils, such as olive oil, flaxseed oil, fish oils, and coconut oil
2. High fiber, high in vegetable protein (dried beans and peas, sprouts, etc),
3. High in vegetables and fruits and whole grains; use olive or coconut oil for cooking
4. Increase fiber rich foods in the diet
5. Drink at least 8 full glasses of bottled water each day (no well water or water containing fluoride or chlorine)
6. Eat at least one serving (two cups) daily of raw/grated beets covered with the juice of one-half of a lemon and two tablespoons of raw, unprocessed flax seed oil.
7. Eat plenty of low glycemic fruits and vegetables.

AVOID THE FOLLOWING FOODS:

1. Dairy products (except butter),
2. Wheat and rye,
3. Fried foods,
4. Hydrogenated fats, partially hydrogenated fats,
5. Cold drinks,
6. Refined carbohydrates, such as white flour, pasta, sugar etc.

AVOID FOOD ALLERGIES:

1. Identify food allergies and avoid the moderate and high reaction foods or do a hypoallergenic diet

HERPES DIET

FOODS TO EMPHASIZE

Especially during active cases of Herpes

- Dairy products if not allergic to them (Cheese, Yogurt, Kefir, Cottage Cheese, Sour Cream, Milk).
- All Fish & Seafood
- Chicken
- Turkey
- Eggs
- Organ Meats
- Potatoes
- Brewers Yeast

FOODS TO BE EATEN WITH DISCRETION

These foods must be balanced with L-Lysine and foods in the first group. During active herpes, these foods must be eliminated.

- Whole grain products (Cereals, Bread, Pasta, Pancakes, Lentils, Barley and other Grains.
- Oats
- Corn
- Rice
- Peas & Beans
- Sprouts
- Chick Peas
- Carob
- Foods containing seeds (Eggplant, Tomato, Squash)
- Fruits and Berries, which contain seeds, may be eaten.
- Citrus Fruits (may irritate canker sores)

FOODS TO AVOID

- Chocolate
- Peanuts and Peanut Butter
- Sugar
- Cakes and Sweets
- Alcohol
- Coffee & Tea
- Nuts (Almonds, Brazil Nuts, Cashews, Filberts, Pecans, Walnuts)
- Seed Meal (Tahini, Sesame Butter)
- Sunflower Seeds
- Coconut
- Bleached White Flour Foods

RECOMMENDATIONS FOR A HEALTHY HEART

1. Eat a good breakfast every day.
2. Eliminate snacks between meals.
3. Remove empty and refined calories from the diet as much as possible.
4. Eliminate or drastically cut down on all visible fats (Crisco, Mazola oil, margarine, salad dressings)
5. Eliminate or reduce use of free sugar found in desserts, jams and jellies, sweetened cereals and other processed foods, or added sugar on dry cereal, in coffee or teas, etc.
6. Eliminate soft drinks (substitute fruit juices)
7. Eat plenty of cold water fish, flaxseed and other sources of omega-3 oils
8. Use unrefined cereal grains. Use brown rice instead of white rice and whole wheat bread instead of "enriched" white bread. Use cooked cereals for breakfast instead of dry cereals.
9. Don't use alcoholic beverages
10. Drink plenty of water
11. Get regular, moderate exercise.
12. Get adequate rest, fresh air, sunshine, and drink pure water.
13. Find ways to manage your stress.

RECOMMENDATIONS FOR A HEALTHY MENSTRUAL CYCLE

DIETARY RECOMMENDATIONS:

Diet plays a major role in both the relief and exacerbation of PMS symptoms. A well-balanced diet of whole foods and grains provides an excellent base. Special modifications designed to decrease the load placed on the liver's detoxification capacity are especially important. This includes decreasing foods containing exogenous estrogen and other challenges to the liver. Other important factors include stabilizing blood sugar levels, and avoiding foods known to be associated with increasing PMS symptoms.

IMPORTANT DIETARY PRINCIPLES FOR PMS INCLUDE:

- Stabilize blood sugar: Eat small, frequent meals, 5 or 6 meals a day by adding a mid-morning and mid-afternoon snack. Limit simple sugars by omitting concentrated sweets, soft drinks. Limit all forms of sugar. Consume sugar foods only with meals.
- Avoid constipation, thereby decreasing estrogen deconjugation by including fiber and water (8 glasses of water per day), whole grain breads and cereals with each meal, fresh, unprocessed vegetables
- Limit dairy intake. Substitute with rice, nut or almond milk. Dairy is constipating and also inhibits magnesium absorption.
- Include small amounts of protein with each meal such as lean meats (preferably organic) and vegetable protein sources from beans.
- Limit intake of red meats (which can contain exogenous estrogens).
- Decrease inflammation by including unsaturated fats such as flaxseed, sunflower & olive oil.
- Other therapeutic foods include garlic, onions legumes kelp, beets, carrots, apples and sesame seeds
- Limit/avoid factors that aggravate symptoms such as caffeine. Eliminate caffeine-containing foods from the diet. Avoid coffee on an empty stomach. Use decaffeinated coffees and teas or other caffeine/sugar-free beverages such as herbal teas, coffee substitutes and WATER.
- Limit chocolate (also aggravates symptoms) intake by using carob in place of chocolate or eat fresh fruits and sorbet for sweets
- Avoid alcohol and tobacco, and decrease water retention by limiting sodium. Use fresh, unprocessed foods and avoid added salt

Stress & PMS: Although emotional stress is not the sole cause of PMS symptoms, it can exacerbate them. If your metabolism is already making you hypersensitive to cyclical changes in your hormones, it is important not to add to the problem by setting up a stressful personal environment. Stress can be managed in three ways. You can choose to go to a qualified professional for counseling, or to restructure your environment to make it less stressful, or to learn relaxation techniques. Many books and tapes are available to help you learn these techniques.

Exercise & PMS: Exercise relieves PMS symptoms by increasing the amount of blood flow and oxygen to the tissues, as well as reducing anxiety and irritability. Increased muscular strength in the back and abdominal muscles can prevent low back pain and cramps. Exercise can also improve posture, which can be one of the causes of PMS. Daily exercise is preferable for general health. To improve PMS symptoms, it is important to increase the activity level of your exercise for a week or two before the onset of your period.

RECOMMENDATIONS FOR CONTROLLING BLOOD SUGAR

Do you feel tired run down or depressed for no apparent reason? In many cases, problems regulating the supply of sugar to your brain and body cells may be the cause.

All cells in the body burn the sugar glucose for energy, similar to the way engines burn gasoline. Reducing the supply of glucose to your brain cells can cause poor alertness, tiredness, difficulty concentrating, and even confusion, loss of memory and emotional depression.

Blood sugar levels can drop for various reasons, producing a variety of symptoms. One of the most common causes is the frequent use of sugar rich foods and beverages in a person's diet.

Sugar in the diet is rapidly absorbed from the gut, causing blood sugar to rise. The body tries to regulate blood sugar by holding it within a normal range, neither too high nor too low. The pancreas gland, for instance, produces insulin to bring the glucose level back down after a sugary meal or snack.

When sugar is consumed on a regular basis, the body often over compensates for the frequent rises in blood sugar -- bringing its levels down lower than it was beforehand. These lowered sugar levels make a person feel hungry, or crave more sweets. Taking that sugar rich snack provides a lift only temporarily, and leaves one feeling drained or tired again shortly afterward.

People caught in this vicious cycle may experience weakness, shakiness or trembling if they go too long without eating. In addition to mental fatigue or depression, they may have periods of light-headedness, coldness of the hands and feet, or a variety of other mental or physical symptoms. These are usually relieved temporarily by eating.

If you have experienced this type of problem, you may find relief by following a few simple dietary guidelines.

1: Eliminate sugars

- Don't eat foods or beverages containing sugar, whether added or natural. Don't eat sweet tasting foods or drink.
- Read labels: Corn syrup, corn sweetener, sugar dextrose, glucose, fructose, brown sugar, cane sugar, beet sugar, turbinado sugar, date sugar, raisin syrup, maple syrup, are all sugar, and should be avoided in even the smallest amounts.
- Avoid the use of artificial sweeteners as a substitution for sugar. Research has shown that artificial sweeteners can cause aggravated hypoglycemia (low blood sugar), loss of diabetes control and precipitation of clinical diabetes in persons who were free from disease. In diabetics, it has caused an aggravation of complications related to diabetes.
- Naturally sweet foods must also be avoided, such as: honey, fruit juice, grapes, raisins, dried fruits, jams and jellies, fruits.
- Avoid all the following: ice cream, cake, candy, carbonated beverages, pies,

pastries, canned jellies, preserves, Jell-O, most cold breakfast cereals, fruit juice, punch, and drink, breakfast syrups, and similar processed food items.

Exceptions allowed: permitted a maximum of one 4-ounce selections daily from list below. Make sure the fruits are fresh and organic whenever possible.

Apple	Papaya	Orange
Melon	Blueberries	Fresh pineapple
Banana	Grapefruit	Pear

Home canned fruit with no added sweetener

2: Eat protein-rich and/or complex carbohydrate rich foods

You will probably feet better if you include some foods rich in protein and/or starch at most meals and snacks. Unlike sugar-rich foods, these provide a "time-released" source of sugar, yielding their glucose slowly and steadily, thereby helping to avoid the "peaks and valleys" of poor blood sugar regulation.

Foods such as eggs, fish and meats are protein rich. So are some types of cheese (like cottage cheese), nuts and seeds, and combinations of various beans and grains. Starch rich foods include whole grains, cereals, and starchy vegetables, such as whole grain breads, crackers, potatoes and squash.

Eating complex carbohydrates and protein-rich foods in small to moderate amounts (e.g.: 1-4 ounces), at most meals or snacks does not mean you should avoid other types of helpful foods which you enjoy, such as vegetables.

3: Eat small frequent meals

Eat small to moderate amounts of food every few hours, particularly if your energy is low. For example, eat 3 moderate meals daily, and one, two, or three between meal smacks as desired, or as needed to keep your energy or concentration up.

SUPPLEMENTS

Many factors besides sweets in the diet influence blood sugar levels. Certain nutrients are also helpful in regulating blood sugar. The mineral chromium is particularly important for the proper utilization of insulin. Brewer's yeast, whole grains, beans and meat are the best food sources of this mineral. Dietary supplements including chromium may be indicated for some people with blood glucose concerns. Each individual is different, and health problems should be considered on an individual basis, whether or not professional treatment is required.

However, the three general guidelines we've discussed have helped many people to reclaim their lost energy and vitality.

In following these guidelines, you may feel worse for a couple of weeks before you begin to feel much better. After a few months or so, you may be able to add moderate amounts of sweets back into your diet without producing the same old symptoms. Patience and consistency bring healthy rewards.

RECOMMENDATIONS FOR DEALING WITH INCREASED THYROID ACTIVITY

1. Get plenty of exercise to use up excess thyroid hormone. Take the exercise in the cool of the day being careful not to overdo it.

2. Apply alternating hot and cold compresses to the thyroid area. Place a hot towel or face cloth over the front of the neck for 3 minutes. Then replace it with a cold towel for 1 minute. Repeat this 3 times. Do this twice daily for seven days, then once in the morning for 30 days.

3. Avoid the use of iodized salt or other high iodine sources. Iodine rich foods include all sea food, kelp, sea salt, clams, oysters, and lobsters.

4. Avoid certain foods, which contain thyroid promoting amines: sauerkraut, wine (histamine), cheese (tyramine), bananas (dopamine, serotonin).

5. Eat at least one RAW serving daily of the following foods as they contain "goitrogens", which suppress the action of the thyroid.

rutabaga	spinach	apples	walnuts
turnip	lettuce	apricots	almonds
green peppers	cauliflower	blackberries	maize
beets	broccoli	raspberries	string beans
carrots	Brussels sprouts	prunes	beans
cassava	collards	cherries	peanut skins
yams	kohlrabi	honeydew	peas
onions	kale	grapefruit	sorghum
radishes	peaches	grapes	bamboo shoots
cabbage	pears	oranges	
celery	strawberries	filberts	

6. Constipation and Diarrhea may be present as the GI tract tends to empty itself periodically and then be unresponsive.

7. Take a neutral bath, the water being neither hot nor cold.

8. Prolonged cold for 15 minutes to the thyroid gland may help suppress the activity of the gland.

9. Drink 8-12 glasses of water daily.

RECOMMENDATIONS FOR DEALING WITH LOW THYROID FUNCTION

DIETARY CHANGES:

- Eating principles: low sugar, low fat, high fiber, low cholesterol
- Calorie percentages: 70% complex carbohydrates, protein 12-15%, fat 15-18%
- Therapeutic foods: oats, kelp, seaweed, artichokes, onions, garlic, dulse, Swiss chard, turnip greens, egg yolks, wheat germ, cod roe, lecithin, sesame seed butter
- Fresh juices: carrot, celery, and/or spinach with powdered kelp or dulse
- Avoid goitrogens (which can reduce thyroid function) unless cooked: broccoli, turnips, cabbage, carrots, kale, rutabaga, soybean, spinach, peanuts, yams, radishes, millet, green peppers, beets, celery, lettuce, cauliflower, Brussels sprouts, collards, kohlrabi, peaches, pears, strawberries, apples, apricots, blackberries, raspberries, prunes, cherries, honeydew, grapefruit, grapes, oranges, peas, sorghum, bamboo shoots
- Avoid known food sensitivities

HYDROTHERAPY:

- Short cold spray to thyroid after warm bath/shower OR
- Cold mitten friction to thyroid after bath/shower
- Alternating hot and cold compresses to thyroid gland daily: Hot compresses molded to neck for 3 minutes hot followed by 30 seconds to 1 minute of cold compresses. Repeat 3-5 times
- Cold shower to middle and lower back to stimulate adrenals
- Constitutional Hydrotherapy treatment to help stimulate digestion

OTHER CONSIDERATIONS:

- Do not use an electric blanket-the body's metabolism will be slightly raised if the body must generate its own heat to keep warm
- Exercise daily to stimulate the thyroid gland and elevate the body's metabolic rate
- Improve overall digestion and assimilation of food

RECOMMENDATIONS FOR DECREASING COLDS, FLU, AND INFECTIONS

When you first feel yourself become sick there are things you can do to avoid becoming ill or to shorten the duration of the illness. These suggestions are especially helpful if you do them early on, as early on as possible. They will help you fend off Flu, colds or minor infections. Call a clinician if your symptoms become severe. These are some steps you can take to boost your immunity:

Eat Very Lightly Or Not At All - With most illnesses the appetite is diminished. This is a natural response of the body. Energy is needed to fight off the "bug" and the body does not have the energy to process food as well. Give the digestive tract a rest!

Get Rest As Soon As Possible - Many people ignore the early warning signs of illness and keep working till they "drop". You will take longer to heal if you allow the illness to get a foothold. If you feel a sore throat, headache, congestion, etc. coming on, **take it easy.** If possible, take the day off from work. This may prevent you from having to take three days off later on.

Drink Plenty Of Fluids - This standard advice works. You can clear the toxins from the "bug" out of your system with large amounts of filtered water and herb teas.

HOME HYDROTHERAPY

Hot Foot Bath

Soak feet in hot water while wrapped in a warm wool blanket. Put a cold cloth on your head and relax while you sit in a comfortable position for 10-15 minutes. Take care to avoid getting chilled after this treatment.

Throat or Chest Compress

Warm the throat or chest with a warm washcloth or hot shower. Dry the skin thoroughly and apply a thin cotton wrap (to Throat) or thin cotton T-shirt (to chest) that has been soaked in cold water and wrung out so that it is not dripping wet. Cover this with a wool scarf (for throat) or wool sweater (for chest). Go to bed this way. By morning the wrap or T-shirt will be dry. This treatment increases circulation and increases the white blood cell activity.

RECOMMENDATIONS FOR DIARRHEA

Fast for 36 hours (a night, a day, and a night). Drink plenty of liquids-dilute fruit and vegetable juices and filtered water to maintain hydration.

Foods to avoid:

- Milk and milk products: butter, cheese, ice cream, etc.
- Sweetened fruit juices
- Sugar, including honey
- High protein foods: meat, eggs, nuts, seeds
- Fats: especially fried or greasy food
- Any gluten containing grains: wheat, rye, barley, oats
- Artificial sweeteners: mannitol, sorbitol, aspartame

Foods to eat:

- High fiber diet
- Ripe mashed bananas
- Rice bran
- Raw foods
- Yogurt (unsweetened)
- Oat bran
- Carrot soup
- Rice or rice cereal
- Toast
- Acidophilus
- Papaya juice
- Applesauce or grated green apples
- Soured products: yogurt, buttermilk, kefir, etc. Barley water: Use 1/2 cup barley in 2 cups water. Simmer for 20-30 minutes. Strain and take the water.
- Carob and amaranth powder (rich in pectin): Mix 1 tablespoon carob or amaranth powder in 1 cup of applesauce or water.
- Carrot and cabbage juice
- Powdered cinnamon: Use 1/4 teaspoon in applesauce or as a tea
- Green drink: Celery or watercress with Cabbage or parsley. Blend together with a little water. Strain. Add a squeeze of fresh lemon juice.
- Sauerkraut and tomato juice: Use equal parts. Take 1 tablespoon of each every hour or 2-4 ounces for each stool passed.

RECOMMENDATIONS FOR KEEPING YOUR LIVER HEALTHY

NUTRITION

Food to Include:

- Dark green leafy vegetables, beets, endive, cucumbers, garlic, onions, artichoke, sprouted seeds, grains, tahini, vegetable products (raw or juiced only).
- Include plenty of fiber rich foods
- Liquid (at least 6-8 cups a day),
- Any type of green juice or drink (can be mixed with some carrot juice).
- Liquid chlorophyll.

Foods to Exclude:

- All processed and refined foods, salt, strong spices, sugar, alcohol, drugs, synthetic vitamins, fats/oils, non-organic meats and dairy (due to hormones), coffee, heavy starches (potatoes, rice, bread, cereal), heavy proteins, chicken, eggs, milk or milk products.
- Condiments except lemon juice and a little salt.
- Avoid hydrogenated oils
- Avoid chemical additives

JUICE/TEA

- Red beet (tops and roots) mixed with carrot (1/2 cup) once a day.
- Dandelion root tea: steep 1 teaspoon in 1 pint boiling water for 20 minutes. Take once a day.
- Lemon juice and hot water
- Grape, radish, papaya and carrot juice

OTHER

- Deep breathing, 30 seconds each time, 10 times a day.
- Brisk walk or other exercises 20-30 minutes a day.
- Drink clean filtered water (at least 2 quarts a day).
- Do not use aluminum cookware.
- Castor oil packs
- Alternating hot and cold spray to the liver area
- Regular sauna

RECOMMENDATIONS FOR THE PROSTATE

DIETARY CONSIDERATIONS

- Eat a diet rich in raw vegetables, fruit
- Bee pollen
- Fasting, and bowel/ colon cleansing are often useful
- Fluid intake should be restricted after dinner to reduce nocturia (especially beverages with diuretic activity, such as alcohol, coffee, tea, and colas)
- Avoid drinking beer, which increases prolactin level which increases BPH
- Increase essential fatty acid consumption. They act as nutritional precursors to protective prostaglandins
- A vegetarian diet helps maintain normal levels of testosterone, estrogen and prolactin
- Avoid saturated animal fat (beef, whole-milk, lard)
- Avoid all sources and forms of hydrogenated fatty acids
- Increase protective carotene-containing foods like green and yellow vegetables, fruits
- Eat foods containing more zinc (nuts - especially walnuts, pumpkin seeds, safflower seeds, and oysters)
- Remove all chemicals and pesticides from diet (eat organic food)

ELIMINATE THE FOLLOWING

Caffeine (Soda pop, coffee, tea and chocolate)
Dairy products
Alcohol
Spicy food

MISCELLANEOUS THERAPIES:

- Cold sitz baths - sit in tub of water 1/2 inch below navel with a temperature of 55-75° F (12-24°C) with feet in a tub of water 105-1110°F (40- 43°C) for 3-8 minutes
- Alternating warm and cool enemas
- Frequent sex - daily ejaculations, but avoid prolonged intercourse
- Frequent urinary voiding
- Avoid prolonged sitting or standing
- Do some form of daily exercise, including Kegal exercise
- Reduce stress (stress increases prolactin levels)
- If overweight, you must lose some weight. Increased abdominal weight causes increased pressure into the pelvic cavity, which puts more stress on the bladder and prostate

RECOMMENDATIONS FOR STRENGTHENING YOUR KIDNEYS

1. **Drink** 6-8 glasses of filtered, spring or bottled **water** daily.

2. Use very little **salt** in your cooking.

3. **Walk barefoot** in the early morning on dew-covered grass for 10 minutes. This stimulates the kidney meridian on the sole of the foot.

4. **Take saunas** 3-4 times a week. This helps improve blood circulation. Stay in the sauna until you are sweating which aids elimination through the skin instead of the kidney.

5. **Take warm salt baths**. Add 2 pounds of any water softening salt (containing sodium chloride) to 24 gallons of warm water in a bathtub. Lower your body into the bath so the water reaches to your neck and stay in the water for 20-30 minutes. If you have a weak heart, don't lower yourself deeper than the level of your heart. Try this on a nightly basis before going to bed. It is important to have the correct concentration of salt/water to create the proper osmotic gradient to help the kidneys eliminate wastes.

6. Ensure that your diet contains an abundant quantity of **minerals**. A diet high in fresh foods, especially fresh vegetables and fruits, contains generous proportions of available minerals.

Books and other Resources from Bear Mountain Publishing

Blood Chemistry and CBC Analysis- Clinical Laboratory Testing from a Functional Perspective- Dicken Weatherby, N.D. and Scott Ferguson, N.D.

Blood Chemistry and CBC Analysis from a Functional perspective- One-Day Seminar on 4 Audio CDs

Quick Reference Guide to Blood Chemistry Analysis- Dicken Weatherby, N.D. and Scott Ferguson, N.D.

In-Office Laboratory Testing- Functional Terrain Analysis- Dicken Weatherby, N.D. and Scott Ferguson, N.D.

Urine Dipstick Analysis and Functional Urinalysis Quick Reference Guide- Dicken Weatherby, N.D. and Scott Ferguson, N.D.

Question by Question Guide to the Nutritional Assessment Questionnaire (NAQ)- Signs and Symptoms Analysis from a Functional Perspective- Dicken Weatherby, N.D.

Complete Physical Exam Reference and Charting System- Dicken Weatherby, N.D. and Scott Ferguson, N.D.

Complete Practitioner's Guide To Take-Home Testing- Dicken Weatherby, N.D. and Scott Ferguson, N.D.

Naturally Raising Your HGH Levels- HGH Secretagogues and the Anti-Aging Diet, Lifestyle, and Exercise Program- Dicken Weatherby, N.D.

Online Functional Blood Chemistry Analysis Training at www.BloodChemistryTraining.com

----

For more information about other titles from Bear Mountain Publishing visit us at: http://www.BloodChemistryAnalysis.com

or e-mail us at info@BloodChemistryAnalysis.com

To receive master copies of the questionnaire and manual assessment form please visit:

www.BloodChemistryAnalysis.com

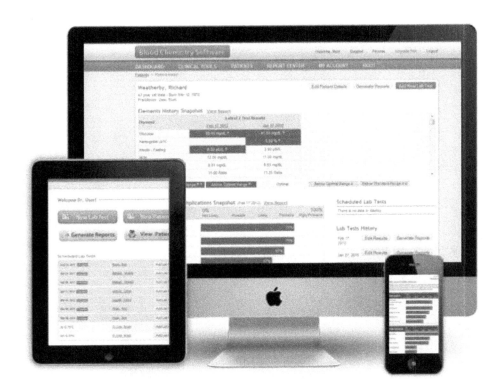

CPSIA information can be obtained
at www.ICGtesting.com
Printed in the USA
FSHW021045150121
77608FS

9 780976 136729